A Colour Atlas and Textbook of

Orthognathic Surgery

The Surgery of Facial Skeletal Deformity

Derek Henderson,
MB, BS, BDS(Lond), FDSRCS(Eng), LRCP, MRCS.
*Consultant Oral and Maxillofacial Surgeon to
St Thomas's Hospital, St George's Hospital and the
Royal Dental Hospital, London. Honorary Consultant
to Charing Cross Hospital. Honorary Civilian Consultant
to the Royal Navy and the British Army.*

Contributions by **David Poswillo,**
DDS, MDhc, DSc, FDS, FRACDS,
FIBiol, FRCPath, HonFFDRCSI
*Professor of Oral and Maxillofacial Surgery,
Guy's Hospital, London*

Wolfe Medical Publications Ltd

Dedicated to
**MY WIFE JENNY
AND TO MY FAMILY**
who will not know how to cope with life no
longer surrounded by slides, diagrams,
and typescript; without whose help and
encouragement this book would never
have seen the light of day

Copyright © Derek Henderson, D. E. Poswillo, 1985
Published by Wolfe Medical Publications Ltd, 1985
Printed by Royal Smeets Offset b.v., Weert, Netherlands
ISBN 0 7243 0760 6

This book is one of the titles in the series of
Wolfe Medical Atlases, a series which brings together
probably the world's largest systematic published
collection of diagnostic colour photographs.
   For a full list of Atlases in the series, plus forthcoming
titles and details of our surgical, dental and veterinary
Atlases, please write to Wolfe Medical Publications Ltd.
Wolfe House, 3 Conway Street, London W1P 6HE.

Cover photograph by R.T. Hutchings

Contents

Section 4: Treatment methods and techniques

Foreword

Hullihen is generally credited with performing the first operation for the correction of mandibular deformity which he described, in the American Journal of Dental Science in 1849, as a 'case of elongation of the underjaw and distortion of the face and neck, caused by burn, successfully treated'. The procedure consisted of a 'V'-shaped ostectomy of the body of the mandible and the release of submandibular scars – a technique which was revolutionary at that time. About one hundred and twenty years later, on the other side of the Atlantic, the introduction of cranio-facial surgery by Tessier of Paris opened up surgical horizons which had, hitherto, never been envisaged. The turn of the century brought about a revival of interest in the correction of jaw deformity both in America and Europe which extended into the period between the two World Wars but problems associated with infection, anaesthesia and stabilisation of the fragments resulted in a limited acceptance of such operations by surgeons and orthodontists.

During the past 40 years there has been an extraordinary expansion of the techniques employed in orthognathic surgery and it is understandable that anyone seeking to become proficient in this field soon becomes lost in a 'maze of methodology' and, but hopefully not too literally, a 'slough of despond'. For far too long there has been a compelling need for a British textbook which would eliminate these difficulties and provide a comforting guide along the tortuous pathway to success. Derek Henderson's superb treatise on orthognathic surgery meets these requirements in the most comprehensive manner possible. Apart from an excellent introductory section on variations and anomalies in the growth and development of the facial tissues by Professor David Poswillo, whose research into these problems has received international acclaim, the entire text, including the line drawings, is based upon the author's extensive personal experience. Within this veritable Cornucopia of clinical expertise it is immediately evident that the extremely lucid and succinct descriptions of the operative procedures, and their logical analysis in relation to pre-operative planning and post-operative prediction, bear the mark of a 'master of his craft' and serve to emphasise his authority derived from a wide range of experience in this highly specialised and complex branch of surgery.

This long-awaited textbook is superbly illustrated throughout with colour prints of exceptional quality that serve to enhance the clinical and operative descriptions of all the techniques which are in current use and have withstood the test of time. This excellent production must immediately become established as one of the major classics in the speciality of oral and maxillofacial surgery; be essential reading for postgraduate students aspiring to higher degrees in the speciality, and provide a pool of knowledge for all those who seek to achieve competence in the demanding, but professionally satisfying, techniques of orthognathic surgery.

Norman Rowe
CBE, FRCS(Eng.),
Hon. FDSRCS(Edin.),
Hon. FDSRCPS(Glasg.),
Hon. FFDRCS(Irel.),

Honorary Consultant in Oral and Maxillofacial Surgery to the Westminster Hospital and Queen Mary's Hospital, Roehampton, London. Emeritus Consultant to the Royal Navy and Honorary Consultant (Retired) to the British Army.

Preface

The purpose of this book is threefold. Firstly, it is intended to present an overall philosophy of case assessment and treatment planning in an area for far too long dominated by technique. If nothing more is accomplished than to stimulate argument about the principles of case management, then the project will have been well worth while. Secondly, it is hoped to provide the trainee with an adequate guide to operative techniques to enable him or her to explore the field and progress to a rational selection of those surgical techniques which are appropriate to the individual patient's needs. And thirdly, it is hoped that experienced orthognathic surgeons will be challenged to justify and possibly expand their surgical approach to long familiar operative procedures. The book is *not* intended to be an exhaustive treatise on all the known techniques of its field of surgery, and some may seek favourite operations unsuccessfully, or at the least find them insufficiently advocated for their taste. This is inevitable in a book which is largely the reflection of one individual's experience, together with his prejudices and limitations. It is hoped that the reasons for the prejudices are apparent in the text, and the reader must subject them to critical analysis and conclude as he will.

I am most indebted to Professor David Poswillo for contributing the whole of Section One, and bringing his unique expertise to bear on the task of setting out the known principles of craniofacial growth and development in so far as these are essential to the practice of orthognathic surgery. There are some areas (for example, the developmental asymmetries) which *demand* to be seen in this context, and the book would be incomplete without this background. Minor differences in terminology reflect the different presuppositions of the experimental pathologist and the clinical operator, and we all have to accept some apparent conflicts when we change hats from the one discipline to the other; time alone, and the research which accompanies it, will eventually harmonise the two languages. In the event, no attempt has been made to bring about uniformity of terminology between Section One and the rest of the book.

Nor has an attempt been made to deal in any depth with the role of orthodontic treatment in the pre- and post-operative phases of management. Proper liaison with the orthodontist is a *sine qua non* in the treatment of deformities of the jaws, and recent trends in the formation of joint orthodontic/surgical teams, particularly in the United States of America, point the way for the future. There are, however, excellent texts covering this area, and the omission of detail in the present volume simply acknowledges this to be so.

The layout of the book is designed to avoid repetition. Surgical approaches to the facial skeleton are therefore discussed together, and reference back avoids unnecessary repetition when skeletal techniques are presented. This leads to the need for some page turning in following particular operative descriptions, but it is felt that the result is a more manageable book in size. The postoperative photographs are all taken between three and six months after operation unless otherwise stated; current evidence suggests that by this time major changes have occurred and the result is more or less stable.

Finally, I am very grateful to Mr Norman Rowe, CBE, for his willingness to write a Foreword and set this book on its way. I personally (along with a host of colleagues) owe a greater debt of gratitude to him than to any other for the initial inspiration and continued stimulus he has provided to my surgical endeavours, and no one has influenced my attitudes more profoundly. If this volume succeeds in propagating the fruits of that influence in some small way I shall be well pleased.

Derek Henderson
London, 1985

Acknowledgements

Section One

The first section in this book includes material collected over many years from different hospitals and many generous colleagues. With the passage of time, the source is often difficult to trace in every case. I therefore acknowledge, collectively, those who have provided illustrations included in this compilation. More specifically, I owe thanks to Dr. Kathy Sulik for permission to use the scanning electron micrographs shown in figs. 1, 2, 3, 4, 63 and 64, and to Mr. David J. David and Mr. Donald Simpson, my co-authors in *The Craniosynostoses*, Springer, 1983, from which figs. 14, 15, 16 and 17 are derived. Figs. 20, 22, 24 and 26 were drawn after Gasson and Lavergene, 1977. The secretarial assistance of Erica Daulman is gratefully acknowledged.

David Poswillo, 1985

Sections Two to Five

The rest of the book similarly contains much clinical material from several hospitals, the management of which involved the participation of many colleagues, and I too acknowledge collectively the assistance and cooperation of all those whose efforts and skills are reflected in these cases, or who generously referred them to me to contribute to their management. With the exception of those specifically acknowledged below, the cases mainly derive from Canniesburn Hospital, Glasgow; St Thomas's Hospital, London; St George's Hospital and the Royal Dental Hospital, London. During my time in Canniesburn Hospital I was fortunate to work closely with Mr Ian Jackson (now Professor of Plastic Surgery in the Mayo Clinic) and latterly with Mr Khursheed Moos, and I am grateful to both for the stimulating cooperation of that period. Due acknowledgement is made in the text where cases were treated jointly, but I wish to establish in general my debt to these two colleagues who cooperated in (or subsequently took over the treatment of) several of the cases presented here.

Inevitably patients treated by more than one person are liable to be presented in different contexts; where this is known to me I have acknowledged the fact; and if any are published elsewhere without my knowledge I hereby pay tribute to the part played by my colleagues from the Canniesburn Unit.

The orthodontic treatment involved has been carried out by several clinicians and their support teams. Specifically I am grateful to Mr A. Cockburn of Stirling (not least for introducing me to the complexities of cephalometric analysis and guiding my early sorties through that maze), and to Mr B. Christie, Mr H.S. Orton, Mr D.A. Plint, Professor W.J.B. Houston, Mr S.J. Powell, and Mr A. Banner, together with their clinical teams, whose skills were essential in the treatment of many cases shown; or who kindly referred cases for treatment over the years.

I gratefully acknowledge the photographic help of the Departments of Medical Illustration in Canniesburn Hospital, the Royal Dental Hospital and St Thomas's Hospital. Most of the dentofacial photography was undertaken by these departments and I am indebted to them; most of the operative photography is my own, as are the majority of line drawings and cephalometric tracings. The latter show many of the faults of the amateur which must be laid at my own door. I likewise acknowledge the indispensable assistance of Mr Walter Smith, and Mr Jim Briggs, my maxillofacial technicians in Glasgow and London.

I am indebted to the Editor of the British Journal of Oral and Maxillofacial Surgery (formerly the British Journal of Oral Surgery) for permission to reproduce material originally presented in black and white photography as follows: Figs. 112–114, 160–165, 178–179, 221, 240, 241, 252, 253, 332–346, 365–368, 374–378, 383–385, 396, 397, 612, 615, 617, 774, 778, 781, 787–792, 794–799, 817, 818, 833, 899, 900, 942, 943, 949–957, 970, 1071–1084, 1125, 1208–1214, 1234–1236; also to the Editor of the British Journal of Plastic Surgery for permission to reproduce material originally presented in black and white photography as follows: Figs. 116–118, 847, 848. I am grateful to Mr H.S. Orton for the pictures presented as Figs. 150–157, 158, 159 (cases in which he provided orthodontic care), 256, 257, 258, 259, 265 and 266; to Mr S.J. Powell for Fig. 270; and to Mr J.S.P. Wilson for permission to include Figs. 507, 525–528, 984–988, all cases originally under his care; to Mr J.C. Mustardé for permission to show the case presented in Figs. 510–512; to Mr Gordon Fordyce for his case shown in Figs. 694–697; to Mr Stephen Plumpton and Mr Peter Clarke for permission to show the case presented in Figs. 682–685; to Mr Derek Wilson and Mr Robin Illingworth who referred and collaborated in the case shown in Figs. 998–1003; to Mr Walter Smith who produced the models shown in Figs. 626, 627 and 908; to Mr Brian Conroy who produced the model shown in Fig. 296; to Mr John Hovell who treated the case shown in Figs. 1041, 1042, subsequently taken over by me. I acknowledge also that Fig. 133 was drawn after Hovell (1965). I am also indebted to Mr Michael Wake for permission to reproduce Figs. 1234–1236, with his medical artist; to Mr Ian Mcgregor for referring the case shown in Fig. 498; and to Mr Murray Foster for permission to reproduce Figs. 775 and 776, together with his medical artist. The cases presented in Figs. 112, 113, 114, 242, 243, 386 and 603 have been presented in black and white in 'Surgical Correction of Dentofacial Deformities', by Bell, W.H., Proffitt, W.R., and White, R.P., Saunders, 1980. To all these, despite the differences in presentation, my acknowledgements. I acknowledge also the kindness of Messrs. McMinn, Hutchings & Logan, and their publishers, Wolfe Medical, for permission to reproduce Figs. 581 and 582 from 'A Colour Atlas of Head and Neck Anatomy', 1981.

I also wish to express my appreciation of the longsuffering toleration of my publishers whose inexhaustible patience and forebearance over many years have been stretched to their limit by my whimsical literary inefficiency during the production of this volume.

Derek Henderson, 1985

SECTION 1

Variations and anomalies in the growth and development of the facial tissues

The normal development of the facial and oral tissues involves complex step-by-step sequences of migration of cells and interaction between cell groups. Based on a genetically determined plan, growth processes lead eventually to an adult appearance.

By the systematic study of human and animal specimens of embryos during those critical periods of morphogenesis which correspond to the 25th to the 45th days of development in man, one can reconstruct, with considerable precision, the sequence of human craniofacial morphogenesis.

To understand some of the abnormalities of development which are corrected by modern techniques of orthognathic and craniofacial surgery it is necessary to comprehend the normal embryological development of the maxillofacial region over this critical period of 4 to 5 weeks.

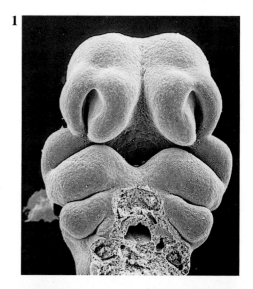

Normal development of the orofacial region

1   In the early somite stage the cranial portion of the embryo develops the first of several mesenchymal elevations, the facial processes. These have a dual origin. Those in the midline arise from the frontal prominence (frontonasal process) while the lateral facial structures arise from the branchial arches. These facial processes surround a central depression, the stomadeum, which is covered at this stage by a membrane. Later, this oropharyngeal membrane ruptures and the cavity becomes the mouth.

2   Initially these facial processes are in contact with the bulging pericardium; as successive branchial arches appear, the pericardium is progressively removed from the boundaries of the stomadeum. These facial processes are covered on their external surfaces by ectoderm which produces skin, and on their internal surfaces by endoderm which develops into mucous membranes. Each has a core composed of mesoderm and specialised ectomesenchymal tissue which has migrated to the processes from the cranial neural crest. From these facial processes arise the soft-tissues and skeletal elements of the craniofacial complex.

It is believed that the frontal process contributes the skeletal elements of the frontal bones, crista galli, ethmoid and nasal bones, the vomer, cartilaginous septum, premaxilla and anterior primary palatine triangle. The skeletal elements derived from the first and second branchial arches include part of the temporal bone, auditory ossicles, zygoma, maxilla, hard palate, mandible and hyoid bone.

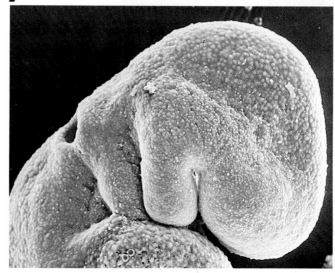

3

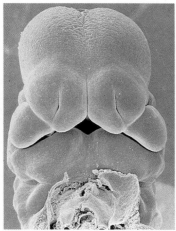

4

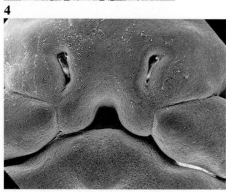

5

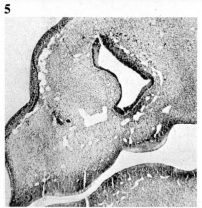

6

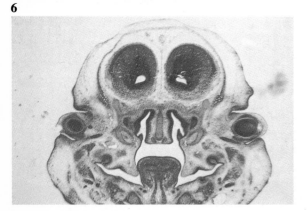

3 By the 5th week of embryonic life all major primordia of the face are easily identified. The frontal process has produced clear medial nasal extensions in the midline rostral* to the stomadeum. The nasal placodes are local thickenings of ectoderm found adjacent to the lateral margins of the frontal prominence.

These nasal placodes, bordered by rapidly-growing horseshoe-like elevations appear to sink beneath the surface, forming depressions known as the nasal pits. The medial nasal processes form the central aspects of the elevations around the nasal pits while the lateral nasal processes form the lateral boundaries. Growing from either side towards the midline are the maxillary processes. The mandibular arches, which also arise from the cephalolateral angles of the stomadeum form the lower border of the oral cavity. Below the mandibular arch, lying on the lateral wall of the pharynx, are the remaining branchial arches and grooves which will eventually form structures in the neck.

*rostral = above, like a beak.

4 During the 6th and 7th week there is marked progress towards the development of the jaws. With differential growth and proliferation of the facial processes, the ectodermal grooves between the processes become obliterated. The contours are smoothed out and the processes merge together. The formation of the arch of the upper jaw is completed by the merging of the two medial nasal processes with each other in the midline and their fusion with the maxillary processes laterally. Thus is established the primary palate or intermaxillary segment. This consists of a labial segment, or prolabium, a gnathogingival component—that part of the premaxilla which will support the incisor teeth and the palatal component or primary medial palatal process.

5 With the formation of the palate the nasal chamber is elongated backwards. The cartilaginous septum and the upper part of the bridge of the nose are probably derived from merging in the midline of the medial nasal processes with the frontal process. The lateral nasal processes form the alae of the nose. Where the epithelial coverings of the nasal and maxillary processes meet there forms an epithelial plate known as the nasal fin. This epithelial wedge eventually disappears as the result of spontaneous programmed death of the redundant cells and the mesenchymal elements of the medial nasal and maxillary processes become continuous.

6 The formation of the palate involves two separate events. The small medial primary palate forms from the fusion of the medial nasal process. The main portion of the hard (secondary) palate and the soft palate is derived from fusion of the palatal shelves which begin as outgrowths of the maxillary processes. At this stage the developing tongue lies between the palatal shelves.

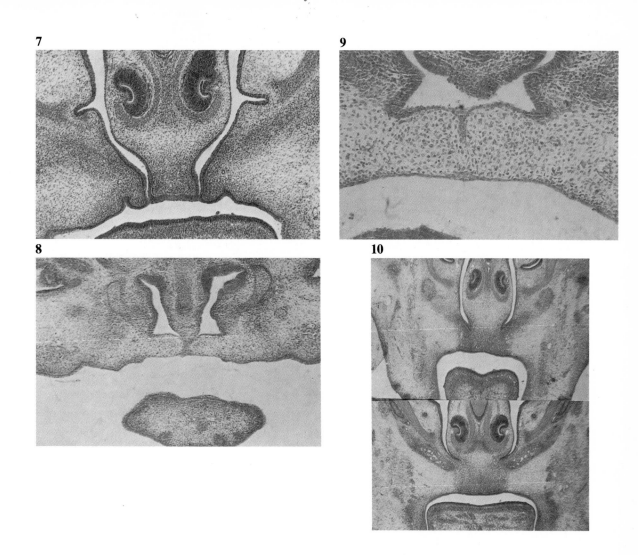

7 The palatal shelves, nasal septum and tongue continue to grow in close relationship until about the 8th week when an extension of the head occurs. This results in freeing the tongue from between the vertical palatal shelves.

8 The enlarging palatal shelves, no longer impeded by the tongue and under the combined influence of turgor-like intrinsic shelf forces and differential growth move from the vertical to the horizontal and fuse with each other and the nasal septum. In the extreme anterior region the primary medial palatine triangle lies between the lateral palatine shelves so that they fuse with it rather than with each other.

9 The palatal shelf epithelium, immediately prior to fusion, becomes glue-like on the opposing edges; on contact, the shelves stick together resisting growth traction forces until the seam of epithelium is broken down by organised cell death and the palate becomes one uniform layer of mesenchyme.

10 Between shelf contact about day 48 and the end of the 10th week, bone expands from two centres of ossification on each side of the maxilla, gradually bridging the gap in the midline of the palate until the central suture forms. The posterior margins of the palatal mesenchyme extend and merge, from anterior to posterior, to produce a soft palate and uvula.

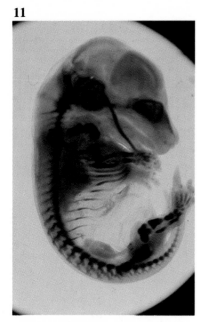

11

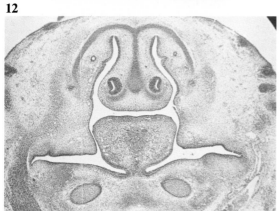

12

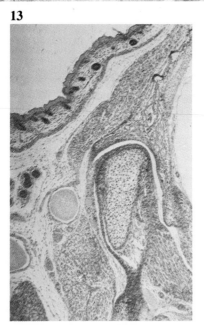

13

11 Prior to the formation of the palate, the mandible exists as a hoop of cartilage (Meckel) which provides a primitive hinge for the earliest mouth opening manoeuvres which commence with the swallowing of amniotic fluid about the 6th week.

12 As the palate is fusing, there develop lateral to Meckel's cartilage, centres of intramembranous ossification which surround the cartilaginous bar and convert the mandibular arch into bone.

13 At the posterior end of the developing mandible, at about the 10th week, the blastema of the mandibular condyle appears as a carrot-shaped cartilage. This grows up towards the lateral aspect of the cranial base to form the temporomandibular articulation. At about 12 weeks the joint cavities appear, separated by a thin central structure, the articular disc.

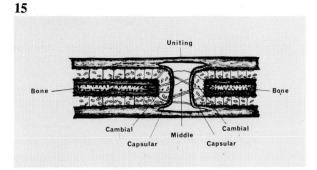

14

15

16

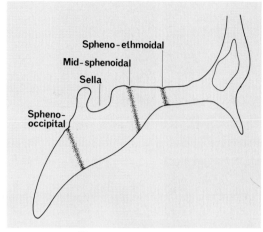

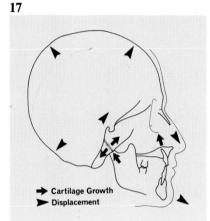

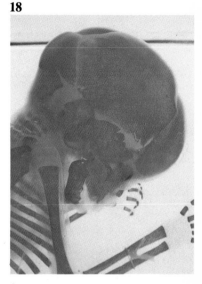

17

18

The development of the cranium

14 The development of the neurocranium is closely related to the growth and development of the adjacent structures of brain, eye, nose and pharynx. The mesenchyme which gives rise to the cranial vault begins about day 45 as a capsular membrane around the developing brain.

15 This later subdivides into inner and outer meningeal layers. Several primary and secondary ossification centres develop in the outer layer to form the individual calvarial bones. As the bones enlarge the intervening mesenchyme becomes compressed to form the sutures.

16 Almost simultaneously with the formation of the neurocranium begins the differentiation of separate cartilaginous centres at the base of the skull which eventually fuse into a single irregular cranial base, much perforated by openings through which pass the spinal canal, cranial nerves and blood vessels which connect the developing brain with the body.

17 By comparison with the rapid expansion of the neurocranium, the cranial base is relatively slow and stable. Thus it maintains a balance between the enlarging cranial bones above and the slower but sustained growth of the facial skeleton beneath. In the first few months of development the face is tucked below the cranium by flexion of the cranial base. Later, extension of this flexure permits enlargement of the neurocranial capacity and prolonged downward, rather than forward, displacement of the facial skeleton as growth proceeds. This feature, more than all others, distinguishes the development of man from that of the apes.

18 At approximately 60 days of gestation the embryo has acquired all of its basic morphological characteristics and enters the fetal period. Until this time, genetic factors determining cell differentiation have played the predominant role in craniofacial development. During fetal life intrinsic genetic factors become less and less important while epigenetic* factors increase in influence. Since both genetic and environmental factors are present, and interact, it is difficult to ascertain the exact role of each. It is the interplay of these genetic and environmental factors on a small scale which accounts for normal variations. These we accept as part of the infinite variety of nature which falls within normal limits.

*relating to progressive differentiation.

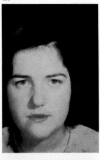
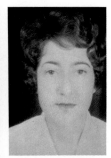
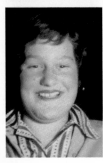
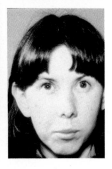

19 **The extent of variation** shown in the form of the human face is remarkable; we loosely classify facial form as roughly square, tapering or ovoid, but in reality a pictorial composite of structurally balanced faces includes a wide variety of facial types. Variations in facial growth occur in amount, timing, rate and direction. Variation is the rule, rather than the exception. It is generally conceded that normal facial growth patterns exhibit certain traits in common, but even so, no single growth pattern can be considered average or ideal.

Craven (1958) has shown that the female face is more protrusive than the male face; Davoody and Sassouni (1978) have demonstrated the differences that can exist between racial groups. One racial group may show a flat skeletal profile because of a retruded maxilla and a protruded chin while another group may exhibit a longer face, with differences in overbite, lip convexity and other features. The significance of these variations should not be lost when planning orthognathic surgery; the cephalometric norms of the race and sex must be taken into account when the range of variability is assessed. In short, while average values or patterns are useful references, individual patients do not always conform to such restricted pathways. Thus the study of variability is of major importance.

20

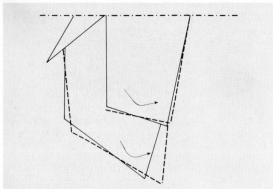

Patterns of individual variation

While the sources of individual variations in growth have not yet been adequately identified, evidence is being accumulated on general patterns of growth which lead to specific facial types. The most productive of these recent studies have been those of Gasson and Lavergne (1977). They have investigated the patterns of rotation of the maxilla and mandible during human growth and have established four principal types of rotation.

21

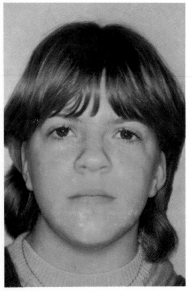

20 and 21 **In the first pattern the maxilla and the mandible** both rotate in an anterior direction. Under normal circumstances there is harmonious growth in sagittal and vertical dimensions and the result is a normal dentofacial appearance. When this growth pattern is abnormal, the short face syndrome may result.

22

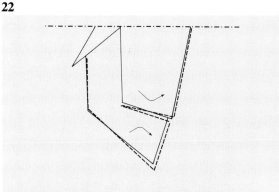

26

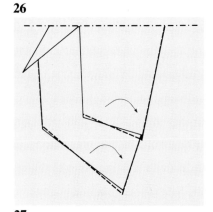

22 and 23   The second combination is that in which the maxilla rotates in an anterior direction and the mandible in a posterior direction. Dysharmony results in a variable degree of opening of the interbasal angle and an increase in the ANB angle. It is easy to see that unco-ordinated growth in this pattern of development leads to anterior openbite.

24 and 25   In the third rotational pattern there is a tendency to a decrease in the ANB angle and the development of a deep anterior overbite.

26 and 27   Finally the maxilla and mandible may both rotate in a posterior direction. When these rotations are harmonious in intensity the vertical and sagittal relationships remain stable. Lack of co-ordinated growth control results in the long face syndrome.

23

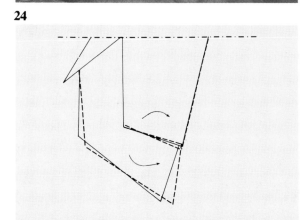

27

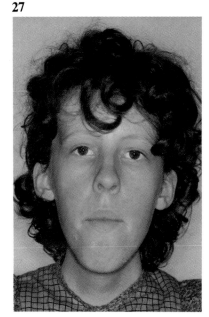

24

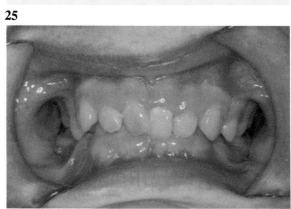

It can be seen therefore that while a harmonious relationship between maxillary and mandibular growth rotation leads to a variety of facial types within the limits of normal variation, the possibility for well defined abnormal patterns of facial development exists when maxillary and mandibular rotation are unco-ordinated. We know that considerable variation occurs between the growth rates of different body parts within a person. When these changes occur in the jaws, under the influence of a wide variety of factors, both endogenous and exogenous, then morphological abnormalities may arise. Since it is so difficult to distinguish between cause and effect, discussions about the respective roles of hereditary and environmental factors in craniofacial development are only of academic interest.

The success of treatment may well depend, to a degree, on the individual factors involved but we will have to wait until much more is known about the factors controlling the variations in growth and development of many craniofacial components before precise conclusions can be made about the absolute cause of many extreme variations in form.

25

The etiopathogenesis of anomalous craniomaxillofacial development

When one studies individual components of the craniofacial complex it is easier to classify and discuss anomalous development. To some extent this evades the complex issues of the extent of interaction which exists between the various parts of the craniofacial complex during their growth and development. Nevertheless, such a simplistic approach has value, if only to assemble, in semi-rigid compartments, those facts which are known. Provided that this is done on the understanding that the domino effect of one part on the other exists at all times in interdependent systems, then the exercise has value.

In the following discussion classification is based on current perceptions of pathogenesis. In Section 3 classification is more clinically based. For clinical description the latter is probably more practical.

Anomalies affecting the mandible

1 Symmetrical malformations: congenital

(a) *Mandibular prognathism*

Prognathism is a common anomaly, and may occur in apparent isolation, sometimes with a family history, or even in association with a recognised malformation syndrome. Recent animal experiments have shed more light on the pathogenesis of variation in mandibular shape and size (Festing and Wolff, 1979). Genetic variation at three loci has pleiotropic effects on mandibular form. External agents such as radiation can induce dominant mutations in mandible shape including prognathism; so also can a teratogenic agent such as heat stress in early pregnancy. The mandible is obviously more susceptible to such influences than other components of the craniofacial skeleton.

28

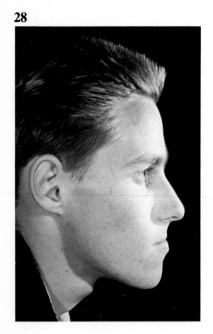

28 The skeletal components of the mandibular body or ramus or both are disproportionately large with a skeletal Class III relationship to the rest of the craniofacial complex. The incisal relationship may vary from edge to edge to severe reverse overjet and little occlusal contact on the posterior teeth. Occasionally anterior open bite exists. (See Section 3, pp. 93 to 96, **299–315**).

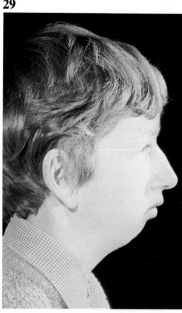

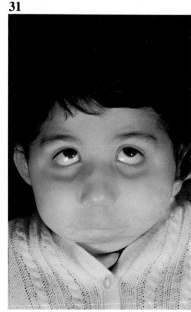

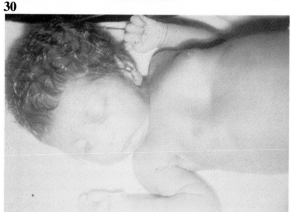

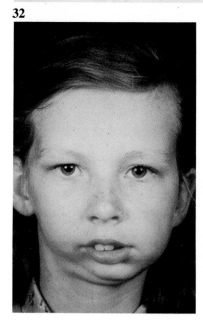

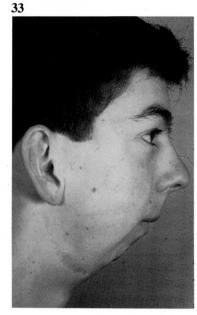

(b) *Severe retrognathism*

29 **This may vary** from a pronounced distoclusion of a mandible normal in form which could be accounted for on the basis of a disturbance in the rotational patterns previously described, or a more severe microgenia. (See Section 3, pp. 97 to 104, **316–350**.)

30 **The Robin syndrome** is first observed at birth when respiratory distress, particularly in the inspiratory phase, may rapidly become apparent. Cyanotic spells with inhalation of saliva lead to pneumonia and death unless great care is taken to prevent the tongue falling back. It is probable that postural problems during intrauterine development lead to compression of the chin against the sternum for long spells with consequent deformation of the mandible during periods of active forward growth. The pathogenesis of the full Robin syndrome including cleft palate will be described in the section devoted to facial clefts.

(c) *Condylar agenesis*

31 **Agenesis of both mandibular condyles** is more difficult to explain. The blastema of the temporomandibular joint arise late in development and it is possible that local disturbances in mesenchyme can result from a failure of inductive or other cell-mediated processes to establish the concentration of chondroblasts which form the condylar heads. In this condition there is severe and progressive underdevelopment of the vertical height of the lower third of the face.

2 Symmetrical malformations: acquired

(a) *Inflammatory disease of the condyles*

32 **Still's disease** (juvenile rheumatoid) can destroy both mandibular condyles, leading to severe retrognathism and all the growth problems associated with loss of posterior facial height.

(b) *Severe condylar trauma*

33 **In rare instances,** improperly treated bilateral fracture-dislocation of the condylar necks can result in the same problems. The condyles serve as an adjustable link between the tooth-bearing alveolar processes and the base of the skull. When condylar form or function is seriously disturbed, by congenital or acquired anomalous development, the effects on the whole mandible can be severe.

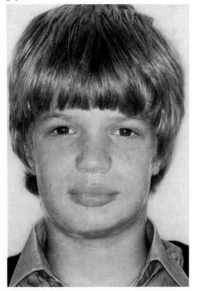

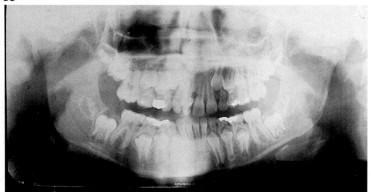

35

3 Asymmetrical malformations: congenital and developmental

Asymmetry often causes more severe disorganisation of the associated structures of the craniofacial complex than does a symmetrical anomaly. This is particularly apparent in the mandible, when dissymetry has wide-reaching effects on the contiguous structures of maxilla, malar and temporal bones.

(a) *Hemihypertrophy of the mandible*

34 Asymmetrical mandibular prognathism occurs in two distinct forms. The more rare is congenital hemihypertrophy which is occasionally familial and may be associated with enlargement of other tissues and organs on the same side. No convincing cause has been proposed for this abnormal concentration of tissues. Whatever the prime cause, it is likely that unequal regulative ability, in the two halves of the developing embryo, has a pronounced effect on the development of the mandibular defect. (See also Section 3, p. 125, **437–443**.)

35 When the mandible appears to be the sole organ affected, the condition is often distinguished by enlarged permanent molar and premolar teeth on the affected side. Patients with any degree of congenital hemihypertrophy have a higher risk than the population at large of Wilm's tumour and adrenocortical carcinoma (Fraumeni, J.F. *et al*, 1967).

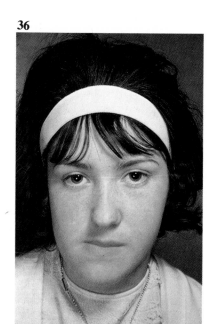

36

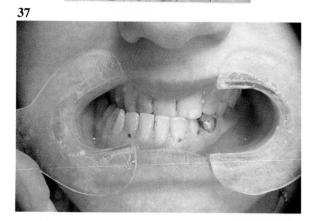

37

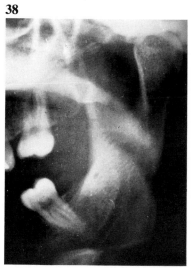

38

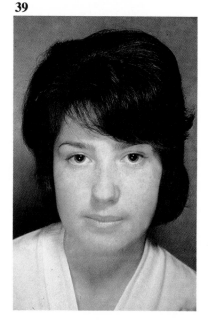

39

(b) *Condylar hyperplasia*

36 and 37 Developmental hyperplasia of the mandibular condyle is much more common. It leads to increasing asymmetry and prognathism. While it is possible that the basic anomaly exists from birth, it is usually at adolescence that the disparity in the jaw becomes obvious. (See Section 3, p. 124, **433–436**.)

38 The condylar cartilage increases rapidly in size but usually retains its capacity for adaptive remodelling. One plausible explanation for the defect is that the secondary cartilage of the condyle assumes the primary growth potential of an epiphyseal cartilage; regrettably, there is no scientific evidence to support this but if the proof of the pudding is in the eating then the case speaks for itself. Excision of the cap of condylar cartilage by high condylectomy arrests the anomalous growth of the condyle and normal development is resumed. (See Section 5, pp. 313 and 314, **1244** to **1248**.)

39 The results, two years after high condylar shave of the left condyle, of the patient shown in **36** and **37**.

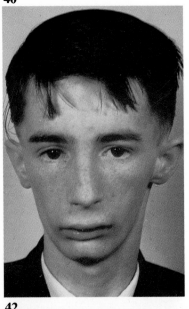

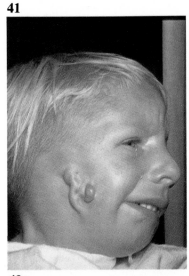

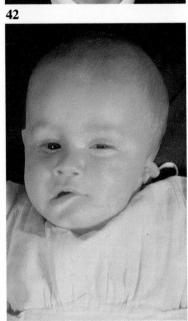

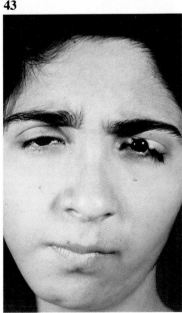

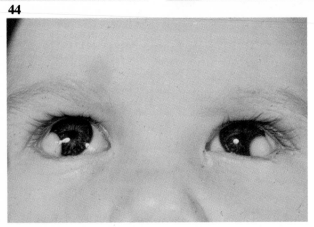

(c) *Craniofacial microsomia*

This is, arguably, the most serious of the asymmetrical malformations which affect the mandible and associated structures. Under this title shelter such conditions described as the first and second branchial arch syndrome, Goldenhar syndrome, and otomandibular dysostosis. These conditions have not been shown to possess any significant family predisposition. In one form or another they occur once in about 3,000 births with a 1 : 1 sex ratio. In about 70% of cases the anomaly is unilateral. When it is bilateral it is always asymmetrical.

40 **In classical craniofacial microsomia** the defects may vary from slight, as seen here, to severe. (See also Section 3, pp. 133 to 135, **483–497**.)

41 **The defects often extend well beyond the mandible** and both primary and derived changes are seen in the form of the auricle, the middle ear, malar, maxilla, squamous temporal bones and many of the associated soft-tissue structures such as the adjacent muscles of mastication, particularly the masseter, medial pterygoid and temporal, and the parotid gland.

42 **There may be paresis** or occasionally paralysis of the muscles of facial expression on the affected side.

43 **In Goldenhar syndrome** ocular defects are also found. These appear as upper lid colobomas.

44 **Epibulbar dermoids** are occasionally found; there may also be associated anomalies of the cervical spine and ribs. Animal and clinical studies support the hypothesis that the causative factor is focal necrosis of tissues in the vicinity of the developing ramus of the mandible at about day 35 of human development (Poswillo, 1973).

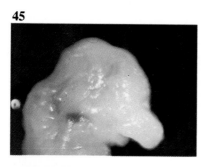

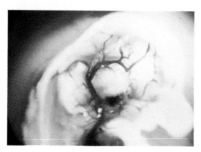

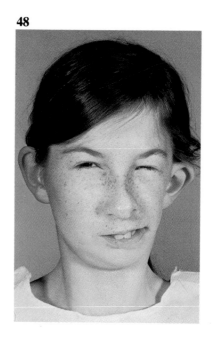

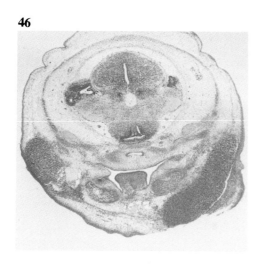

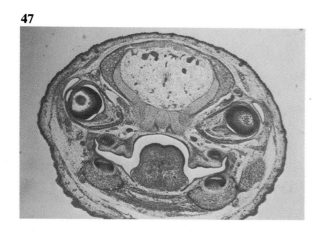

45 **An expanding hematoma** arising from the stapedial arterial system destroys and disorganises actively differentiating mesenchyme in a localised area of the face unrelated to embryologic boundaries.

46 **The blood clot, centred on the developing ear,** and seen here in a frontal section of the animal model, encroaches variably, depending on size, on many structures adjacent to the condyle and ramus. In this bilaterally affected case a large hematoma is seen on the right side and a smaller lesion on the left. The hematoma is thus quite unselective in its effects and clinical cases vary in severity according to the degree of primary destruction and the capacity of the disorganised tissues to effect catch-up repair. Not only are skeletal tissues affected by this embryological accident but so also are the soft-tissue components of the functional matrix unit described by Moss (1968) as the prime mover in facial growth.

47 **In this frontal section** of the animal model in which only the right side has been affected one sees the loss of the masseter muscle and zygomatic arch and a significant reduction in size of the body of the mandible.

48 **The end result** of this embryologic accident is insult added to injury, for the disturbance of the functional periosteal matrix may have a severe and lasting impact on the growth and development of the affected face. A series of secondary growth disturbances adds to the problems of form and function in the mandible and contiguous structures. This disparity can continue to affect development until active growth ceases late in adolescence, thus causing the dilemma for the reconstructive surgeon who must attempt to find the optimum time for stable repair of the residual defects.

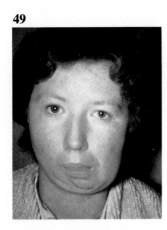

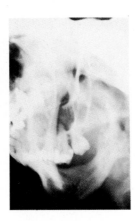

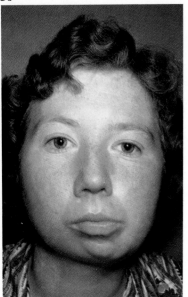

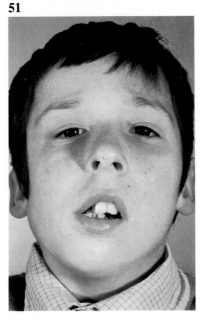

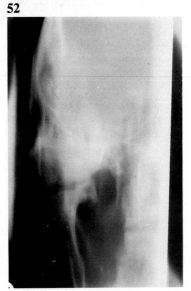

4 Asymmetrical malformations: acquired

Acquired anomalies of the mandible may be asymmetrical and severe. The etiopathogenesis of these conditions is usually obvious. (See also Section 3, pp. 131 and 132, **471–482**.)

49 **The most common cause** is an infective process which spreads from the middle ear to the temporomandibular joint with subsequent lysis of the condyle.

50 **This causes disturbances** in facial growth closely comparable with those found in less severe cases of craniofacial microsomia where all or most of the muscles of mastication are present and functional. The condition usually arises in the first two years of life; it has also been termed condylysis but the name gives little extra information in terms of the pathological process.

51 **Trauma to the mandibular condyle** with subsequent infection, especially in childhood, may lead to progressive ankylosis of the affected joint and gross disturbances in facial growth.

52 **The condylar head** is frequently flattened or misshapen and there are corresponding changes in the radiological architecture of the glenoid fossa. Early surgical excision of the ankylosis and reconstruction with a costochondral graft is seen to restore function and growth. (See Section 5, p. 324, **1313** and **1314**.)

Summary

All of the acquired conditions which lead to asymmetrical anomalous development of the mandible are found, in practice, to impose severe restrictions and limitations on the functional matrix growth unit. The end result, in terms of anomalous facial development, may be closely akin to that found in the congenital malformations. The determining difference may be the possibility which exists to restore to normal form and function those parts which have been lost or distorted by disease or trauma.

Where nature has failed to provide, as in facial microsomia, the reconstructive problem during the period of active growth may be insuperable. On the other hand, where the problem is acquired, as in ankylosis, the opportunity for surgical repair may be first class. On such pragmatic variables as these depends the success or failure of measures taken to restore the growth potential and reestablish normal development (Poswillo, 1974).

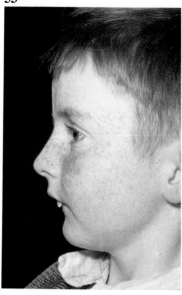

53

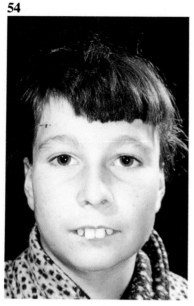

54

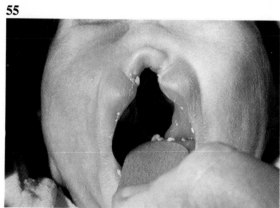

55

Anomalies affecting the maxilla

Many maxillary anomalies are not easy to classify or quantify. They occasionally exist in isolation, but more often are associated with anomalous development of other components in the craniofacial complex. This is especially true of the syndromic patterns of anomalous development which will be discussed later. (See Section 3, pp. 105 to 122, **351–423**.)

53   Premaxillary protrusion. It is generally accepted that this results from disharmonies of skeletal growth leading to a Skeletal 2 base; these growth disturbances are complicated by functional activity of the tongue and lips. (See Section 2, pp. 48 to 55, **140–170**.)

54   Maxillary alveolar hyperplasia is more difficult to explain. Alveolar development is ill-understood. The apparent alveolar prognathism observed in children is masked as the face gradually drifts forwards. If mandibular alveolar bone growth does not keep pace or maxillary alveolar bone growth is excessive then maxillary alveolar hyperplasia will result.

55   Maxillary hypoplasia is a more complex phenomenon. In cases of severe frontonasal deficiency such as those which arise in gross examples of the fetal alcohol syndrome, all or most of the mesenchyme of the frontonasal process would appear to have failed to form.

56   In less severe defects it is not clear what developmental disturbances are involved, although numerous environmental teratogens such as alcohol and drugs with related effects may disturb the flow of ectomesenchymal cells into the developing face.

57   Those cells from the cranial neural crest which migrate over the frontal region into the midline facial processes are obviously vulnerable at critical stages of morphogenesis. Death or diversion of these cells will disorganise, to a greater or lesser degree, those structures which form from the frontonasal prominence and the medial nasal processes.

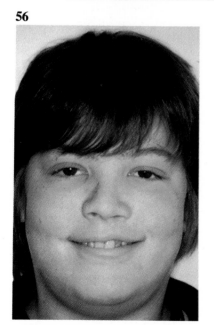

56

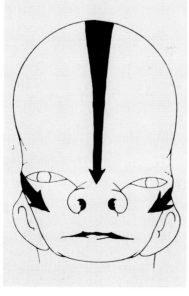

57

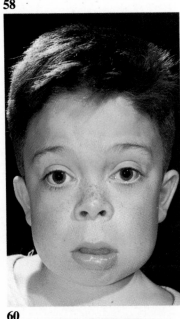

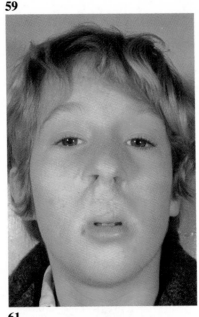

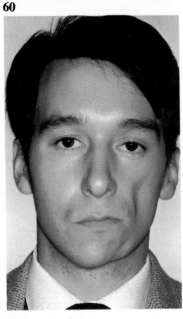

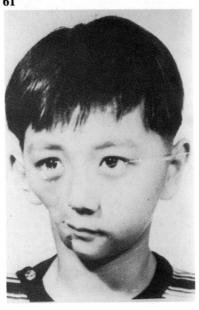

58 **Congenital dish-face deformities** may possibly arise as a result of asynchronous development between the calvarium and the cranial base. Any reduction in the growth of the cranial base as a result of chondrodystrophy may lead to maxillary hypoplasia and rounding of the neurocranium. We see examples of this in achondroplasia, cretinism, and Hurler syndrome, one of the mucopolysaccharide disorders, which is illustrated here showing the gargoyle-like facies.

59 **The growth and development** of the maxilla can be severely affected by trauma. The effects of surgery for cleft lip and palate play an important role in the development of maxillary hypoplasia. The pathogenesis of cleft lip and palate will be discussed later, but it is important at this point to note the role of surgical trauma in the pathogenesis of maxillary hypoplasia in the cleft lip and palate patient. Untreated or mistreated mid-face injuries may also have lasting effects on the growth of the maxilla, producing hypoplasia and anterior openbite.

60 **Hemifacial atrophy** (Romberg disease) is a slowly progressive condition in which one half of the face, particularly the maxilla, becomes atrophic sometime in the first decade. The degenerative process slowly spreads from dermis to facial muscle to underlying bone and cartilage. (See also Section 3, p. 138, **508–512**.)

61 **The condition often begins** in the area covered by temporal or buccinator muscles and can extend to the brow above and the angle of the mouth below. The disease often burns out after three or four years.

The relationship between this disease and scleroderma has long been debated; some authors contend that the *coup-de-sabre* form of scleroderma is only a variant of hemifacial atrophy. Although many afflicted patients give a history of previous trauma, more emphasis has been placed on changes in the sympathetic nervous system as likely precursors of the atrophic process. Experiments in rats in which unilateral cervical sympathectomy has been carried out have resulted in facial changes which resemble those in man. However, it is difficult to account, in man, for contralateral Jacksonian epilepsy or trigeminal neuralgia, which often accompany hemifacial atrophy, on the basis of degeneration in the peripheral sympathetic system (Moss and Crikelair, 1960).

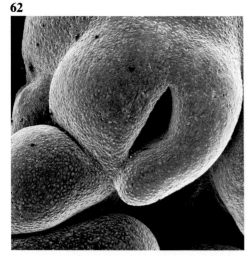

62

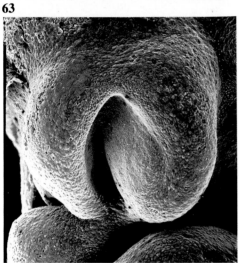

63

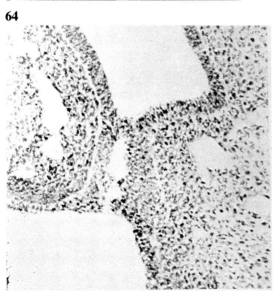

64

Clefts of the lip and palate

Normal facial development depends on two principal inter-actions. First, there are genetic instructions for morphogenesis. Second, there must be the capacity in the local tissues for the unhindered completion of complex metabolic processes which are necessary for cell replication, cell survival and programmed cell death. Complex malformations may arise in many different ways. Morphogenesis and growth may be influenced by factors as diverse as chromosomal anomalies at one end of the spectrum and interacting environmental factors at the other. Genetic and environmental factors may combine to affect, in subtle ways, single developmental processes such as palate closure or more complex morphogenetic activities such as the establishment of sutures or the organisation of joints.

There are many enigmas when one studies the etiopatho-genesis of craniofacial deformity. For example, similar orofacial malformations may arise from substantially different etiological agents which have only one property in common; the capacity to initiate a particular causal mechanism of malformation. Para-doxically, however, similar causal mechanisms do not always produce identical malformations. This was obviously apparent in the case of facial microsomia. Where the developmental pathway is long or involves the interaction of many different processes the pathological events can be exaggerated, modified or ameliorated by changes in the balance between the com-peting forces of cell death and repair.

The most common serious orofacial anomaly is cleft lip and palate. It is considered to be a problem in which genetic susceptibility is influenced by multiple and probably cumulative environmental factors. Neither the genetic nor the environ-mental factors have been well documented as yet, but there is some evidence to suggest that diazepam and phenytoin are but two of the drugs which, taken in early pregnancy, may shift the developmental threshold towards cleft lip and palate. (Safra and Oakley, 1975, Slone et al, 1976.)

The incidence of cleft lip and palate varies from 1 : 700 live births in Caucasians to about 1 : 3000 in the Negroid races. The incidence is very much higher, about 1 : 400, in the Japanese and certain American Indians. Cleft lip and palate is slightly more common in males than females among Caucasians but in the Japanese the incidence is much the same.

62 The critical stage of lip formation is when the medial and lateral nasal processes contact each other before coalescence. At this stage teratogenic insults may produce disturbances in the mesenchyme which vary the size of the lateral nasal processes (Sulik et al, 1979).

63 A severe reduction in size, such as is produced in the mouse by maternal doses of phenytoin or dexamethasone, may lead to failure of the process to make contact with the adjacent medial nasal process and result in cleft lip.

64 Additionally, at the time of consolidation of the facial processes there is a concurrent programme of spontaneous cell death involved in the removal of epithelial debris from the developing nasal placode (Warbrick, 1960).

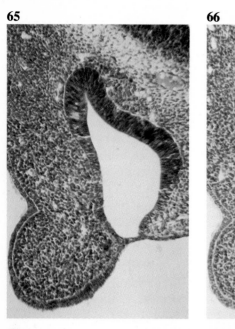

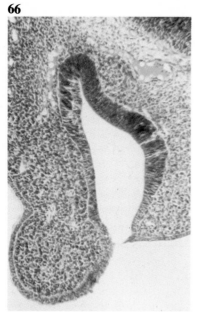

65 When this cell death is more extensive than necessary and repair of mesenchyme is disturbed, a weakness develops in the forming lip and alveolus.

66 The continued action of growth traction forces may further disrupt the association of the facial processes with the lip margins being pulled apart.

67 Under such circumstances it is not difficult to envisage that complete disruption would produce a severe cleft which extends from the margin of the lip into the floor of the nose.

68 Likewise, a lesser injury may produce an incomplete tear in the precursor tissues, leaving only an incomplete cleft of the lip.

69 In the simplest cases there may be only a line or sign of dysymmetry on the lip tissue proper.

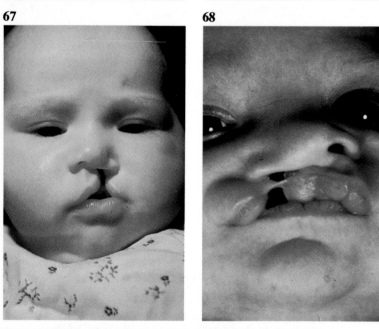

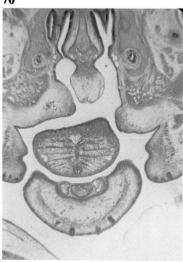

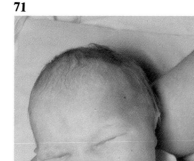

70 **There is a frequent association** between clefts of the lip and cleft palate. Animal studies suggest that following the failure of lip closure there is an overgrowth of the prolabial tissues which then diverts the tongue into the nasal cavity. The mechanical obstruction of the tongue can delay the movement of one or both palatal shelves so that opportunities for palatal fusion are lost.

71 **The abnormal position** of the tongue may still be seen at birth, high in the palate between the margins of the cleft, effectively sealing off the cleft of the lip to facilitate the process of swallowing—a process which commences, in utero, about the time that the lip is formed and before the palatal shelves have moved from their vertical to the horizontal position prior to fusion.

72

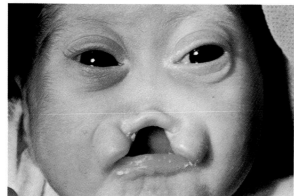

Rare facial clefts

72 **The median cleft** probably represents the failure of the paired primordia of the medial nasal processes to fuse into a single globular process. The frequent association of this anomaly with bifid nose and orbital hypertelorism suggests that there is a common link between all these anomalies. Avian studies in which small punch grafts of neural crest tissues have been removed from the mesencephalon have led to the conclusion that disturbances in the central flow of neural crest-derived ectomesenchyme may be responsible for these defects.

73 **Oblique facial clefts** are probably the result of disruptive forces applied to the formed face by swallowed strips of amnion. These strands are attached to the fetal sac at one end and enter the oesophagus of the fetus at the other. The amniotic bands ulcerate through the tissues of the lip and cheek during fetal movements. Subsequent repair of the margins produces bizarre congenital clefts which follow no natural junctions of the facial processes.

In the description of normal facial development it was pointed out that the sequence of lip and palate formation extends over 15 days in man. It is not surprising, therefore, that in many syndromes cleft lip and palate should accompany anomalies of other parts of the body. Many developing systems can be disturbed simultaneously by teratogenic influences which operate over a long period of morphodifferentiation.

73

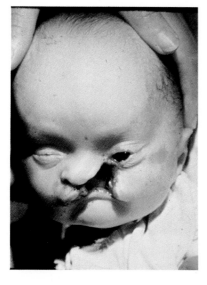

Isolated cleft palate

Isolated clefts of the posterior palate are distinctly different in etiology from those that accompany cleft lip. They differ in incidence, sex predisposition and their relationship to associated birth defects. In Caucasians the incidence is approximately 1 : 2000 live births and the male/female ratio is 40 : 60.

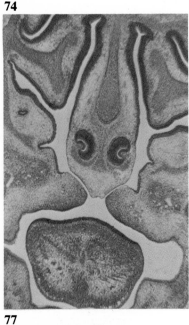

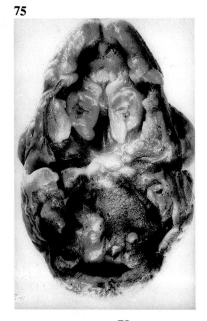

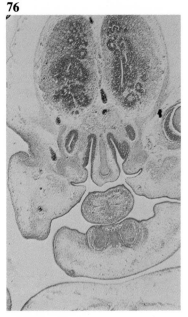

74 **Interference with elevation** of the palatal shelves by delaying the onset of the intrinsic shelf force by maternal dosing with vitamin A leads to a characteristic form of cleft palate.

75 **Here the palatal shelves are large** but there is a small V-shaped central cleft.

76 **Radiation with ionising rays** can delay the differentiation and growth of the palatal shelves sufficiently long to produce stunted, small shelves which fail to meet each other or the nasal septum after shelf rotation, leaving a wide cleft.

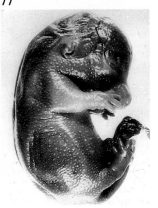

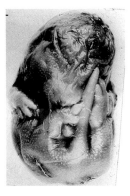

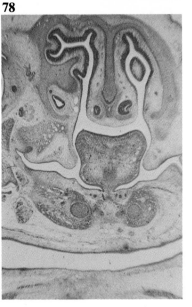

77 **Induced loss of amniotic fluid** from the fetal membranes immediately prior to palate closure prevents the essential extension of the cranial flexure which releases the tongue from the space between the palatal shelves (Poswillo, 1966).

78 **The vertical palatal shelves** are prevented from rotating to the horizontal position essential for fusion by the mechanical obstruction of the tongue.

The pathogenesis of isolated cleft palate

Fusion of the palate depends on shelf adhesion, death of the midline epithelial seam and fusion of ectomesenchyme between one shelf and the other. Thus there exists in the developing palate a variety of phenomena which must act in harmony over a relatively short time span to produce normal palatogenesis.

Animal experiments have shown that a number of situations can be induced in which palatal shelf fusion fails to occur.

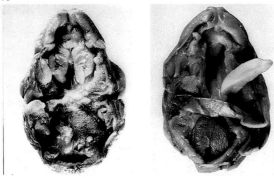

79

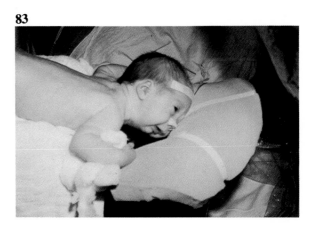

83

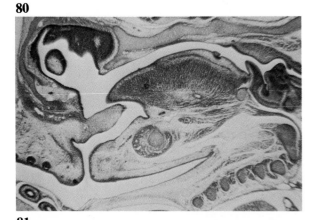

80

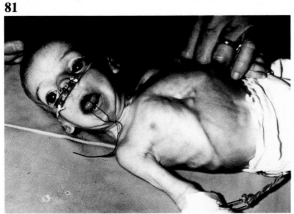

81

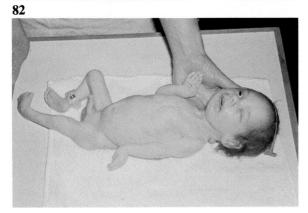

82

79   **The resultant cleft** is U-shaped rather than V-shaped.

80   **There is also marked microgenia** and a high obstuctive position of the tongue identical with that seen in the human Robin syndrome.

81   **In the Robin condition** the tongue frequently becomes wedged in the characteristic U-shaped cleft in the neonatal period, leading to respiratory crises, asphyxia and inspiration pneumonia.

82   **Because the defects** in the Robin syndrome are caused by postural moulding, with associated postural defects such as congenital hip dislocation and talipes, there exists the possibility that much of the abnormal moulding will disappear with growth provided that attention is paid to the basic principles of catch-up development.

83   **Prone postural nursing** of the Robin baby permits the partial or complete recovery from microgenia and restores normal tongue-hyoid-mandible activity essential for trouble-free respiration.

The most common facial clefts are submucous clefts of the hard palate which occur in 1 : 1200 births and bifid uvula, 1 : 100.

Both submucous cleft palate and bifid uvula can be regarded as microforms of isolated palatal clefting and are probably the result of disturbances in the local mesenchyme at the time of ossification of the palatal bridge and merging of the margins of the soft palate. These phenomena occur late in morphogenesis, between the 7th and 10th weeks of human development; all the more reason for protecting the embryo from teratogenic insults until well into the second trimester of pregnancy.

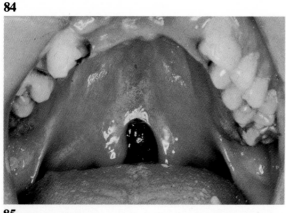

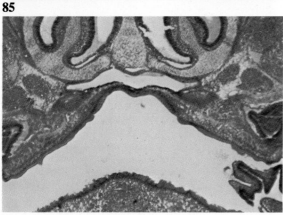

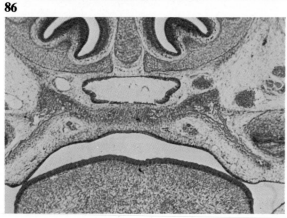

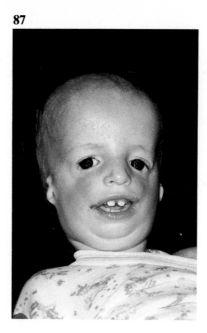

87 Hemifacial microsomia and mandibulofacial dysostosis. In both there are obvious but distinctly different eye anomalies. While anti-mongoloid slanting of the eyes is common to both conditions, in Treacher Collins there are bilateral colobomas of the outer half of the lower eyelid and absence of eyelashes in the medial portion of the lower lids. The maxilla and mandible, especially the condyle, are underdeveloped and the zygomatic arch is frequently missing. The auricles are malformed and hypoplastic, and conduction deafness is common.

84 Submucous cleft is characterised by thin transparent mucosa over a V-shaped cleft in the posterior third of the hard palate.

85 This condition can be induced in animals by agents such as phenytoin which disorganise the differentiation of the bony palatal plates. Disturbances in inductive processes result in thin attenuated palatal shelves, arched high into the palatal vault, with incomplete bridging of the gap in the posterior third of the hard palate. The terminal margins of the soft palate fail to merge into a single uvula (Poswillo, 1974).

86 By comparison, the normal palate at the same stage of development has a flat bony reinforced vault with a well defined median suture.

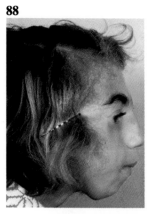

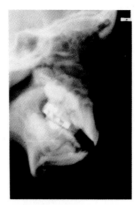

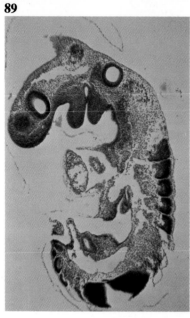

There are many other syndromic patterns of anomalous craniofacial development. Indeed the list seems to grow longer year by year. It will not be possible to discuss all of these syndromes but certain significant examples can be taken as indications of other developmental phenomena which lead to craniofacial deformity.

There are a number of symmetrical syndromes characterised by dysplasia of first and second branchial arch derivatives. Some of these closely resemble facial microsomia. The most common of these unusual conditions is Treacher Collins syndrome or mandibulofacial dysostosis. Treacher Collins is an autosomal dominant trait with total penetrance and variable expressivity. Within a family, all graduations of the condition may be found.

It has not been exclusively established that environmental factors play a part in these symmetrical craniofacial anomalies in man, nevertheless it has been possible to construct animal models of identical malformations by the use of exogenous teratogens and there is the suggestion in man that variants in expressivity of the autosomal dominant gene which is responsible for Treacher Collins syndrome in man is a result of modification of the abnormal genes by exogenous factors. Observations made during embryogenesis of the animal model of Treacher Collins syndrome indicate that the anomalies arise as a result of destruction or disturbances of migration of the preotic neural crest ectomesenchymal cells which normally migrate to the facial and auditory primordiae (Poswillo, 1975).

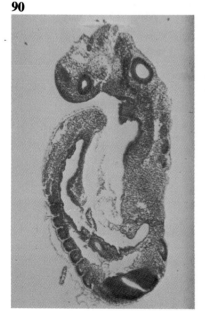

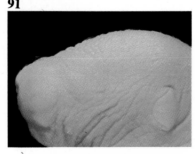

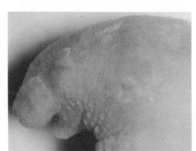

88   The nose may be beaked, with narrow nostrils and loss of the nasofrontal angle. The lower border of the mandible is concavely curved, anterior openbite is common and the chin is retruded. Cleft lip and palate may also be present. The craniofacial defects are invariably symmetrical.

89   The branchial arches in the normal animal are full of ectomesenchymal cells which contribute greatly to the skeleton and soft-tissues of the developing face.

90   Failure of these cells to migrate into the branchial arches reduces the normal volume of mesenchyme participating in morphodifferentiation and leads to hypoplasia of the musculoskeletal derivatives of these arches.

91   As a result of cell death in the mesencephalon there is a flow of adjacent tissue into the defect. The otocyst migrates upwards into the territory of the first branchial arch so that the eventual position of the pinna is closer to the angle of the jaw, as is seen in the normal and affected animal models of mandibulofacial dysostosis. Despite the deficiencies in musculoskeletal development and the symmetrical anomalies in the ear, malar, maxilla and mandible there exists in Treacher Collins syndrome an intact but modified functional periosteal matrix.

31

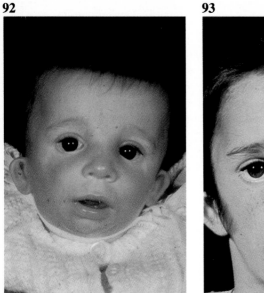

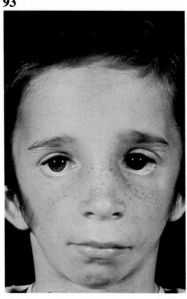

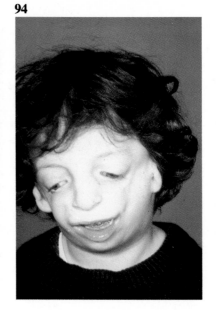

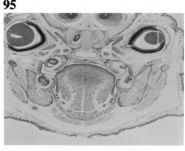
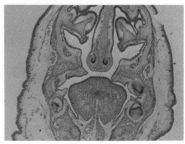

In the Treacher Collins model there is no evidence of masseter or medial pterygoid. These two muscles are found as a single muscle band behind the angle of the mandible. The marked bowing of the lower border of the mandible in this syndrome results from the abnormal interplay of muscle forces in the absence of the stabilising effect of a normal masseteric attachment.

92 and **93**   **The infant with mandibulofacial dysostosis** grows symmetrically into the adolescent.

94   **The extreme variation in craniofacial form,** however, leads to considerable variations in the pattern of growth and the clinician should appreciate that surgical reconstruction of the facial skeleton may not restore a normal or near normal pattern of growth in these syndromes. As they are malformed, so shall they grow.

95   **In the frontal section** through the angle of the mandible in the normal animal the usual morphological relationship of masseter-mandible-medial pterygoid is observed. In the Treacher Collins model below the masseter-medial pterygoid attachment is not seen at the angle of the jaw.

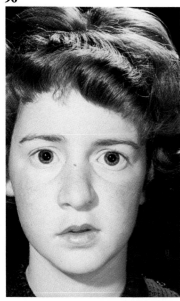

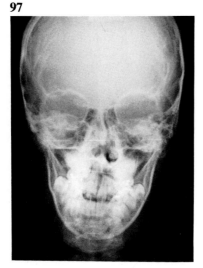

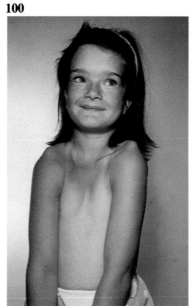

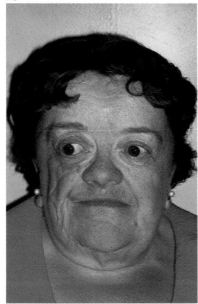

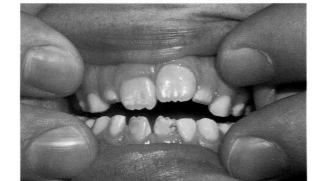

Anomalies affecting the cranium

Craniostenosis syndromes are many and varied; the majority occur rarely and many are associated with severe mental retardation or premature death. Thus only a small number are suitable for surgical reconstruction (David, Poswillo and Simpson, 1982).

More severe distortion of skull and facial shape may follow extensive changes in the timing of closure of sutures in the calvarium. When sutural fusion is delayed, as in the syndromes of Down and progeria, there is usually a broad forehead and a degree of hypertelorism.

96   Plagiocephaly most commonly arises from premature unicranial fusion of the coronal suture. Localised calvarial recessions and bulges are commonly found and the face shows three-dimensional asymmetry, occasionally comparable to the orbital and maxillary changes found in craniofacial microsomia. More than any other simple calvarial deformity, frontal and hemicranial plagiocephaly are craniofacial problems.

97   Radiological views show asymmetry of the orbits both in the horizontal and the vertical planes.

98   A similar pattern is found in cleidocranial dysostosis where the anterior fontanelle may never close, producing a broad skull and facies.

99   There are serious delays in the eruption of the teeth in this syndrome with many permanent teeth remaining fully covered by alveolar bone for most of the life of the patient. This condition is transmitted by autosomal dominant inheritance and is best recognised by the partial or complete absence of clavicles.

100   The affected patient is frequently asked to attempt to approximate the shoulders to demonstrate the clavicular deficiencies.

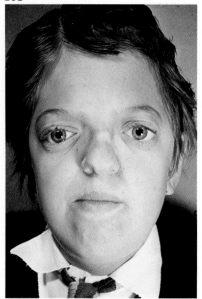

Syndromes which involve the incomplete development or premature fusion of the coronal, sagittal and lambdoid sutures are of the greatest interest to craniomaxillofacial surgeons. Especially so are those in which modern techniques of intracranial and extracranial surgical intervention have permitted near-normal reconstitution of the cranio-orbitofacial appearance and prevented the onset of blindness and other severe morbidity previously associated with severe cases.

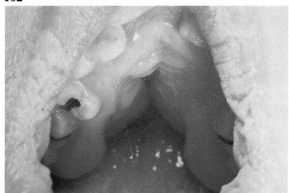

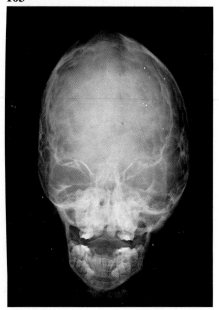

101   Crouzon syndrome. This condition is characterised by cranial synostosis, bilateral exophthalmos with external strabismus, a parrot-beaked nose and relative mandibular prognathism with drooping of the lower lip. It is inherited as an autosomal dominant trait with incomplete penetrance. Sporadic cases represent new mutations.

102   The hypoplastic maxilla, high V-shaped palate and malocclusion compound the craniofacial deformity.

103   The 'beaten-copper' skull. Radiographs show the classical pattern caused by progressive adaptive remodelling of the inner table of the calvarium in the absence of expansion of the skull bones in the sutural regions.

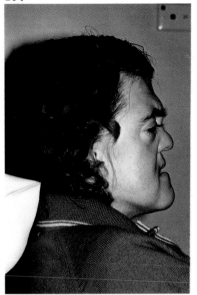

104

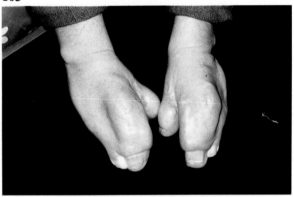

105

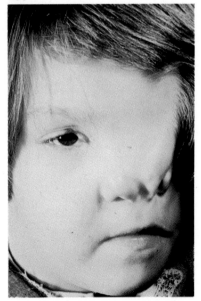

106

Premature fusion of many cranial sutures is said to occur in the Crouzon syndrome but as yet there is no valid evidence to support this hypothesis. There may be an equal likelihood that sutural abnormalities arise *ab initio* by incomplete sutural development at the time of calvarial ossification. Removal of the complete superficial calvarium from the supraorbital margins to the superior nuchal lines of the occipital bone permits regeneration of the calvarium with normal sutural junctions if performed before the 6th post-natal month. This exhibition of catch-up potential adds support to the hypothesis that inductive errors at the time of morphodifferentiation may lead to abnormal calvarial growth in many of the syndromes characterised by oxycephaly, turricephaly and acrocephaly. Removal of the calvarial bones in the neonate permits a second chance of normal induction and morphodifferentiation and the possibility of normal sutural development the second time around.

104 Apert syndrome (acrocephalosyndactyly) is a rare variant among the craniostenoses with turribrachycephaly comparable to that found in Crouzon syndrome.

105 Syndactyly of the hands and feet accompany the skull defects. The syndrome may be transmitted as an autosomal dominant disorder but most cases are sporadic. The co-existence of calvarial and limb defects in this anomaly would suggest that a basic disorganisation of the induction or morphodifferentiation of mesoderm may be responsible for the spectrum of defects.

106 Frontonasal dysplasia is a non-genetic congenital disorder in which the defects may range from ocular hypertelorism alone to severe defects of the nose, mid-face and upper lip and palate. In many severe cases of hypertelorism there is associated disorganisation of the frontal lobe of the brain with an increasing risk of neurological deficit as the morphological defects increase in number and severity.

It is probable that disturbances in the central flow of ectomesenchyme into the frontal prominence produce disturbances in the maxillary processes at the time that the developing orbits wedge together from their early lateral to their definitive central positions in the mid-face. Any disturbance in mitotic activity which keeps the optic primordiae separated could prevent normal differentiation of the frontonasal mesenchyme and lead to defects of the mid-face ranging from simple ocular hypertelorism to the median cleft face.

Many mysteries remain in the understanding of the etiology and pathogenesis of craniomaxillofacial malformation. Little is known of the histological and biochemical details of normal fusion of the cranial sutures; even less is known regarding the determinative role of the cranial base in establishing the matrix on which the whole complex is constructed.

Despite all the information which has been accumulated on normal growth and development and the pathogenesis of craniofacial anomalies, very little is known about the determinants of individual patterns of facial growth.

Orthognathic surgeons must learn to predict patterns of craniofacial growth in the various congenital and acquired anomalies. In this way they will become more competent in the treatment planning of surgical reconstructive procedures.

As the scientific basis of malformation is clarified it will be easier for surgeons to advance the quality and stability of treatment. Research efforts in both basic science and clinical practice will, hopefully, provide the answer, eventually, to many of the problems of abnormal development in the craniomaxillofacial region.

John Hunter, the Father of Scientific Surgery, proposed, in 1775, the significance to surgeons of the pathogenesis of deformity. He wrote "In treating (the deformed) it cannot be necessary to give a minute description of all the preternatural formations constituting them; however, some of their structures may explain two states, namely that state before birth and that after, both of which are of considerable consequence." These consequences remain our concern today and provide the basis for a continuing search for knowledge and perfection.

SECTION 2

Assessment and treatment planning of facial disproportion

Introduction – the approach to treatment planning

The surgical treatment of facial dysharmony has three main objectives—the correction of dental malocclusion, improvement of facial appearance, and the longterm stability of the results achieved. These reflect the three constituent elements of the facial complex, dental, skeletal, and soft tissues. If anatomical correction is to be achieved within physiologically stable limits, diagnostic assessment and treatment planning must embrace each of these three elements for any individual case.

This Section and Section 3 are concerned with general principles essential to proper clinical assessment, and with the systematic application of these principles to the evaluation of particular cases, including to some extent also the choice of alternative treatment methods or techniques. Each clinician will develop a personal system of case analysis; the following discussion is set within the framework of the author's own method principally as a means of bringing out the background logic and the known data to which that logic must be applied.

The formulation of a treatment plan must consider a series of questions which combine patient motivation with the objective clinical definition of abnormality.

Assessment scheme

(a) Appearance versus occlusion
   (Why is this patient seeking treatment?)

(b) Clinical examination and radiological analysis
   (What is the diagnosis in all its aspects?)

(c) Profile and occlusal planning
   (What would we like to achieve for this patient?)
   | Tests of Profile Prediction
   | Tests of feasibility (model surgery)
   | Tentative treatment plan
   ↓ (Can we achieve what we would like?)

(d) Definitive treatment plan

The motivation of the patient is of primary importance. Presenting complaints fall into two categories:

(a) *Disturbances of function*, which may be actual or potential. The commonest are reduced ability to masticate food, temporomandibular joint dysfunction, speech defects, nasal airway obstruction, or ocular disturbances (including inadequate bony protection of the globe). These may reflect dental malocclusion outside the scope of orthodontic correction alone, or the anatomical expression of midfacial hypoplasia. Ocular problems often arise in association with the more severe deformities of the facial skeleton.

(b) *Disturbances of appearance* have both objective and subjective results. A particular individual's reaction to cosmetic defects may reflect his own personality, the influence of friends or relations, or the type of job to which he aspires. Some people undergo corrective facial surgery, not so much to satisfy themselves as to render them more acceptable to an imperfect society which rates outward appearance more highly than strength of character or personal ability. Equally, many inadequate individuals seek to compensate for their personality defects by changes of body image, commonly by alteration of facial appearance. This type of patient may move from surgeon to surgeon, operation to operation, in a hopeless and misdirected quest for self-fulfilment. He (or more often, she) should be identified and referred for skilled psychiatric assessment before being accepted for surgery; otherwise both patient and surgeon may bitterly regret embarking on treatment together.

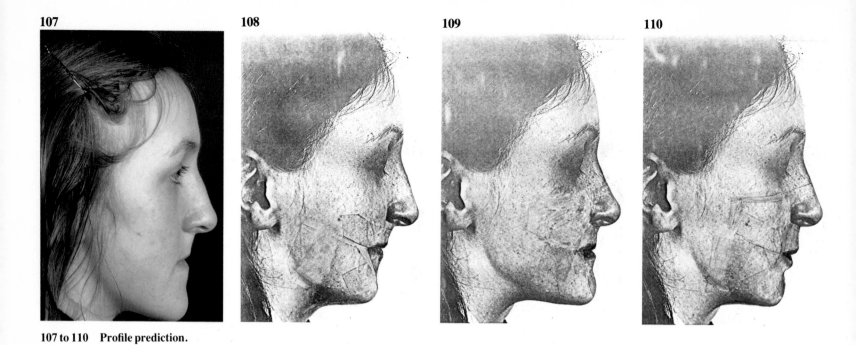

107 to 110   Profile prediction.

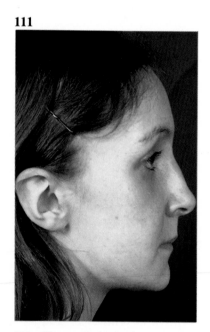

111   The result obtained.

The relative importance of appearance and function must be established at the outset, and is largely related to patient motivation. The answer to the question 'Why is this patient seeking treatment?' not only serves to identify the neurotic but also directs the surgeon's attention to the proper treatment objective. The illustration shows a typical case of moderately severe skeletal prenormality in profile (**107**), together with three predictions of profile after alternative osteotomies (**108**, **109** and **110**). Each result would have identical occlusion of the teeth, but the facial appearance in both profile and frontal views is quite different.

Some years ago the only surgical option would have been mandibular set-back (**108**) resulting in this case in bimaxillary retrusion characterised by a sloping profile settling into the neck. The chin is inadequately projected and the features of maxillary hypoplasia are not corrected. With the development of improved methods of maxillary surgery an alternative would have been maxillary advancement at the Le Fort 1 level until the occlusal correction was obtained. The prediction (**109**) shows an improvement in profile but there is once again a lack of harmony between the component thirds of the face produced by a bimaxillary protrusion. A series of possibilities is opened up by operations on both jaws, varying the proportion of the correction obtained by mandibular set-back and maxillary advancement respectively. The prediction shown (**110**) represents a fifty/fifty proportion and accords well with the actual result obtained by this method (**111**).

If restoration of occlusion is the prime objective then (provided postoperative stability is likely) the surgeon may well choose the simplest procedure. If appearance is the prime objective then the finest of occlusions will not deliver the result the patient seeks, and a complex bimaxillary procedure would be more appropriate. Incidentally, the value of methods of profile prediction can be seen in this case (p. 63 *et seq.*).

Determination of patient motivation may take time. Many are loathe to admit their readiness to undergo major surgery for reasons which may be seen by others as pure vanity. The true reasons for consultation must be brought out. It is much more commonly the case that patients undergoing orthognathic surgery are primarily interested in their appearance, and this accounts for much of the emphasis of this Atlas.

Clinical and radiographic analysis

The object of clinical and radiographic assessment is full diagnosis in all its aspects, including the *site* and *extent* of all skeletal and soft-tissue abnormalities both primary and secondary, together with a judgment of those aetiological and physiological factors which will bear on the timing and type of surgery to be undertaken, and its probable postoperative stability.

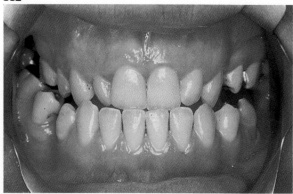

Abnormal skeletal anatomy can usually be defined fairly precisely by clinical and radiographic examination. Cephalometry yields invaluable information, but must only be used as a guide. The occlusion by itself may be most misleading. Compare the two cases shown in Figures **112** to **115** and **116** to **120**. Both cases present with similar Class 3 malocclusions. The girl, however, shows the classic features of nasomaxillary hypoplasia (see Section 3, p.112 *et seq.*), both clinically and cephalometrically. The man is a much more complex diagnostic problem. Underdevelopment of the maxilla is associated with a prominent but humped nose, vertical overclosure of the jaw in occlusion, mild mandibular protrusion, marked progenia, and transverse narrowing of the mandible in relation to cranial width.

113   **114**

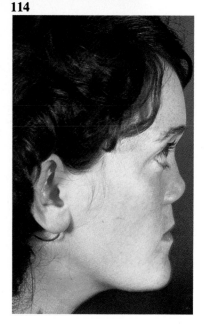

115

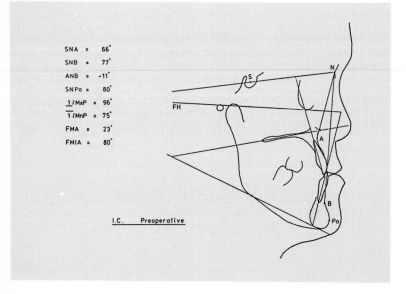

SNA =	66°
SNB =	77°
ANB =	-11°
SNPo =	80°
$\overline{1}$/MxP =	96°
$\overline{1}$/MnP =	75°
FMA =	23°
FMIA =	80°

I.C.   Preoperative

112 to 115   Abnormal skeletal anatomy. Nasomaxillary hypoplasia.

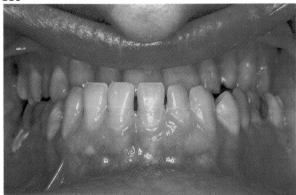

116

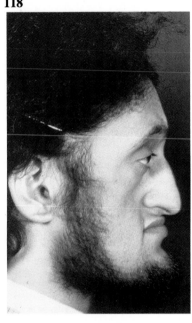

117   **118**

Identifying the sites of abnormality is the first guide to treatment, as it is technically possible to correct all the features identified in these two cases. Cephalometric analysis is especially helpful in distinguishing maxillary hypoplasia (or enlargement) from mandibular enlargement (or hypoplasia) and in identifying compensatory changes in the dentition or bone. Examples of the latter are retroclination of the lower incisors unduly influenced by lower lip pressure in prenormal occlusions, and lateral hypoplasia of the maxilla in cases of unilateral mandibular hypoplasia.

Soft-tissue anatomy is important in relation to its displacement or distortion when the associated hard-tissues are moved. The environment within which the corrected skeletal tissues must establish physiological balance will determine whether the surgery will be stable during the postoperative months and years. The hard and soft tissues are linked with the physiological environment by both growth and soft tissue activity, especially muscular activity. We shall start our assessment, therefore, with the soft tissues.

119

116 to 120   Abnormal skeletal anatomy. Panfacial disharmony.

120

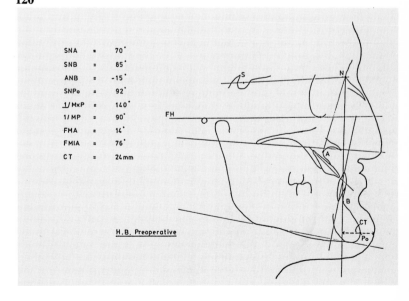

SNA	=	70°
SNB	=	85°
ANB	=	-15°
SNPo	=	92°
1/MxP	=	140°
1/MP	=	90°
FMA	=	14°
FMIA	=	76°
CT	=	24mm

H.B. Preoperative

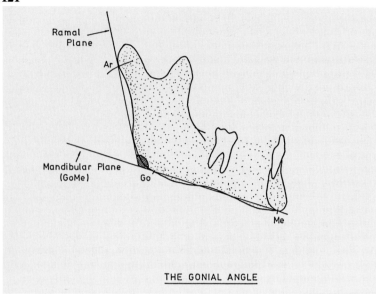

THE GONIAL ANGLE

121   The shape of the mandible.

The soft-tissue environment of the facial skeleton

Morphology and behaviour

The soft tissues which invest the facial bones vary quite considerably in their form and take part in infinitely variable behaviour patterns. They may or may not be involved in the excess or deficiency of tissue which characterises the skeletal abnormality, and in some cases (for example masseteric hypertrophy (**312 to 315**)) may constitute the prime abnormality. In general those skeletal patterns usually associated with soft-tissue deficiency or excess are those of congenital or developmental origin; soft tissue deficiency causes the greatest clinical difficulties.

Bone is affected during growth and adult life by a continual process of resorption and deposition in response to soft-tissue forces and humoral stimulation, resulting in moulding of the skeletal architecture to produce a structure in dynamic equilibrium with its soft tissue environment. Similarly, the position of individual teeth and the shape of the dental arches reflects the balance of these pressures, mainly (but not exclusively) muscular. Just as these forces affect the stability of orthodontic treatment, so they affect skeletal surgery. Both the anatomical contribution of the soft tissue to the condition itself, and the effect of the proposed alteration in the bone/soft tissue relationship must be considered. Three functional groups are involved—the pterygomasseteric tissues, the linguovestibular musculature, and the suprahyoid group.

1   The pterygomasseteric group of soft tissues

This includes not only the masseter, internal pterygoid, temporalis and external pterygoid muscles, but also the skin, subdermal tissues, fascia, ligaments, and periosteum. All these contribute to soft tissue tension during growth or after surgery.

The shape of the mandible (**121**) reflects the influence of the soft tissues on a genetically determined basic pattern, thus giving many clues to the nature of those soft tissues.

The *gonial angle* is formed by the ramal plane and the mandibular plane and has a mean value of 126°. It expresses the proportion between the height of the face anteriorly (say from nasion to menton, N–Me) and posteriorly (say from sella to gonion, S–Go), being large where the anterior face is relatively long, and vice versa. This in turn reflects the balance of growth between the pterygomasseteric soft tissues and the posterior facial skeleton, especially the mandibular ramus and the posterior maxilla.

A large angle indicates posterior rotational growth of the mandible with condylar growth directed more posteriorly, and is likely to be associated with excessive vertical facial growth patterns. A small angle is indicative of anterior rotational growth patterns in the mandible with more vertical condylar growth.

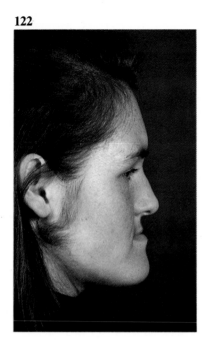

122

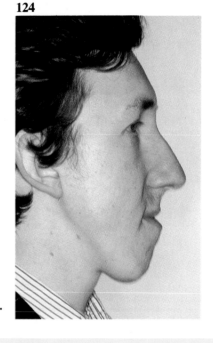

124

122 to 125   Mandibular enlargement.

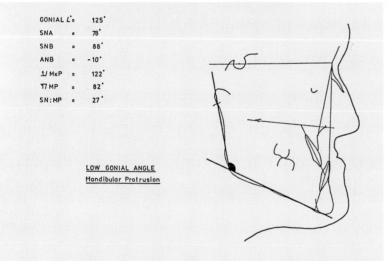

123

GONIAL L°=	125°
SNA =	78°
SNB =	88°
ANB =	-10°
1̲/MxP =	122°
1̄/MP =	82°
SN:MP =	27°

LOW GONIAL ANGLE
Mandibular Protrusion

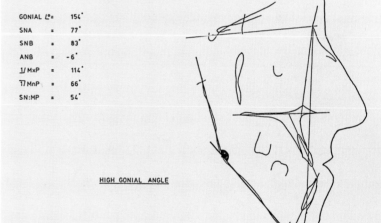

125

GONIAL L°=	154°
SNA =	77°
SNB =	83°
ANB =	-6°
1̲/MxP =	114°
1̄/MnP =	66°
SN:MP =	54°

HIGH GONIAL ANGLE

Mandibular enlargement presents in two characteristic shapes. In the first patient (**122** and **123**), the enlarged lower jaw is of approximately normal shape, the gonial angle within normal limits, the ramus is normal in relation to anterior facial height, and the appearance is of a normally shaped but disproportionately large mandible. In some variations the ramus may actually be long in relation to anterior facial height and the gonial angle smaller than normal. The pterygomasseteric tissues appear to be involved in the lower-facial enlargement, being concomitantly increased with the bone. If the functional matrix theories of Moss are correct (Moss, 1968), the primary abnormality may well be a soft-tissue one with secondary stimulation of mandibular growth in an overactive muscular environment; alternatively the growth of both soft tissues and bone may be genetically determined.

In the second clinical type (**124** and **125**), the gonial angle is large and the ramus short in relation to anterior facial height.

There may be an anterior open bite, as here, or alternatively the anterior alveolar processes may increase in height to bring together the incisior teeth. The latter adaptation tends to occur mainly in the mandible and results in increased anterior lower dental height (see p. 58). Whether the soft-tissue relationship is causal or secondary is again arguable, but the resulting facial skeleton exhibits increased growth of bone in the areas not constrained by the pterygomasseteric tissues which appear not to be involved in the excess tissue growth. Ramal development is consequently restricted within this relative shortage of soft tissues and posteriorly directed rotational growth proceeds in a downward and forward manner resulting in a high gonial angle prognathism, where the anterior open bite is more evident than the protrusion. This gives rise to the commonest form of 'long face syndrome' and contrasts with the the first type of mandibular enlargement where protrusion is the main feature.

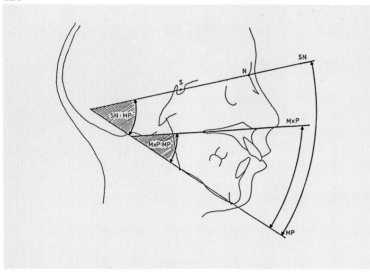

126 Antero-posterior planes and angles between.

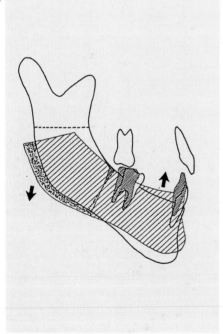

127 Effect of sagittal split correction on case of anterior open bite (high FMA).

The inclination of the mandibular plane (**126**) to the rest of the skull is best stated in terms of the angle it makes with the anterior cranial base (SN), forming SN–MP°. In the past the Frankfort Horizontal Plane was used (FH) and the angle FMA° quoted, but it is generally agreed that the Frankfort Horizontal Plane is subject to an unacceptable degree of plotting error. Nasion and sella are both reliable points to plot and hence SN–MP° a good index of the slope of the mandibular base. The mean angle is 32°. The term 'high angle' or 'low angle' case in this book will refer primarily to the SN–MP°.

The maxillary plane extends from anterior nasal spine (ANS) to posterior nasal spine (PNS) and is also sometimes called the palatal plane. It can be used to relate the angulation of the mandible to the maxillary base (MxP–MP) sometimes called the 'basal plane' angle, and having a mean of 25°. This in turn is divided by the occlusal plane into an upper and lower part, having mean values of 11° and 14° respectively. Where the SN–MP° is large and the basal plane angle is also large, the abnormality probably lies in the lower-face (ie below the Frankfort level). However, evidence must be sought to confirm that the slope of the maxillary base is within normal limits, as this will also affect the MxP–MP°.

The surgical significance of relative pterygomasseteric shortage lies in stability (**127**). Any corrective procedure which involves lengthening the mandibular ramus without at the same time increasing the length of the pterygomasseteric tissues, for the most part impracticable without introducing tissue from elsewhere in the body, inevitably raises the tension exerted by these tissues on the ramus. Postoperative relapse usually follows. The temptation occurs in high angle cases associated with an anterior open bite. If full sagittal splitting, for example, is undertaken in this situation the ramus stretches the investing tissues as it lengthens, tissues which include the masseters and the internal pterygoids as well as the others previously mentioned. Relapse is inevitable.

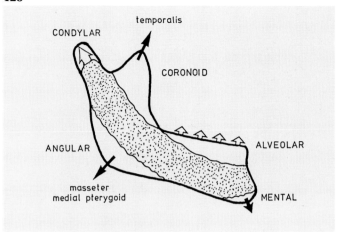

128 Basic shape of mandible.

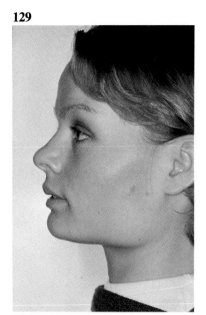

129 to 132   Bilateral masseteric hypertrophy.

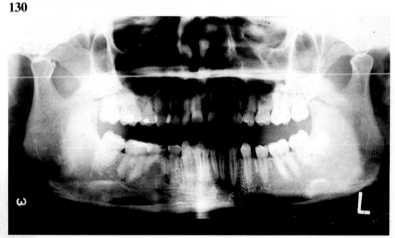

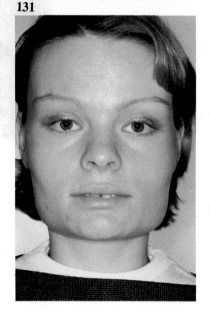

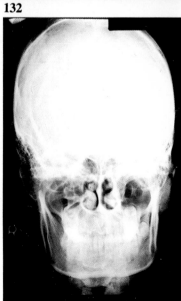

The basic shape of the mandible at birth (**128**) is modified during growth in a number of ways, the mechanism of which is still controversial. While some believe that the condyle is a growth centre others consider its growth to be secondary to mandibular development in the body and ramus. According to this latter view the proliferation of the condylar cartilage leads to upward and backward extension which maintains the spatial relationship of the growing jaw to the temporal bone, while the muscular processes (angular, coronoid) the alveolus and indeed the body itself grow by association with dynamically functional tissue areas—the 'functional matrices' of Moss (1968). Hence the coronoid process is associated with function of the temporalis muscle, atrophying when this muscle is destroyed during development or failing to develop if the muscle is congenitally absent. Overactivity of the temporalis leads to coronoid enlargement, usually as elongation. The masseter muscle is associated with the mandibular angle, which is enlarged when the muscle is overactive and reduced when the muscle is under-developed or absent.

This is well illustrated in bilateral masseteric hypertrophy (**129** to **132**). The shape of the angle is palpable and can be seen on the radiograph, enlarged and square in profile, flared laterally on AP view. Clinically the enlargement of the muscle can be seen and palpated during contraction (teeth clenched). Ramus and angle development are also associated with the medial pterygoid, the alveolar process with the dentition, the condyle to some extent with the lateral pterygoid, and growth of the mandibular body is possibly in functional equilibrium with growth of the neurovascular bundle, and with the suprahyoid musculature.

133

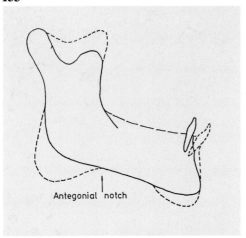

133 Development of muscular processes. Note the characteristic shape of the mandible in localised skeletal growth inhibition.

134

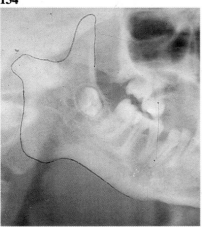

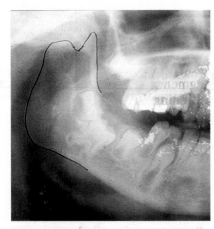

134 Hemifacial microsomia. Top: The case above shows a good notch and clinically active masseteric function. The reverse is true of the case below.

135

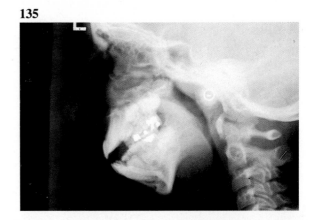

136

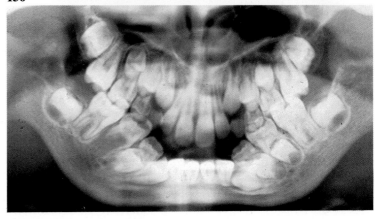

135 and 136 The Treacher Collins syndrome.

The importance of mandibular shape (**133** and **134**) as an ~~~~catio~~ ~~f~~ the presence of normal or near-normal muscular ~~~~~~~~~~ ~~~~~articular importance in dealing with cases of ~~~~~~~~~ ~~ral mandibular hypoplasia, most often in the ~~~~~~~~~ group. Hovell (1965) pointed out that the ~~~~~~~~ s of diagnostic significance in these cases. ~~~~~~~~~eric and medial pterygoid function is present ~~~~~~~~ ess develops, leaving the hypoplastic 'basic ~~~~~~~~~igher level thus creating a notch. The notch is a ~~~~~~~~~rygomasseteric activity, giving some hope of a ~~~~~~~~ active matrix within which elongation of the man-~~~~~~~ ar ramus by bone grafting might succeed during the ~rowing period. Absence of the notch points to inadequate muscular function to support ramal elongation and relapse is almost certain.

In the Treacher Collins syndrome (**135** and **136**) there is always good, symmetrical antegonial notching, indicative of adequate pterygomasseteric soft tissue investment, both anatomically and functionally. Clinically palpable, this is well demonstrated both on lateral radiography and on orthopantomography; it has been argued that early reconstruction is not only desirable but essential to restore the dimensions of the functional matrix (Poswillo, 1974).

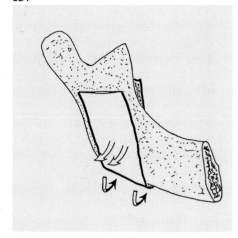

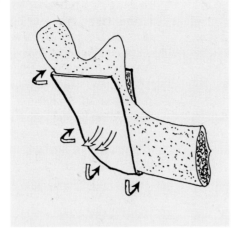

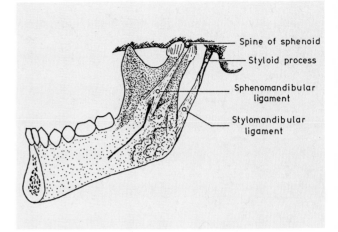

137 Concept of the pterygomasseteric sling.

138 Reality of the pterygomasseteric envelope.

139 Anatomy of stylomandibular and sphenomandibular ligaments.

The attachment of the masseter and pterygoid muscles to the mandible is through the periosteum which is inelastic. If during surgery this is detached from the underlying bone the muscles remain attached to its soft tissue surfaces. There is thus a continuous investment of muscle and periosteum around the ramus, which is erroneously described as the 'pterygomasseteric sling', (**137**). The term is in fact dangerous. It was formerly taught that during forward or backward sliding osteotomies of the mandible, the sling should be detached and the mandibular elements slipped through the resulting loop to their correct positions. The muscles would then reattach to the mandible in the new position without lengthening of the muscle fibres or alteration of the direction along which they exert, either of which would produce relapsing. In reality the periosteal envelope invests the whole including the posterior aspect of the ramus. fragments 'through the sling' tensions the periosteal envelope drawing the lateral periosteum (and masseter) posteriorly and also displacing the medial posteriorly (with its attached medial pterygoid, stretching of muscle fibres and the alteration of their may still occur, though to a lesser extent.

The question thus arises 'should the periosteal envelope be divided along its posteroinferior borders during mandibular set-back procedures involving the ramus?' This will be discussed further in Section 4.

The deep cervical fascia is reinforced as it passes medial to the parotid gland to form the *stylomandibular ligament* (**139**). This passes from the tip of the styloid process and the stylohyoid ligament to the angle of the mandible. As it is an inelastic and inextensible sheet of fibrous tissue, it limits the forward and upward movement of the mandibular angle to an arc having the styloid tip as its centre of rotation, unless it is detached from the mandible during surgery. Similarly, the *sphenomandibular ligament*, derived from the perichondrium of Meckel's cartilage, stretches in a triangular sheet from the spine of the sphenoid to the lingula of the mandible. Where necessary it is possible to increase the distance between the proximal and distal bony attachments of these structures, but only after separation of one end of the ligament from bone. In practice this means separating the distal attachment of the stylomandibular ligament from the angle of the mandible, and of the sphenomandibular ligament from the lingula.

2 The linguovestibular group of soft tissues

This includes the tongue, cheeks and lips. The tongue is a muscular organ, continually active during speech, deglutition and facial habits. This continual activity makes it a powerful acting on the teeth and dental arches, which lie in a zone of muscular neutrality between the pressures of the directed laterally and labially on the one side, and the of the cheeks and lips directed lingually on the other. orthodontic alterations of the position of teeth or segments change this balance. Stability will depend on positioning the segments in a new state of physiological equilibrium, or on predicting the direction or magnitude of the equilibrating forces so that allowance may be made for the extent to which these forces may be harnessed to move the teeth into the required position afterwards.

Linguolabial and linguobuccal forces are not alone in influencing the position of teeth and their supporting bone. The relative sizes of the maxillary and mandibular skeletal bases, their relationship to each other, and the degree of occlusal interlock all play an important part in the stability of the segments. Fortunately these are factors which can be modified by the surgeon or orthodontist; this alone makes skeletal surgery feasible.

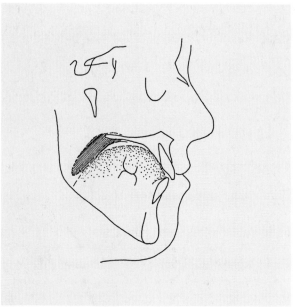

140

140 Normal tongue position.

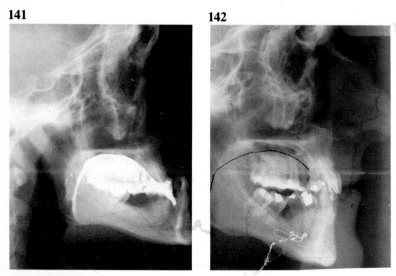

141

142

141 and 142 A case (**141**) treated by bilateral body ostectomy, and (**142**) the postoperative tongue position (see also **260**).

The tongue tends to procline the incisor teeth and widen the dental arch. Hovell (1961) has drawn attention to the importance of tongue position and tongue size in the prognosis for prenormal skeletal disproportion. Normally (**140**) the resting tongue lies high in the mouth, in contact with the soft palate posteriorly, the hard palate anteriorly, and the lower incisal tips. A small space exists between the lingual dorsum and the mid-palate above.

The normal relationship of tongue to surrounding structures also occurs in some patients with a prenormal occlusion, and mandibular set-back might be expected to cramp the tongue severely, increasing lingual pressure on the dentition and inducing skeletal relapse or incisor proclination (dental relapse). In practice, however, this occurs less often than might be anticipated and it appears that the tongue moves backwards slightly and that the floor of the mouth moves downwards to compensate. The body of the hyoid bone is thus seen to move further backwards and downwards than the chin, only partly repositioning in the postoperative months (**141** and **142**).

Nevertheless, the tongue exerts a pressure against the lower incisors and shows a tendency to cause incisor proclination. This tendency is greatest when the mandibular set-back is performed in the body of the mandible rather than the ramus, a fact which can sometimes be used in cases requiring correction of incisor axial inclination (ie decompensating incisor retroclination in Class 3 cases by allowing for proclination under tongue pressure after body ostectomy). Equally, maxillary advancement increases tongue space in these cases. We will call this 'normal' tongue position in skeletal prenormality a Type A position. It is not common and indicates a greater likelihood of postoperative incisor proclination, and a lesser chance of maxillary contraction (orthodontically or surgically) being stable.

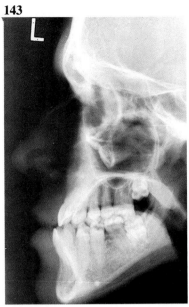

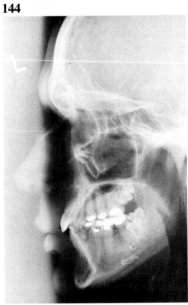

The more usual tongue position in skeletal prenormality, which we shall call Type B position, is shown in **143** and **144**. The tongue adopts a low, forward resting posture with its upper surface lying almost parallel to the occlusal plane. The tip reaches forward to contact the lower incisor edges when the lips are closed, achieved by contraction of the intrinsic muscles which narrow and lengthen the organ. To a lesser extent the extrinsic muscles also contract to posture the whole structure forwards. Narrowing of the tongue reduces the outward pressure it exerts on the buccal segments of the lower arch, which may therefore move lingually. More important, the maxillary arch is subjected to a reduced tongue pressure and tends to become narrowed with an increase in the height of the palatal vault.

After mandibular set-back in these patients the tongue is restored to the more normal, higher position further back in the mouth. It widens and rises into the palate so that the postoperative effect on the lower incisors is less and incisor proclination less likely to occur. Conversely the lingual pressure on the narrowed dental arches is restored which assists in stabilising preoperative orthodontic expansion, or (where this has not been performed) may expand the arches postoperatively by muscular pressure alone.

143 and 144 Usual tongue position in skeletal prenormality – **143**, preoperative position; **144**, postoperative position.

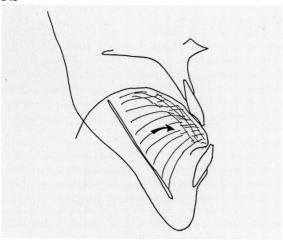

145 Effect of mylohyoid slope on tongue posture.

146

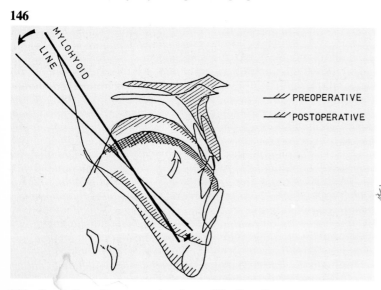

—— PREOPERATIVE

—— POSTOPERATIVE

146 Correction of tongue posture by modification of mylohyoid slope.

147

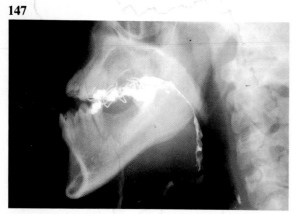

147 Sloping mylohyoid line in a high angle case with anterior open bite.

The baseline from which the tongue is projected forwards may slope very acutely in high angle cases, because the mylohyoid muscle is the effective floor of the mouth and tongue. The tongue is then tilted in the same downward and forward direction as the mylohyoid line on the medial aspect of the mandible, thus facilitating forward posturing and increasing the lingual influence on the anterior dentition, often contributing to the development and maintenance of anterior open bite. The hyoid bone tends to be positioned relatively nearer to the cervical spine in these cases (**145**). The reverse occurs in low angle cases. Hence the impact of the tongue is considerably affected by the skeletal pattern (or itself reflects the skeletal pattern of growth) (**147**).

Either way, it follows that in the established case surgical alteration of that skeletal pattern must have a secondary effect on the tongue behaviour. The aim should be to rotate the mylohyoid line (or, put another way, to reduce the high angle to nearer normal magnitude) and this certainly modifies the *postural* behaviour of the tongue. It will not affect an endogenous tongue thrust. Figure **146** shows a correction involving Le Fort 1 maxillary advancement and elevation, bilateral mandibular osteotomy (angle ostectomy to control ramus height) and reduction genioplasty in the vertical direction. Note the new position of both tongue and hyoid bone (3 month postoperative tracing).

The influence of the lower lip on the dentition tends to bring about lower incisor retroclination which is in turn resisted by lingual counterpressure (**148 & 149**). Both labial and lingual muscle activity and bulk contribute to this result, seen most clearly when the pressures become unbalanced, as for example in a Class 3 incisor relationship. Here the lower incisors have been carried away anteriorly from the influence of the tongue by skeletal prognathism, and thus into an area of increased lip pressure. The usual result is retroclination, sometimes quite severe. The upper lip only rarely has a significant effect on the lower incisors, apart from its indirect effect through interincisal contact.

The influence of the lips on the upper incisors depends on the relative lengths of the two, and on the overjet. If the lower lip is able to get behind the upper incisor teeth during function it will tend to procline them, a situation seen in many Class 2 Div 1 malocclusions, and illustrated here (**150 to 153**). When the lower lip is long enough to cover the lower part of the upper incisor crowns it will tend to control the upper incisors into good interincisal contact, the upper lip also contributing to this effect.

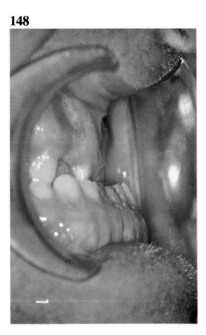

148 Lower incisor retroclination.

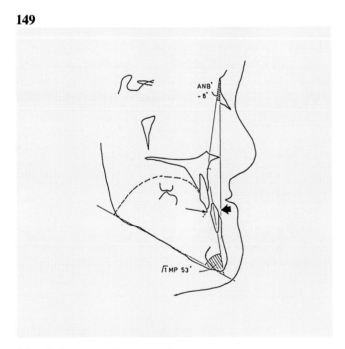

149 Incisor retroclination under
increased labial pressure (Class 3).

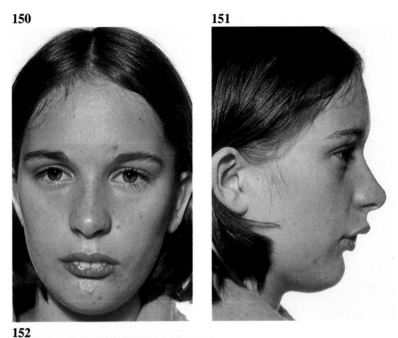

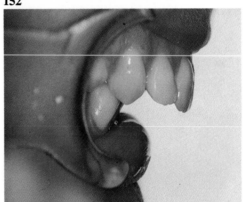

**150 to 153 Influence of
the lip on upper incisors.**
The lower lip is behind the
upper incisors, which are,
as a result, proclined
(Class 2, Div. 1 case).

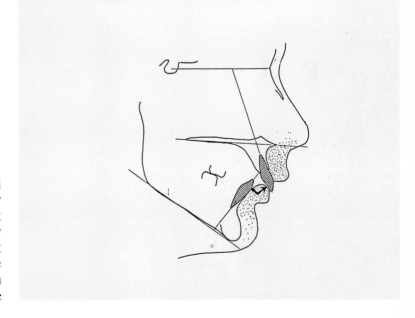

The probable lip/incisor relationship should be considered during the planning of all orthognathic surgery. A short lower lip which cannot control the upper incisors may be a point against correction of a Class 2 Div 1 malocclusion by premaxillary set-back and a point in favour of mandibular advancement possibly combined with premaxillary setdown to improve the relationship and the chances of stability. Other factors will often decide the choice of surgery, but the attainment of a stable lip/incisor balance is mandatory (**154** to **157**).

51

154 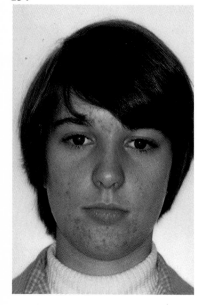 **155**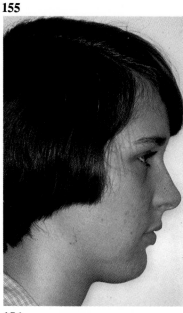

156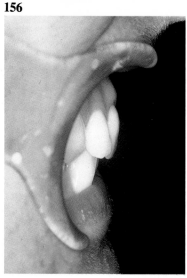

Excessive upper incisor display may indicate shortness of the upper lip in itself, or relatively excessive anterior maxillary height. The latter is correctable while there seems to be no acceptable method of lengthening the upper lip without scarring. In the case illustrated (**158**) the upper lip is able to exert hardly any pressure on the upper incisors which are therefore subject to unopposed proclining forces (both lingual and lower labial). The proper incisor/lip relationship at rest should allow a display of about 3 mm of tooth crown. Figure **159** shows the proper exposure. The amount of tooth shown during laughing or smiling brings in many factors not necessarily amenable to correction. The width of the mouth, the personality reflected in the broadness of smile, and the extent to which the upper lip curls towards the nose during function are all variable. In some patients the characteristics of the smile may force a modification of the 3 mm at rest guideline.

158 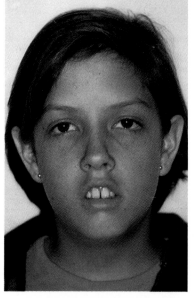 **159**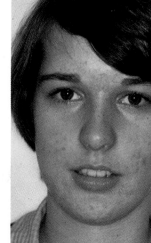

154 to 157 The case (150 to 153) postoperatively, treated by forward sagittal split mandibular osteotomy and premaxillary set-back (Wassmund technique).

157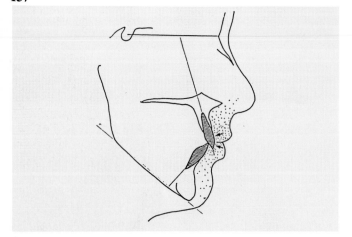

157 Restored labio-dental balance. One year after operation.

158 Excessive upper incisor display.   **159 Proper exposure.**

Lip competence depends on several factors. The length of the lips, their intrinsic muscle tone, patient motivation and understanding, and basic skeletal patterns all affect it directly, while pseudoincompetence may result from an obstructed nasal airway.

In high angle cases the height of the lower-third of the face is increased anteriorly. The height of the lower lip (even if intrinsically normal) is therefore relatively short in relation to the anterior lower-facial height. This makes it difficult for the lips to be kept in contact at rest, and there may be lip incompetence. The case illustrated (**160 to 162**) exhibits several factors causing incompetence—a high angle skeletal pattern

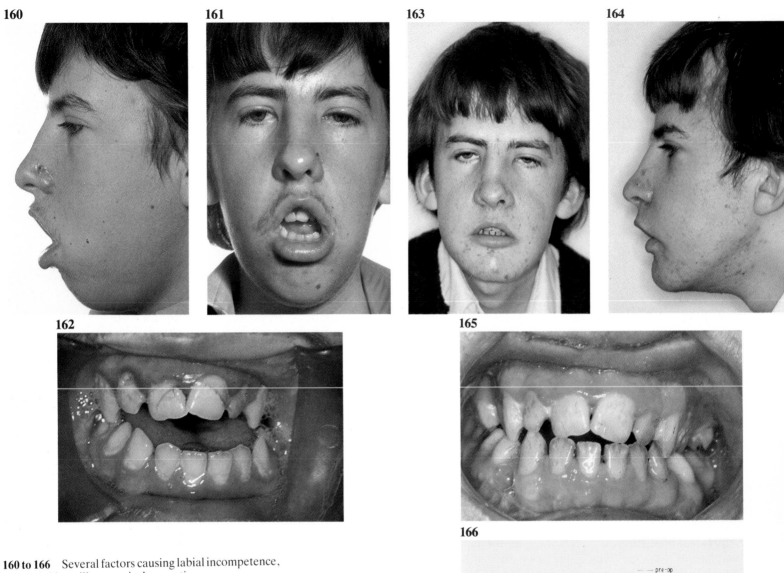

160 to 166   Several factors causing labial incompetence, and their bimaxillary surgical correction.

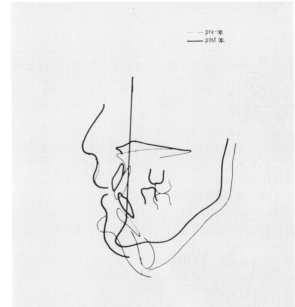

with anterior open bite, a short upper lip, and myotonia. The appearance is misleading, however, and improved seal is obtained after bimaxillary surgical correction of the underlying skeletal disproportion (**163 to 165**). The postoperative tracing (**166**) shows the result after Le Fort 1 maxillary osteotomy with upward repositioning of the anterior maxilla, and anterior mandibuloplasty incorporating vertical reduction genioplasty with advancement.

While the congenital facial myopathy is still reflected in the postoperative facies, the improved lip competence corrected continual salivary drooling, and restored quality of life. The case illustrates planning directed to the correction of lip competence as a primary objective. Orthodontic finalisation was impracticable.

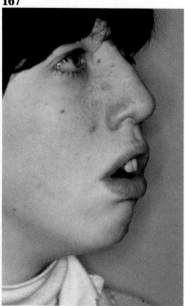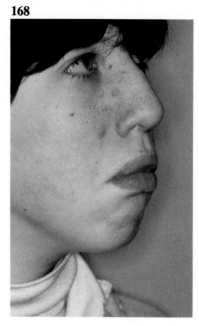

167 and 168 **Contraction of the mentalis muscle. 167** – lip at rest. **168** – during swallowing the mentalis contracts to facilitate lip to tongue seal.

Tongue behaviour. Two distinct patterns of lingual behaviour must be defined. They differ in aetiology, effect and prognosis, and despite the clear descriptions given they can be difficult to distinguish with certainty. In summary the two types are:

(a) *Tongue to lip posturing.* This is common, and is essentially a persistence into adult life of an infantile pattern of activity directed to the maintenance of an anterior oral seal, a pattern normally discarded when active lip competence is achieved. Tongue posturing is especially likely to occur where lip incompetence is associated with a high gonial angle, when it may contribute to the development of anterior open bite. As it is not the prime cause, however, it will not cause the open bite to recur after surgical correction of the underlying skeletal abnormality. The same type of tongue posture occurs in many cases of skeletal prenormality and will also disappear after skeletal correction.

(b) *Endogenous tongue thrusting* is quite a different problem, occurring rarely and caused by a basic abnormality in the neuromuscular control of the tongue (hence 'endogenous'). For this reason it persists into adult life and cannot be altered by any form of treatment. The resulting anterior open bite always recurs whether treated orthodontically or surgically.

Anterior oral seal is achieved in infancy in many cases by compensatory thumb-sucking, and later by posturing the tongue forward to meet the lip, which increasingly learns to assist by contraction of the mentalis muscle and sometimes also by orbicularis contraction circumorally. The latter is recognisable on casual swallowing and is usually associated with endogenous tongue thrusting, but the former is common in association with the features of lip incompetence described.

Figures **167** and **168** show mentalis contraction during swallowing while the slope of the mylohyoid line allows the tongue to be brought forward easily to occupy the space between the anterior teeth, thus establishing one form of anterior open bite (or at the least assisting in its maintenance).

In the low angle case, however, the tongue is able to effect a posterior oral seal by contact with the soft palate. Fortunately, most low angle cases have competent lips because the height of the lip is in proportion to that of the anterior lower-face, and the imbalance between the lingual and labial pressures (with increased lingual pressure) is more likely to produce bimaxillary alveolar protrusion than anterior open bite.

The thrusting can be recognised by three features, which should all be present to make the diagnosis with any confidence.

1. *Changes in the dentition.* Both upper and lower incisors are proclined, although this is modified in some skeletal patterns. In skeletal postnormality, or where a normal skeletal base relationship exists, the upper incisors are more proclined than the lowers. In a prenormal skeletal relationship the thrust may be directed wholly below the upper incisors retarding their full eruption, but producing marked lower incisor proclination. These are distinctive dental changes.

2. *Muscular contraction of the circumoral tissues* occurs during casual swallowing. This sign must be observed, not solicited, and must be distinguished from mentalis contraction in tongue posturing (which is confined to the area below the lower lip).

3. *A special type of sibilant lisp* occurs and can be recognised with experience. The anterior open bite case illustrated shows the dental changes, produced marked circumoral contraction during casual swallowing, and had a sibilant lisp (**169** and **170**).

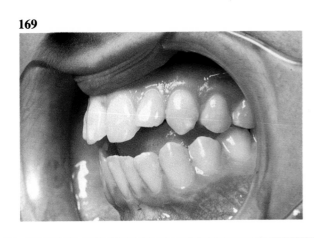

169

develop relapsing muscle forces in the postoperative phase. Division or separation of these muscles from the mandible (suprahyoid myotomy) has been recommended (Steinhauser, 1973) in high angle retrognathic or anterior open bite cases. In all mandibular advancements *division of the periosteal envelope* and wide *detachment of the facial integument* from the underlying anterior, lateral, and inferior surfaces of the mandible will reduce tension on the advanced chin, and this is a mandatory step in advancement genioplasty. *Suprahyoid myotomy* is more controversial and will be discussed further in Section 4.

170

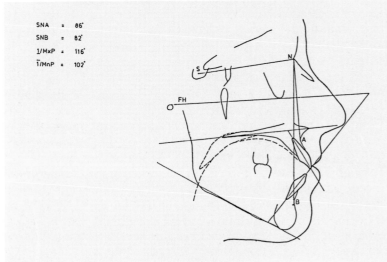

SNA	= 86°
SNB	= 82°
1/MxP	= 116°
1̄/MnP	= 102°

171

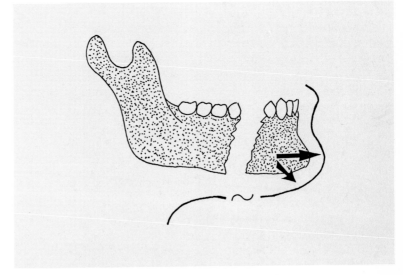

169 and 170   A case of endogenous tongue thrust

171   Relief of tension. A = Periosteal division; B = Soft tissue detachment; C = Supra-hyoid myotomy.

3 The suprahyoid group of soft tissues

This is important in relation to procedures designed to advance the anterior mandible, either totally or at the lower border only (advancement genioplasty). The suprahyoid muscles, comprising the geniohyoid, mylohyoid and anterior belly of the digastric attached to the mandible and the hyoglossus attached to the tongue, together with the overall lower-facial integument resist forward translation of the anterior mandible, irrespective of the site chosen for osteotomy. The greater the distance the chin is advanced the greater the forces of resistance (**171**).

The problem is maximal in the severely retrognathic mandible of the so-called bird-face deformity (**172 and 173**). It is also significant in any anterior open bite case involving upward movement of the anterior lower border, especially the high angle type of case. The proximity of the chin and the hyoid bone results in short, tight suprahyoid muscles. Their elongation must

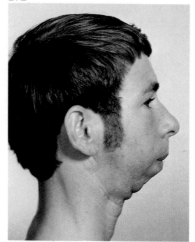

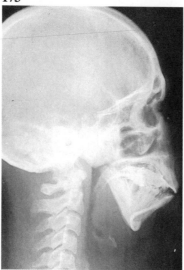

172 and 173   Bird-face deformity.

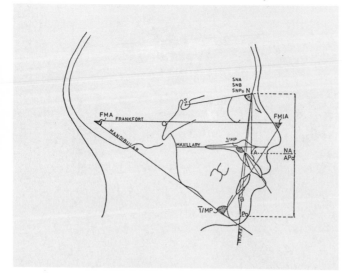

174   Cephalometric analysis.

Note the proximity of the chin to the hyoid bone in **172** and **173**. This case suffered trauma to the condyles in infancy with resultant ankylosis. Several operations were required to maintain some jaw opening, at one stage metal joint prostheses being inserted. Unfortunately these became infected with ultimate loss of much of both mandibular rami, and the case presented for treatment in late adolescence with a severe bird-face deformity.

Cephalometry

Patient orientation in the cephalostat, plotting and tracing errors all contribute to inaccuracy. Most important of all no single linear or angular measurement can be assessed by itself; the whole analysis must be seen as one before the significance of individual figures can be related to the known normal ranges, mean figures, and even standard deviations for a particular ethnic group. Nevertheless, guidance from quantitative analysis is helpful in planning surgery provided that the clinician allows his clinical assessment and judgment to override the figures where necessary.

Any of the cephalometric analyses in common use among orthodontists can be applied to surgical planning, and all have their place in diagnostic radiology. Whether Downs (as here), Sassouni, Ricketts or Tweed are followed, or any of their more recent successors, the process of predictive photocephalometry can be readily adapted to the analysis. The parameters found most useful by the author in surgical planning will be briefly indicated, but the reader is referred to works on cephalometry for background reading (eg Rakosi, 1981; Krogman and Sassouni, 1957; Broadbent and Golden, 1975 are recommended).

Figure 174 shows the important points, lines, and angles on the standard lateral cephalogram.

SNA is an indication of the relationship of the maxilla to the cranial base, in the sagittal plane. Normal range 78°–84°. Mean value 81°.

SNB is an indication of the relationship of the mandible to the cranial base, in the sagittal plane. Normal range 77–82°. Mean value 79°.

ANB is an indication of the relationship of the maxillary and mandibular bases to one another. Normal range 1°–3°, A lying anterior to B.

SNPo is an indication of the relationship of the pogonion to the cranial base. This is important as it establishes chin to cranial base relationship by comparison with SNA and SNB, but must be related to total chin thickness (see **189** to **193**).

NPo is the *facial plane*, and establishes an important plane of reference for facial convexity (or concavity).

FH, the Frankfort Horizontal plane, which passes through orbitale and both porion points of right and left, has already been discussed (**126**).

SN, the Sella-nasion line, is a reference against which other horizontal lines may be assessed. Hence the FMA is little used

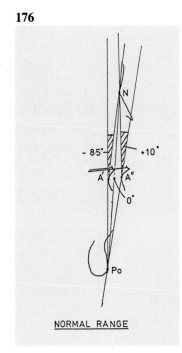

NORMAL RANGE

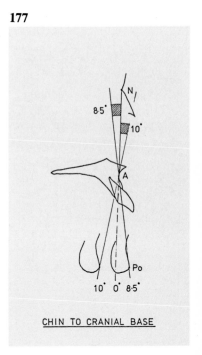

CHIN TO CRANIAL BASE

(Mean value 22°) and the SN:MP° angle has superseded it (Mean value 32°).

MP, the Mandibular Plane, is taken in this book to run from Gonion to Menton (GoMe).

Tweed's Triangle (made up of the angles FMA, FMIA, IMPA – the latter marked 1̄/MP in the figure) is therefore also subject to the errors of FH plotting. It is important in that it emphasises an aspect of facial profile of great significance. The axial inclination of the lower incisors compensates for increasing mandibular plane angulation (in the triangle this is the same as an increasing FMA) to maintain a pleasing labiomental relationship; if the FMA is within normal limits (say 22° to 25°) then the lower incisors should form approximately a right angle with the mandibular plane (ie an IMPA of 90°) to project the lower lip to a pleasing contour. As the FMA increases, in a high angle case, such an angulation would result in unsightly projection of the lower lip. Hence the need for compensatory retroclination. With two interrelated internal angles of a triangle bearing an inverse relationship to one another the third angle (here the FMIA) is a useful guide. The FMIA is normal (ie indicative of lower incisal angulation likely to produce pleasing lower lip projection given the value of FMA as fixed) between 65° to 68°. The FMA is of course alterable during surgery. Hence in prediction the final mandibular plane should be estimated; and hence an estimate of the degree of lower incisor compensation (or decompensation) required is obtained. In rough terms the FMA can be used for this as the final result of incisor angulation cannot be estimated very accurately; alternatively the lower incisors may be related to the SN:MP (Mean value 53°).

Downs Angle of Convexity is of considerable use in surgical planning. The angle NAPo (**175**) is an indication of the protrusion or retrusion of the maxilla in relation to the facial plane NPo. Downs recorded a mean of 180° (angle of convexity = 0), the A point lying on the facial plane. If A lies behind the facial plane a negative angle is recorded, if in front a positive one.

For simplicity of measurement the reciprocal angle (**176**) is actually recorded and this gave a range in the Caucasian population with which Downs worked (1948) from +10° to −8.5° in 'normal' people. This includes many individuals at each end of the range whose faces would not generally be regarded as aesthetically pleasing. Downs himself liked a flat (orthognathic) profile; Reidel (1957) preferred a slightly positive angle of convexity (his ideal being +1.6°), and Petraitis (1951) opted for +3.0°. These figures resulted in varying studies of those whose facial profiles were good, including several popular figures publicly noted for their fine appearance.

The variations indicate the essentially personal nature of beauty or good looks from the beholder's viewpoint; they also indicate general acceptance that facial convexity must be narrowed considerably within the 'normal range' if good facial profile is to be obtained. When dealing with patients of obvious maxillomandibular disproportion, the angle of convexity is an excellent guide to the relative manipulation of mandible and/or maxilla. The author aims for an angulation between 0° and 4°, greater convexity being more acceptable in women than in men. SNPo must be established in planning before the angle of convexity can be given predictive value as the facial plane must be used for reference. In other words the values given (0° to 4°) are only of value after the correct chin to cranial base relationship for that patient has been estimated (**177**).

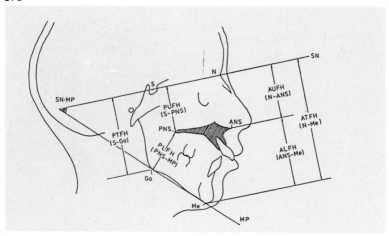

178 Vertical facial height.

179

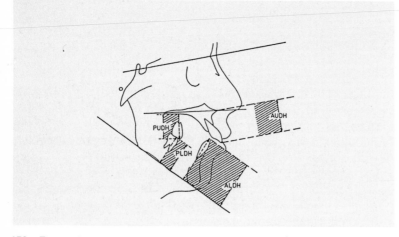

179 Dentoalveolar height.

The vertical dimension is increasingly important and its cephalometric assessment very helpful in managing cases of vertical facial dysplasia. The simple 'in clinic' guide, advocated by McIntosh (1970) is useful but subject to great error. This estimates the balance between upper and lower components of the mid and lower face by the measurement of NA relative to APo, which should be about 8:7. If any clinical suspicion of vertical dysharmony arises it is wise to undertake a full vertical analysis (**178** and **179**).

The A point and the pogonion are both subject to plotting error in the vertical plane and considerable errors may be compounded into the proportion NA:APo. Both anterior nasal spine, ANS, and menton, Me, are reliable vertically, although the spine may be disproportionately displaced in some vertical dysplasias (eg the short face syndrome). It should be noted also that the ANS is most unreliable in the anteroposterior plane.

In vertical cephalometry a plane of reference must be adopted to which anterior and posterior facial height may be measured.

The Frankfort Horizontal is rejected for reasons already discussed, and the SN plane, while reliable for plotting, inclines variably upwards from the horizontal. However, it is the most reliable and norms are available from the Bolton Standards (Broadbent *et al*, 1975). Vertical abnormalities must be studied in lateral cephalograms as the site(s) of abnormality may be in the anterior or posterior face (eg maxilla tilted down at the back and up at the front). The analysis rapidly determines the type of facial development (horizontal or vertical) and the rotational direction of growth in both upper and lower parts of the face (Lavergne and Gasson, 1978). There are three sets of measurements and two derived proportional relationships (**178** and **179**).

Linear measurements

Table 1

Linear measurements in vertical cephalometric analysis

	Mean	S.D.
Anterior total facial height (ATFH)	119.8mm	7.00
Anterior upper facial height (AUFH)	54.3mm	3.48
Anterior lower facial height (ALFH)	65.4mm	4.96
Ramus height (RH)	56.3mm	3.92
Posterior total facial height (PTFH)	79.0mm	
Posterior upper facial height (PUFH)	46.0mm	
Posterior lower facial height (PLFH)	43.0mm	
Anterior upper dental height (AUDH)	28.5mm	
Anterior lower dental height (ALDH)	39.0mm	
Posterior upper dental height (PUDH)	21.0mm	
Posterior lower dental height (PLDH)	32.0mm	

After Broadbent *et al*, (1975)

The anterior facial height (ATFH) from N to Me is divided into anterior upper facial height (AUFH) and anterior lower facial height (ALFH) in the proportion 45:55, measured at right angles to SN. The posterior total facial height (PTFH) is similarly measured from SN plane to Go. Posterior upper facial height is also measured at right angles to SN as far as PNS, giving PUFH, while posterior lower facial height is measured at right angles to the mandibular plane (PLFH). Ramus height (not shown) is measured from gonion to the uppermost point on the condylar tracing.

The dentoalveolar measurements are also divided into anterior and posterior (**179**). Anterior upper dental height (AUDH) is from ANS to the tip of the upper incisor, at right angles to SN plane. Anterior lower dental height (ALDH) is measured from the lower incisor tip to the mandibular plane, at right angles to that plane. Posterior upper dental height (PUDH) is measured from the mesiobuccal cusp of the first upper molar to the lower tracing of the hard palate along the long axis of the molar. Posterior lower dental height is measured from the mesiobuccal cusp of the lower first molar to the mandibular plane at right angles to that plane (PLDH).

Proportion

The two proportional relationships derived from the figures are the SN:MP angle already discussed and the facial proportion index FPI, introduced by Opdebeeck and Bell (1978). This is a useful way of expressing upper and lower anterior facial height in proportion to total anterior facial height, normally the ALFH being 55% of the total and the AUFH being 45%. The FPI is calculated as ALFH expressed as a percentage of ATFH minus AUFH expressed as a percentage of ATFH (normally 55% minus 45%) and should about equal 10, regardless of the absolute measurements. The FPI is less than 10 in short faces and more than 10 in long faces.

Profile analysis

This is closely related to lateral cephalometry and plays an important part in the assessment of individual cases as well as in treatment planning. However, it is true that the patient rarely perceives himself in profile, and is usually regarded by onlookers in full face and varying oblique face views. The importance of the profile lies in its ready analysis and comparison with 'normal' or 'good-looking' faces. It is not always true that good profile implies good facial appearance from other aspects (Powell and Rayson, 1976) especially where there is some asymmetry, but it is always true that good profile is an important aim of treatment and that bad profile is a potent cause of patient dissatisfaction.

The following profile analyses of Ricketts, Steiner, Merrifield and Holdaway are all based on studies of good faces, many of them including those whose appearance has won public approval (film and television stars, beauty queens, etc). They apply principally to Caucasian races, and other ethnic groups require careful consideration in relation to these criteria. As always commonsense must override science—there are many most attractive faces which do not accord with these criteria. Despite all these notes of caution the analysis of profile is essential in case assessement and within the variable accuracy of profile prediction the method of photocephalometric planning is an indispensible aid to treatment planning generally. Tweed (1954) defined facial normality as 'that balance and harmony of proportions considered by the majority of us as pleasing in the

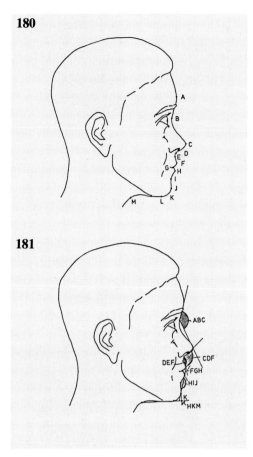

180 and 181   Profile reference points.

human face'. Profile analysis seeks to identify more precisely what that balance and harmony is about.

The analysis of profile requires that reference points be established on the profile itself, and many theoretical points have been proposed. The figure shows the commonly noted reference points (**180**) and the angles which have been used most often to assess profile contour (**181**). An excellent review of the literature is given by Waite and Worms (1974) and by Rakosi (1981). In this book the points shown here will be used in profile discussion.

Ricketts described an aesthetic plane (**182**) extending from the soft-tissue chin (J) to the nasal tip (C). The lips should lie behind this line, but not substantially, the upper being a little in advance of the lower (as measured by the skin/vermilion borders F and H). In the adult the upper lip should lie about 2 mm to 3 mm behind the line, the lower lip 1 mm to 2 mm behind it. In the early adolescent (12-year-old) the upper lip will lie on the aesthetic line and drops back during growth (Ricketts, 1957). Reidel (1957) found that the upper lip, the lower lip and the chin commonly fall on one plane but never does the nasal tip fall on this same plane in good profile, despite the teaching of some art schools to the contrary.

182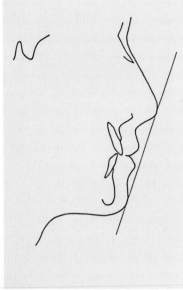

183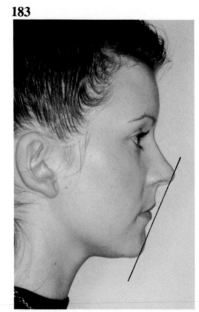

The cases shown illustrate normal good profile by this analysis (**183**), and the two extremes of abnormal variation (**184** and **185**). It should be noted that the aesthetic line defines a relationship or series of relationships; it does not in itself establish a diagnosis. The operator should concentrate on the *shape* of the Cupid's bow lying between the line and the nose-lip-chin profile, and ask where abnormality exists and why there is a departure from the ideal. The latter question will require further clinical and cephalometric information before it can be firmly answered.

186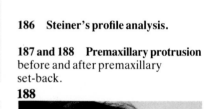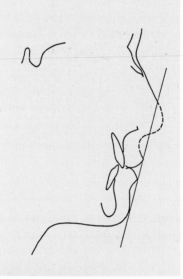

184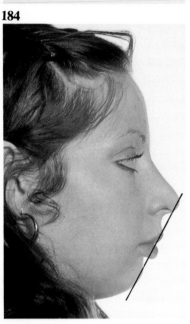

185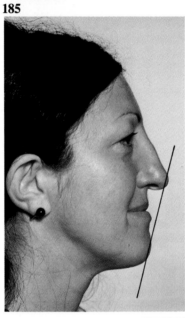

186 Steiner's profile analysis.

187 and 188 Premaxillary protrusion before and after premaxillary set-back.

187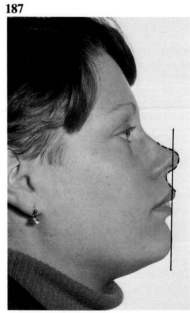

188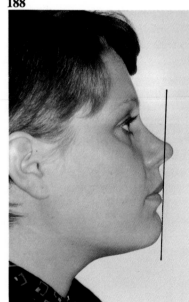

182 Ricketts' profile line.

183 Normal good profile.

184 and 185 Two extremes of abnormal profile.

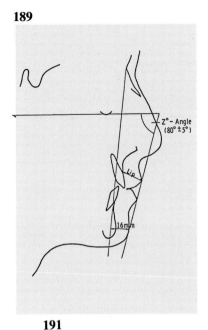

189

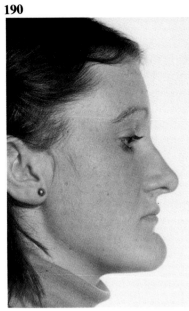

190

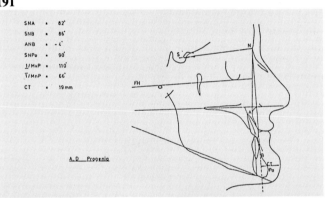

191

SNA	=	82°
SNB	=	86°
ANB	=	-4°
SNPo	=	90°
1/MxP	=	110°
1/MnP	=	66°
CT	=	19 mm

A.D Progenia

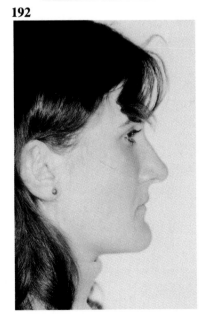

192

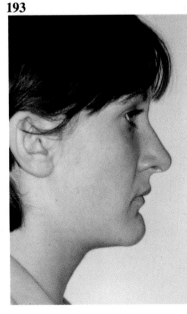

193

Steiner (1953) projected a line from the soft tissue chin, J, to the middle of the nose so that it bisected the S shaped curve formed by the nasal tip and the upper lip (shown in the diagram as a broken line (**186**)). The proximity of the lips to this line is used to measure their fullness; should they fall in front of it they are too full, or behind they are too flat. Ideally the lips should lie on this line, but the analysis presupposes a pleasing nasal tip projection. A case of premaxillary protrusion is shown before and after premaxillary set-back (**187** and **188**) to illustrate the help provided by this simple analysis.

Merrifield (1966) described a line tangential to the soft tissue chin and to the most anterior part of either upper or lower lip, whichever was the most prominent (**189**). He extended this line upwards to intersect the Frankfort Horizontal plane at an angle he designated Z angle. The line expresses the amount of lip protrusion, reflecting the influence of the underlying dentition.

In good profiles both the upper and lower lips frequently lie on this line. Most important in Merrifield's analysis is the further observation that the thickness of the chin in total (soft tissue plus hard) may be expressed in millimetres anterior to the plane NB projected inferiorly. This excludes any contribution to chin prominence made by mandibular protrusion or retrusion (indicated by SNB and therefore posterior to the chin measurement), and measures the bony chin (NB to Po) plus the integumental overlay at this point (Po to J). In good profiles this combined measurement usually approximates 16 mm (smaller or larger in proportion to the overall head size on the cephalometric image). Sometimes the most prominent point of the chin is too high in relation to pogonion and a composite correction is required, both re-establishing the correct thickness and the correct level of maximum projection.

The case shown (**190** and **191**) is a patient of mixed prognathism and progenia who opted for correction of the chin only (**192**) initially, later having a mandibular set-back (**193**), and illustrates the importance of correction of both elements of the too prominent chin. The Z angle is a useful measure of lip protrusion and should equal $80° \pm 5°$, tending to be greater in men than in women. The chin thickness should also equal or slightly exceed the thickness of the upper lip.

189　Merrifield's profile analysis.

190 to 193　**A patient with mixed prognathism and progenia;** after correction of the chin only (**192**); after mandibular set-back also (**193**).

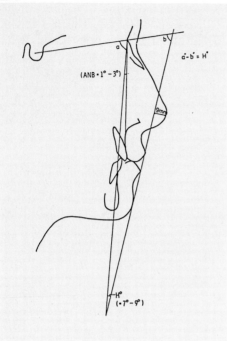

194 Holdaway's profile analysis.

Holdaway (1976) projected a similar line from soft-tissue chin, J, to the upper lip, F, and extended it superiorly to intersect with SN through the nose, and inferiorly to intersect the projected line NB at an angle (the H angle) (**194**). The H angle expresses the relative prominence of the upper lip to the slope of the underlying facial skeleton, and its value is related to the value of ANB. Where ANB lies between 1° and 3°, the normal value, then the H angle should be between 7° and 9°, both lips should lie on the profile line, and the nasal tip should project approximately 9 mm anteriorly to this line. There should be no lip tension, defined by Holdaway as existing where the difference between the soft-tissue thickness, A–D, and the border of the upper lip exceeds ±1°. The 9 mm nasal-tip measurement reaches normality at 13 years of age.

Photocephalometry

Photocephalometric prediction imposes the discipline of cephalometry on the use of lateral photographic techniques formerly used empirically. Data derived from postoperative studies are used to predict the most likely changes in profile to result from specific surgical procedures. **Profile planning** is defined as 'reasoned prediction of the probable effects of alternative facial osteotomies (or other hard tissue corrections) on facial profile, and the use of the resulting predictions to formulate a treatment plan' (Henderson, 1974).

Two notes of warning are necessary. There is a considerable variation in the soft tissue changes which accompany some movements of bone and teeth, for example in the movement of the upper lip after maxillary advancement. Therefore, the most that can be claimed is that an average prediction is possible; nevertheless, this is most valuable in establishing in general terms the balance of change the face will undergo. Second, prediction is not concerned with stability. If a procedure is chosen which is likely to be unstable postoperatively, then an additional movement may be built into the planning so that the eventual result approximates the predicted aim. Overcorrection for this reason is a separate and deliberate stage of surgical planning; with proper case selection it is less often necesary than formerly, but there are still indications for overcorrection (see Section 5).

195

196

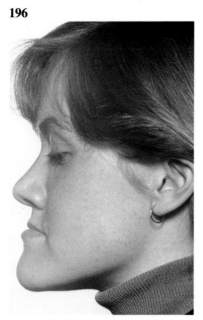

197

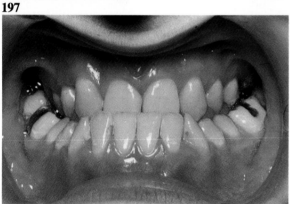

198

SNA	77°
SNB	88°
ANB	-11°
SNPo	90°
1ˈMxP	120°
1ˈMnP	70°
SNˈMP°	28°
NAˈAPo	60:58 mm
CT	17mm

P.C PREOPERATIVE

195 to 198 Patient with gross abnormality in the lower facial profile.

The technique of photocephalometric planning

Photocephalometric planning will be illustrated by reference to this patient complaining of an unacceptable appearance and a prenormal incisor relationship (**195** to **198**). In profile the upper face and orbital region is well proportioned but there is a little para-alar hollowing in the lower midface. The nasolabial angle is acute and there is too little vermilion exposure in the upper lip by comparison with the lower lip. The lower lip projects too far forwards, the labiomental curve is not displeasing, but the anterior mandible and chin project too far.

On any of the profile analyses described above there is a gross abnormality present in the lower-facial profile. In full face view the upper face and upper mid-third are again seen to be pleasing, the alar flare is adequate but there is para-alar hollowing, the lips are out of balance and the lower-third is clearly projected forwards. The occlusion of the teeth shows a Class 3 incisor relationship with a bilateral molar and premolar crossbite and retroclination of the lower anteriors. Cephalometrically there is an ANB difference of −11° (ie 13° of disproportion).

With an SNB of 88°, an SNA of 77° and a flat cranial floor this is clearly largely caused by mandibular protrusion (a view supported by the clinical findings), but the disproportion is too great to accept readily that there is no maxillary underdevelopment in real terms. The upper incisors are a little proclined and the lower incisors retroclined in dental compensation for the underlying skeletal discrepancy. The angle of convexity is −27° and the ratio NA:APo is 60:58. The chin thickness is within normal limits at 17 mm. The Z angle is 100° and the H angle is divergent. The malocclusion could be corrected by mandibular set-back, maxillary advancement at the Le Fort 1 level, or by a combination of the two. The extent of disproportion argues for the desirability of distributing the correction between both jaws for reasons of stability. The steps in photocephalometric planning are as follows:

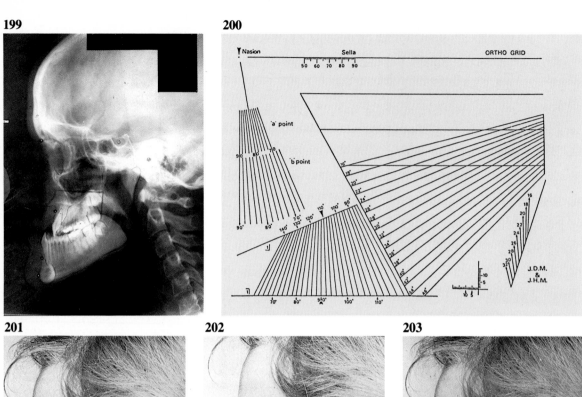

199 and 200   Photocephalometric planning: step 1.

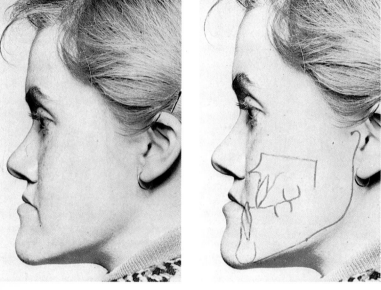

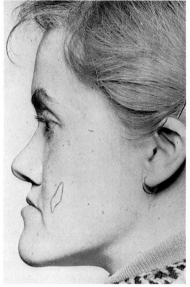

201 to 203   Photocephalometric planning: step 2.

Step 1. (199) The relevant data are marked on the cephalogram directly (a separate cephalogram or duplicate is used for record tracing). The points are marked with a pin through the radiograph, and the lines are scratched onto its surface with a stylus. The profile is traced with a chinagraph pencil as is the outline of the upper and lower incisor teeth, the first standing molars, the lower jaw (as this may be under consideration for surgery) and the upper jaw at the Le Fort 1 level. In the clinic rapid cephalometric assessment may be undertaken by the use of a transparent protractor of the kind designed and described by McEwen and Martin (1967) (200).

Step 2. A profile transparency is produced (201). This is a positive photographic image printed on a transparent base and enlarged to allow accurate superimposition on the soft tissue profile of the cephalogram.

The patient is normally photographed in the 'tooth together' position with the lips in repose, the back erect and the head straight. Both cephalogram and photograph are thus taken in the same pose for a true lateral view—ideally both photograph and radiograph being exposed on the same apparatus, but this facility is rarely available. If there is a marked freeway space, then the process is repeated with the patient in the rest position of the mandible for both views.

A fine-grain film and an illuminated white background are used. The negative is printed onto a thick-based photographic film enlarged to the same line as the cephalometric profile. After superimposition the relevant data are traced from the radiograph to the transparency, pins being used through both to mark the points. This allows easy relocation of the transparency on the radiograph at will (202). An additional transparency is also

204 **205**

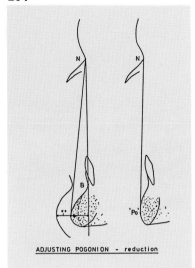

ADJUSTING POGONION - reduction

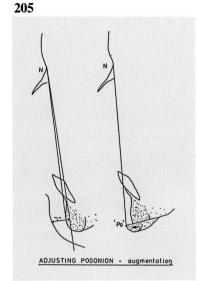

ADJUSTING POGONION - augmentation

206

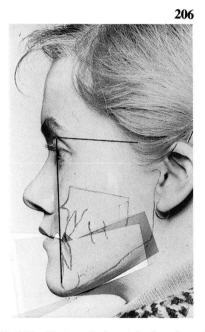

204 to 206   Photocephalometric planning: step 3.

marked out showing the anterior facial points, N, Or, A, B and Po plus the full outline of the upper central incisor (**203**). This is the Reference Transparency and is laid to one side for use in Step 5.

Step 3. At this stage the transparency has been marked with points S, N, Or, A, B, Po, the incisor outlines, the molar outlines, the mandibular outlines and the Le Fort 1 maxillary outline. The reference planes may be etched in (left out of the figure for clarity) and the occlusal plane is seen. The latter is compared with the study models which should be trimmed so that the bases are parallel to the occlusal plane. The next move is

to relate the mandible to the cranial base in what is likely to be a good relationship in the anteroposterior plane. The transparency is sectioned, care being taken to keep the incisor outlines on their respective segments.

The chin is considered first. Total chin thickness, measured anterior to the line NB projected inferiorly (**189**) may be excessive and then the bony prominence will have to be reduced (**204**), or on occasion augmented (**205**). This will result in a new position of pogonion. Therefore, an assessment is made at this stage to determine whether the bony chin itself is likely to require augmentation or reduction, and if so the extent of this change is estimated. From then on the corrected position of Po is used in the ensuing stages of planning. As the angulation of the line NB may itself be altered by surgery the assessment is a provisional one and may require to be revised at the conclusion of planning. In the case under consideration the chin thickness is within normal limits at 17 mm, and no alteration is necessary.

The mandible is next related to the cranial base using the angle SNPo (and its clinical equivalent, as assessed 'artistically' from the photograph) as a guide (**206**). As the mandible is set back the changing value of SNPo and SNB may be monitored with the transparent overlay protractor. In this case the SNPo is set at 85° and the SNB at 84°. The amount of set-back is partly artistic and partly cephalometric; it is partly determined by the desire to distribute the correction evenly between the mandible and the maxilla. Note that the soft tissues, the dental relationship and the mid-third are ignored at this point. There is a tilt in the mandibular set-back which will be discussed later. At this stage it would be logical not to produce a tilt but to move back along the occlusal plane. The section is fixed down with sticky tape. This stage establishes the facial plane, NPo, against which the rest of the facial skeleton will be assessed.

The relationship of the lower incisor tips to the facial plane should be examined. Ideally when the incisor axis is both stable and aesthetically pleasing (predictive indications of which are sought in the interincisal angle, Tweeds triangle—especially the FMIA—and likely labiolingual balance) the tip should rest on the facial plane. To achieve this may call for adjustment of the whole mandibular position (as the correct relationship of the chin to the cranial base must be maintained this may require a compensatory rotation of the entire anterior mandible or a genioplasty), or movement of the incisors by subapical segmental surgery or orthodontic movement preoperatively or postoperatively. Allowance may be made for postoperative orthodontic or physiological changes in incisor angulation. In this patient such an allowance for decompensation of the preoperative lower incisor retroclination has been made, and there is room for proclination to bring the tips onto the facial plane.

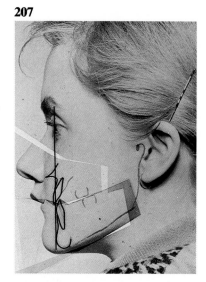

207 Photocephalometric planning: step 4.

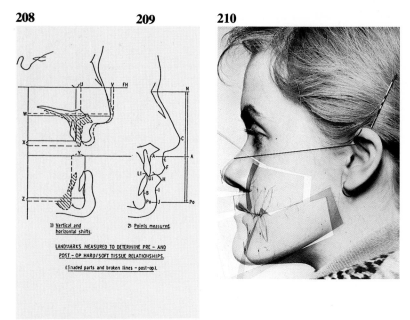

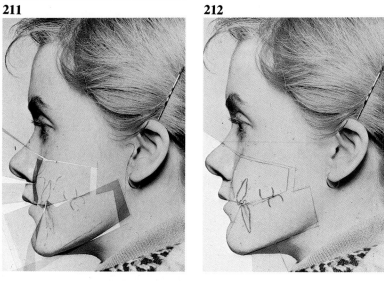

208 to 212 Photocephalometric planning: step 5.

Step 4. The maxillary base is next adjusted to the facial plane. Ideally the maxilla should be advanced until the A point is on or anterior to the facial plane, thus establishing a good angle of convexity. The transparency is sectioned so that all parts which will move with a Le Fort 1 advancement are included on the maxillary segment to be repositioned. Thus the line passes through the nasal profile just below the mid-dorsum, and includes the dentoalveolar segment with the upper incisor outline.

Again, rotation, segmental correction or orthodontic treatment may be necessary to correct incisor axial inclination. The aim is to bring the incisor tip to a point 1 mm or 2 mm anterior to the facial plane. The correction at this stage (and the process is similar for higher levels of maxillary advancement) is intended to correct the skeletal relationships while allowing for compensatory occlusal changes. This step must be carried out with due regard to the study models and the possible occlusal relationships, with or without orthodontic correction.

In this case advancement is impracticable to bring the A point right up to the facial plane and the compromise shown is adopted. When the models are positioned as indicated by the interincisor and intermolar outlines it is seen that the model bases are no longer parallel but tilted towards one another anteriorly. It is at this stage that the decision is made to rotate the mandible rather than the maxilla, and in practice the rotation would require repositioning the mandibular outline on the transparency. For clarity in a complex situation this rotation was introduced ahead of time in the figure accompanying Step 3.

Step 5. Allowance for soft tissue changes. Finally it is necessary to know what soft tissue changes will accompany each of these osteotomies. Both qualitative and quantitative information is needed—or the *pattern* and *magnitude* of change.

Quantitative evidence is sought from careful studies of pre-operative and postoperative tracings of the kind illustrated in **208** and based on observation of the points shown in **209** (Henderson, 1976). Cephalograms are superimposed on cranial base structures, and from the study of multiple cases certain patterns of change can be predicted. The hard and soft tissues do not move in a one-to-one relationship, as we see clearly from Figure **207**. For example, bringing the maxilla forward at the Le Fort 1 level usually brings the nasal tip forwards one-third of the distance the A point is advanced, and elevates it slightly. If the movement of A point is known (as in the prediction under consideration) the position the nasal tip, C, will adopt may be plotted.

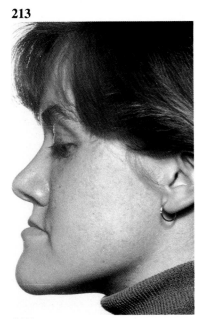

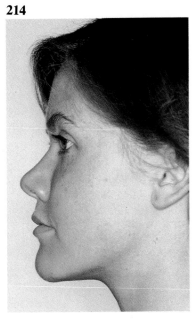

215

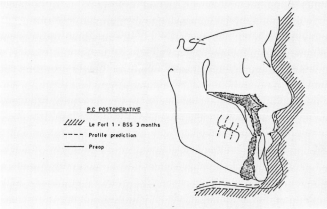

P.C POSTOPERATIVE

⟋⟋⟋⟋ Le Fort 1 + BSS 3 months

---- Profile prediction

⎯⎯ Preop

216

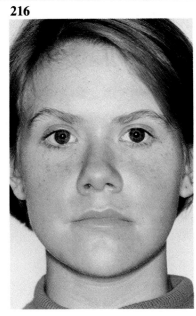

Similarly certain qualitative patterns of change accompany specific osteotomies. In the Le Fort 1 for example the nasal profile hinges forwards from a point just below the mid-dorsum (where the transparency has been sectioned in **207**). By combining the qualitative and quantitative information fairly reliable predictions of change are usually possible. In practice the soft-tissue profile of nose, upper and lower lips is cut from the plan arrived at in **207**, and the residue of the plan is superimposed on the Reference Transparency already prepared in step 2.

This allows comparison of the fixed bony points in the original and after proposed movement. Thus the movement of the A point, for example, is seen by comparison and a vertical line is scribed on the underlying Reference Transparency one-third of this movement in advance of the nasal tip. The nasal profile can then be repositioned so that it is advanced to this line with slight elevation, bending from the original just below mid-dorsum. Similarly the upper lip and lower lip can be positioned and simulated, given the relevant data (see below). The transparencies are shown (**210**) after repositioning of the soft tissue outlines on the original, but still attached to the Reference Transparency, and the arrows show the movements of A, B, Po and upper incisor tips.

The vertical lines scribed on the underlying transparency indicate the levels to which C point and F point will be advanced, and I point and J will be set back. The Reference Transparency is then separated and the plan looks as shown in **211**. Defects are sketched in, and if desired overlaps can be excised, gaps filled by cutouts from a third transparency, and irrelevant data rubbed off where chinagraph pencil was used (**212**). A realistic prediction is obtained. For quicker results the plan may be photostated at the stage shown in **211** and gaps pencilled in, excess painted out. Figures **108** to **110** were produced this way.

The result of treatment as planned in this patient can be seen (**213** to **217**). The preoperative and postoperative profiles are shown together and may be compared with the prediction; the tracings show what has happened and the extent to which the prediction was accurate, and the full face and occlusal views complete the picture.

The requirements of profile planning are: (a) That it must realistically, although not necessarily in detailed accuracy, predict the changes produced by surgery; (b) It must be readily appreciated by the planner, and (c) It must be meaningful to the patient. In the latter respect it affords an excellent medium for communication between the surgeon and his patient which helps both to define their objectives. It also serves as an excellent means of teaching, compelling detailed discussion of the several aspects of the patient's profile problems.

213 to 217 Photocephalometric planning: result of treatment.

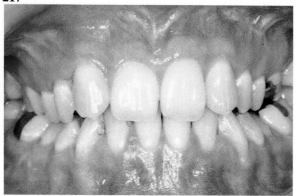

217

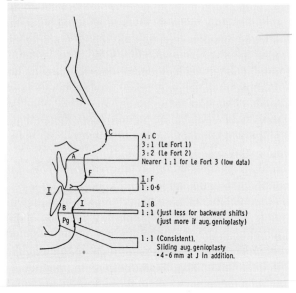

218

218 Quantitative criteria for profile prediction.

Soft tissue changes after surgery

Only in recent years has interest focused on the detailed changes in the soft tissues which accompany hard tissue surgery; yet these are the changes actually observed by patients. Two questions need to be answered before reasonable predictions can be made. Are there any consistent quantitative relationships between hard and soft-tissue movement? Is it possible to establish reliable qualitative patterns of change in facial contour which accompany specific osteotomies or combinations of osteotomies? It must be understood that quantitative statements are all the means of ranges of observation, and individual variation may occur. The guidance presented here is based on personal work (Henderson, 1976) put together with the observations of Robinson *et al* (1972), Bell and Dann (1973), Hershey and Smith (1974), Lines and Steinhauser (1974), Dann *et al* (1976), and Freihofer (1976, 1977).

Quantitative data reliable for profile prediction are summarised in **218**, for the non-cleft palate/hare-lip case. All the data refer to horizontal movements; to date no usable information relating to vertical movements has been presented, there being much greater variability in the associated factors, although the qualitative changes are more clearly defined.

(a) *The movement of the nasal tip* (Point C). This moves with the A point one unit for each three units of movement in Le Fort 1 procedures, two units for each three in Le Fort 2 procedures where there has been no associated columellar surgery or nasal tip bone grafting, and one-to-one for Le Fort 3 procedures.

(b) *The movement of the upper lip* (Point F) is best seen by comparing with the tip of the upper incisor. The subnasale is unreliable and reflects several other changes which vary from procedure to procedure. The F point will move about one-third of the advancement of the incisor tip in orthodontic movement of the tooth, and from one-third to one-to-one movement in surgical advancement. A usable average is two-thirds advancement of F compared with incisor tip advancement (or set-back). The important clinical factor to watch is the 'stretchability' of the lip, the bulk of soft-tissue in it. The thick, fleshy lip is thinned more readily as the teeth are advanced below it, and therefore the advancement is less (say one-third). The average lip will advance two-thirds, and the tight or scarred lip will often approximate full one-to-one movement.

(c) *The movement of the lower lip (H point)* reflects many factors and does not follow the lower incisor teeth in any predictable fashion. The B point and the overlying soft-tissue supramentale (I) move in almost a one-to-one relationship; a little less if the mandible is set back and a little more if there is an associated augmentation genioplasty. Genioplasty alone advances the I

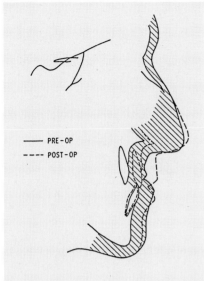
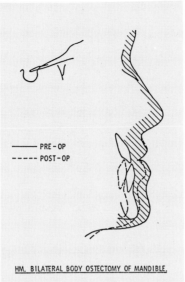

219   Typical pattern of change produced by Le Fort 1 maxillary advancement.

220   Pattern of change typical of mandibular set-back.

point by about 1 mm in standard augmentation procedures. The amount of vermilion of the lower lip which is displayed is reduced as the mandible is set back and increased as it comes forwards, but the movement is affected by the relative lengths of the lips in relation to the upper and lower incisor teeth, and is therefore not predictable with accuracy.

As a general rule the lower lip will move back about 60% of the movement of the supramentale in mandibular set-back operations, but in advancement procedures will depend on whether or not it starts from a position of entrapment behind the upper incisors. If so then advancement brings it in front of the upper teeth and the deep labiomental furrow is converted into a smoother curve, with a greater degree of forward movement of the lower lip. If not there may be relatively little forward movement of the vermilion of the lip.

(d) *The movement of the chin* is the most consistent of all. Pogonion (Po) and soft tissue pogonion (J) move consistently in a one-to-one ratio when the whole mandible or anterior mandible is advanced or set back; sliding augmentation genioplasty will add 4 mm to 6 mm to the chin for each standard slide (ie a double-sliding genioplasty will add between 8 mm and 12 mm, depending on the anteroposterior thickness of the anterior lower border). Reduction genioplasty is less predictable and less

satisfactory. About two-fifths of the set-back of Po may be expected at J.

Qualitative patterns of change are specific to particular osteotomies and quite consistent. The different patterns will be presented with the descriptions of the osteotomies in Section 4. Suffice to note here that each osteotomy will produce a specific type of change which may be varied by additional factors which the planner will learn to recognise.

Figure **219** shows the typical pattern produced by Le Fort 1 maxillary advancement, and the details are discussed with **924** to **927**. However, if the maxilla is superiorly repositioned, or tilted, then this pattern will be modified (see pages 281/2). Similarly **220** shows the change typical of mandibular set-back except that there is no effect on the upper lip. This is because there is not only set-back but also slight elevation of the anterior segment, in this case part of a bilateral body ostectomy. This elevation has cancelled out the normal effect of set-back on the upper lip (slight elongation and flattening, slight set-back of the F point, a drop down and back of the stomion). This subject will be expanded in the discussion of vertical changes, but the factors most likely to modify the basic patterns of change are: (a) The relative lengths of the lips in relation to the teeth; (b) Alteration in the vertical dimension, and (c) Rotational movements in the positioning of underlying bony fragments.

Full face analysis

The analysis of the face as viewed from the front is much more qualitative than quantitative. As will be seen in considering facial asymmetry the PA cephalogram yields important information when determining the site of asymmetrical growth, but the clinical examination of the full face is relatively much more important than the X ray film. This contrasts with the profile cephalogram in the study of the side face view.

The face should be studied in full face, oblique and profile views (these cannot be separated in this part of the assessment) for: (a) Total facial proportion; (b) Orbital balance; (c) Symmetry; (d) Infraorbital recession; (e) Paranasal hollowing and its relation to nasal projection; (f) Alar and oral commissural width, and (g) Vermilion exposure in the upper and lower lips.

Dentally the importance of lip competence, and of lip to incisor length, has already been stressed (see pp. 50–53). Finally the face should be observed during muscular action, in laughing, speaking and habit as abnormalities in these areas can be readily confused with structural abnormalities by the patient.

Total facial proportion. The well proportioned face is divided into three thirds, comprising the cranium, the mid-third (from eyebrows to oral commissure), and the lower-third. There are several proportions which are clinically useful as markers of vertical balance (**221**):

(a) The distance from the outer canthus of the eye to the angle of the mouth should about equal the distance from the nasal columella to the chin, ie A should equal B.

(b) The lateral edge of the alar rim should lie vertically below the medial canthus of the eye, or slightly lateral to this position.

(c) The medial limbus of the eye should lie vertically above the angle of the oral commissure.

(d) The vermilion exposure of the lips should be equal, ie a should equal b.

Some authors emphasise that the distance from the subnasale to the lip stomion should be one-third of the distance from the stomion to the menton, but this appears to be quite variable in faces otherwise apparently well proportioned, especially in non-Caucasian races. The intrinsic size of the lip itself and the tone of the orbicularis muscle should be noted before imbalance is blamed on the underlying dentoalveolar structures. Vertical or anteroposterior abnormality can both affect the vertical balance of lips and chin in the lower-third.

221

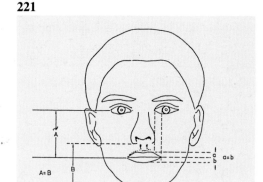

221 Vertical proportion.

Orbital balance (222) exists only where the orbits are symmetrically positioned, lying on the same horizontal plane and also at equal distances from the midline. The interpupillary distance should approximate 63 mm, the intercanthal distances 98 mm (outer canthal distance) and 35 mm (inner canthal distance), in the adult; for children and early adolescents tables exist for age variations from these norms.

Too much attention should not be paid to these figures in absolute terms, as the clinical impression of balance and proportion is more important than the measurements. However, the distances should be noted, especially to determine whether there is asymmetry and of what degree. Even in the correction of hypertelorism it is better to remove an apparently excessive amount of median bone rather than rely on careful bony measurement. This probably reflects the influence of the medial canthal position which is not readily predictable, especially if detached during surgery. In profile the supraorbital ridge should lie about 12 mm anterior to the globe, the nasal bridge 5 mm to 8 mm anterior to the globe, and the infraorbital rim from 2 mm posteriorly to 2 mm anteriorly. All these are subject to considerable individual variation, but are useful guides. Figure **223** shows a case well within normal limits while **224** shows one with grossly inadequate supraorbital support and the same in the infraorbital region.

A good example of orbital dystopia with three-dimensional displacement of the orbital blocks in relation to each other is seen in the case of Apert's Syndrome (**416** to **423**).

Facial symmetry is rare, if indeed it ever occurs. Most individuals show some degree of right/left variation which can be demonstrated by dividing full face photographs vertically through the mid-face and printing composite pictures composed of two right sides and two left sides. Quite different faces result; but the exercise has little clinical value in assessing individual patients.

222

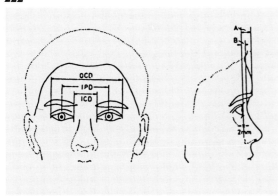

222   Orbital balance OCD = Outer Canthal Distance; IPD = Inter Pupillary Distance; ICD = Inner Canthal Distance; A = Globe to glabellar; B = Globe to nasal bridge; X = Infraorbital margin.

223

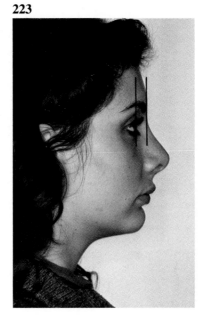

223   A case well within normal limits of orbital balance.

224

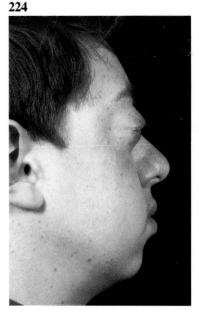

224. Grossly inadequate supraorbital and infraorbital support.

Most significant asymmetry is immediately obvious as such, and it then becomes necessary to define the areas of abnormality and the sites at which the two sides differ from one another. A midline must be established and a useful method is to mark the mid-glabellar, the nasal tip, the subnasale, the midline of the Cupid's bow of the upper lip, and the mid-chin; or a selection of these (**225**). In this patient the chin is clearly deviant to the left, evidence of mandibular asymmetry. With experience the marks need not be made but imagined. More widespread aysmmetry is determined by careful and systematic examination of each facial area, and for this it is helpful to have a full face photograph and PA cephalogram taken in the 'natural head' position, with the jaw in the 'rest' rather than the 'tooth together' position.

Analysis of the photograph is directed to the assessment of whether or not there is any real asymmetry, and to the determination of the sites and magnitude of that asymmetry

225

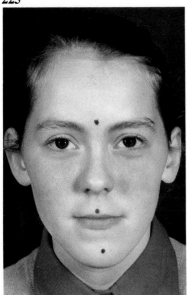

225   Marking of a midline to determine areas of asymmetry.

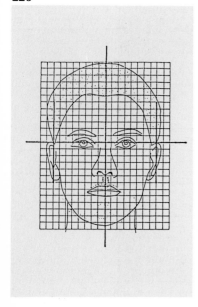

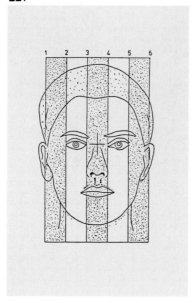

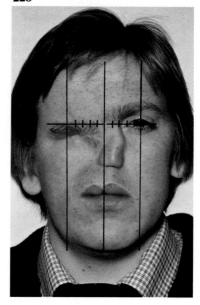

226   Symmetry grid.

227   The Rule of Fifths.

228   Use of overlay grid on an asymmetrical face.

A simple overlay grid on acetate paper with a central cross superimposed on a 'graph paper' type of grid (226) may be centralised over the face and the squares counted laterally to compare various levels of facial width, together with an assessment of the distances all the facial features lie from the midline. There are sometimes problems with even this, as the face may be difficult to centralise under the grid. Usually the cross axis may be centred over the interpupillary line with the intersection at the centre of the nasal bridge. This presupposes that the eyes and orbits are level and that the nasal bridge is central. Some commonsense is necessary in using the grid but it certainly helps to make left/right comparisons rather more accurately than by inspection alone.

The use of the Rule of Fifths (227) is also helpful in comparing different features of the face. The five vertical sections shown should be approximately equal in a well balanced and symmetrical face. (Bell *et al*, 1980).

The very asymmetrical face shown in 228 is overlaid with a transparent grid and also divided into fifths and makes interesting study. This case illustrates the need to judge the correct centralisation of the grid, as one eye is absent with a reduced right orbit at a lower level than that on the left.

Mandibular displacements commonly complicate the symmetry of the face. An abnormal path of mandibular closure is usually the result of occlusal abnormality and any lateral deviation may accentuate asymmetry, especially of the lower-third of the face.

229

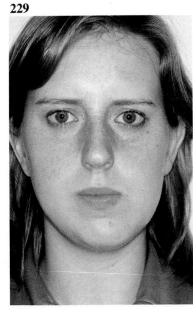

231

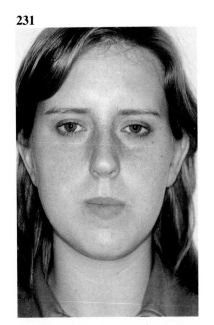

229 to 232   Apparent asymmetry.

230

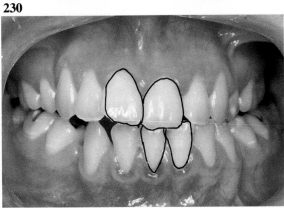

232

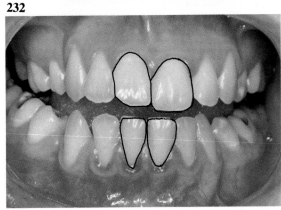

One of the first steps in determining the nature of asymmetry must be to decide whether there is any lateral mandibular displacement. Plint and Ellisdon (1974) draw attention to the fact that an asymmetry may be entirely the result of mandibular displacement, there being no skeletal asymmetry present. This is called *apparent asymmetry* and can be detected by observing the face (and the PA radiograph) with the jaw at rest, at the point of initial dental contact, and in full cuspal interdigitation.

The case shown in **229** and **230** is in full occlusal closure and appears to present mandibular asymmetry with the chin to the left. When examined at the point of initial dental contact (**231** and **232**) the incisor midlines coincide and the chin is central. The case is one of apparent asymmetry and treatment must be directed to the occlusal abnormalities. The importance of

relating the incisor midlines to one another and to the midline of the face is seen here; this assessment is also brought out in the PA cephalogram.

Plint and Ellisdon classify apparent asymmetries in relation to the cause of the mandibular displacement: (1) Skeletal anteroposterior disproportion, eg Class 3 cases with bites of accommodation; (2) Skeletal transverse discrepancies with maxillary alveolar narrowing; (3) Maxillary narrowness associated with atypical soft tissue behaviour, eg thumb-sucking, and, (4) Local factors, eg one or more teeth in crossbite or malpositioned.

Where there is an eccentric incisor midline, other causes must be excluded—unilateral loss of teeth in crowded arches, developmental anomalies of eruption, and habits.

233

235

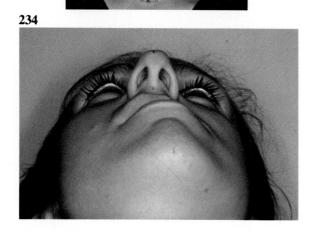

233 to 236   Real mandibular asymmetry exaggerated in occlusal closure.

234

236

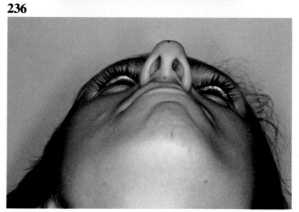

Mandibular displacements also commonly complicate real skeletal asymmetries of the mandible or maxilla. The case shown in **233** and **234** is in full occlusal intercuspation. Compare this with the appearance when the initial tooth contact is made (**235** and **236**). There is no doubt that real mandibular asymmetry exists, but the magnitude of that asymmetry is greatly exaggerated in occlusal closure.

It should be noted that mandibular deviations also occur symmetrically by protrusive deviation in anteroposterior disproportions, and may mislead the unwary in studying the facial profile with the teeth together. Where this occurs, the cephalogram and the lateral profile transparencies must be taken in the position of initial dental contact.

The PA skull radiograph should be taken in the cephalostat, and both rest position and 'tooth together' position should be posed, to assist in the determination of mandibular displacements in occlusion.

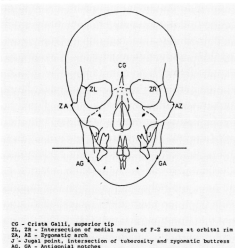

237

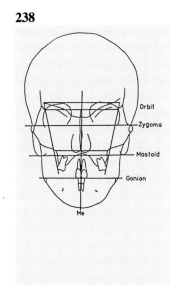

238

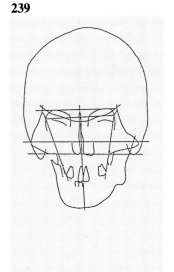

239

CG - Crista Galli, superior tip
ZL, ZR - Intersection of medial margin of F-Z suture at orbital rim
ZA, AZ - Zygomatic arch
J - Jugal point, intersection of tuberosity and zygomatic buttress
AG, GA - Antigonial notches

237 PA radiograph: Rickett's
frontal analysis (diagrammatic).

238 PA radiograph: Sassouni's
tracing analysis.

239 Tracing of a typical asymmetry.

The subject of PA cephalometry has developed a considerable literature but the assessment for treatment purposes should be kept simple. The tracing may be studied in any way which allows comparison of those structures represented bilaterally, and as with the full face photograph the object is to determine the sites and magnitude of asymmetry. As an aid the points which make up the basis of Rickett's frontal analysis are shown in **237**, and Sassouni's recommendation for tracing analysis is shown in **238**. A typical asymmetry is shown traced out in **239**. Simple overlay grids, like those used over the photographs, will often provide as much information. The importance of detailed and systematic examination of the PA cephalogram must be emphasised (see Sassouni, 1964; Ricketts, 1972).

Infraorbital recession (240–246)

This varies greatly in cases of mid-third hypoplasia, sometimes affecting only the medial part of the infraorbital rim (**240** and **241**) when it may be necessary to detect the abnormality by palpation rather than inspection; sometimes affecting most of the infraorbital rim when there will be increased scleral exposure between the cornea and the lower lid, together with obvious lack of bony support below the globe in profile (**242** and **243**); and sometimes amounting to gross lack of protection for the globe around the whole of the periorbital rim (**244** and **224**).

240

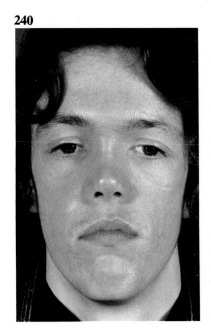

241

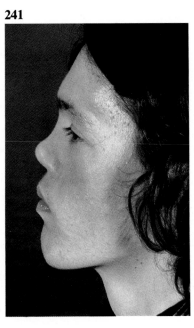

242

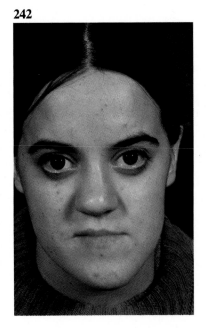

243

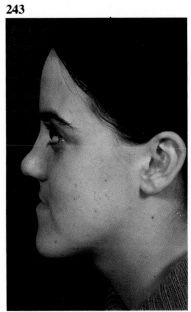

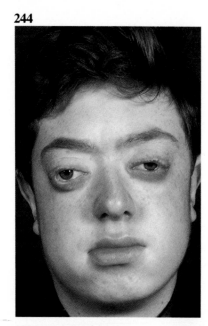

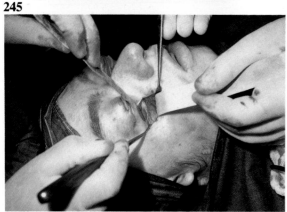

244 and 245   Gross orbital rim recession (see also **224**).

246

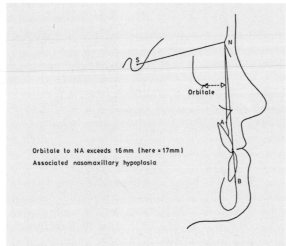

The underdevelopment of the infraorbital region can be quite dramatic as shown in the operative exposure (**245**). The clues to this problem are often to be found in the full facial examination. Thus the patient in **240** and **241** shows nasomaxillary hypoplasia with a short, upturned nose and profile recession in the upper mid-face; the patient in **242** and **243** also has mid-facial recession in her case involving the dentoalveolar segment with a Class 3 incisor relationship (and incidentally a severe mandibular deviation to the left); and the patient in **244** exhibits severe upper mid-face and frontal recession necessitating early tarsorrhaphy to protect the globe before advancement of the frontal bone and mid-face.

The extent of inferior orbital recession will determine the extent of inferior orbital rim advancement or augmentation, and therefore the choice of osteotomy lines in Le Fort 2 and 3 advancements. Cephalometrically some indication of the extent of infraorbital recession is given by the distance of the orbitale from the line NA, measured at right angles to it. This is normally 10 mm to 16 mm in Caucasians (Leonard and Walker, 1977) and a distance in excess of 16 mm should raise the question as to orbital rim advancement (**246**). Where there is a low SNA (or maxillary advancement at the Le Fort 1 level is under consideration) a projected correction of the A point is made. The distance the orbitale lies behind this new NA line is then measured on the profile cephalogram, and this may determine whether the correct level of osteotomy is based on the Le Fort 1 or 2 pattern. However, the author finds clinical assessment to be of greater value in this area than measurement.

Paranasal hollowing and its relation to nasal projection

Paranasal hollowing or recession in the area lateral to the lower part of the nose is an indication of maxillary hypoplasia (**247** and **248**). Correction is by maxillary advancement (at all levels) or by onlay augmentation.

Most cases require a Le Fort 1 advancement, but the hollowing must be compared with the *projection of the nose* (as distinct from the shape of the nose in itself). Comparison of **247** with **249** makes the point. The former case combines marked hollowing with a definite protrusion of the nasal skeleton. Le Fort 1 maxillary advancement will further project the nasal tip by only one-third of the advancement of the bony maxilla and therefore tend to reduce the discrepancy between the two, in addition to the intrinsic reduction in the hollowing which the operation brings about, especially when combined with bone grafting in the para-alar region.

The second case (**249**) also shows paranasal hollowing but here the nasal skeleton is recessed relative to the rest of the face and a Le Fort 2 advancement is indicated, bringing the whole nose forwards by about two-thirds of the maxillary advancement (see **967** to **968**), as well as restoring the hollowed area in proportion. Le Fort 2 advancement in **247** would overproject

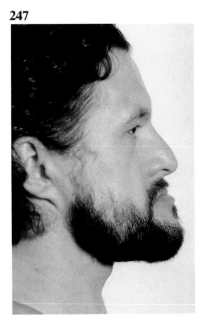 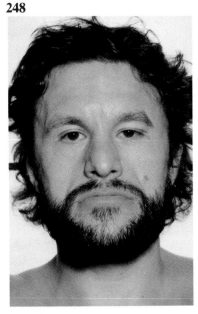 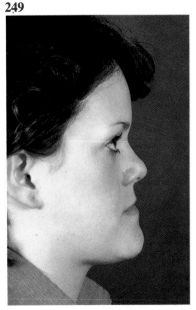

247 to 249   Paranasal hollowing.

the nose, and the degree of infraorbital recession requires more than a simple Le Fort 1 for its correction; Küfner's modified Le Fort 2 is indicated for correction as the best compromise between the competing demands of different parts of the face.

Alar and oral commisural width

Alar width also reflects maxillary hypoplasia, or vertical disproportion. Assessed as in **221** the alar width should equal the intercanthal distance or slightly exceed it. Also the slope of the nasal columella should result in the nasal tip being a little above the horizontal; therefore the columella and nasal vestibule should be visible to a small extent in full face view.

The patient in **250** shows narrowness of the alar flare and inadequate exposure of the columella. Correction by Le Fort 1 osteotomy widens the flare and raises the nasal tip (**251**) correcting the area. Similarly in **252** (a long face syndrome, see **365** to **368**) there is even greater reduction in alar flare, and here also the *width of the oral commissure* is reduced. Correction of the vertical discrepancy by Le Fort 1 maxillary elevation and bilateral mandibular set-back widens the nose and the mouth to restore balance (**253**). Maxillary lengthening also affects the alar flare and oral commissure, in this case decreasing both.

250   **251**   **252**   **253**

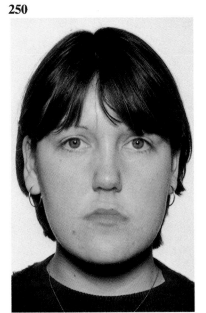 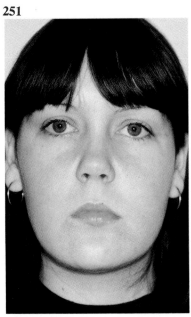 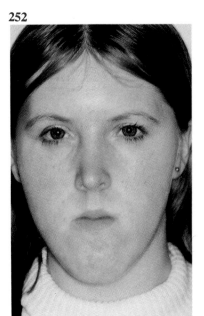 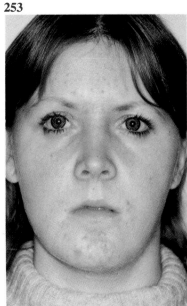

250 and 251   Narrow alar flare and inadequate exposure of the columella corrected by Le Fort 1 osteotomy.

252 and 253   Long face syndrome corrected by Le Fort 1 maxillary elevation and bilateral mandibular set-back.

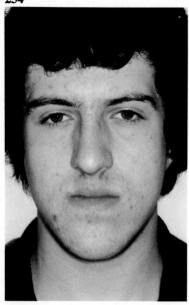
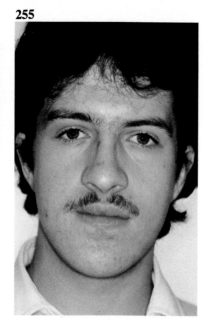

254 and 255   Vermilion exposure of the lips.

Vermilion exposure of the lips

Throughout this book examples abound of the imbalance in *vermilion exposure* of upper and lower lips which accompanies maxillomandibular disproportion. Case **254** exhibits all these features as part of gross anteroposterior maxillomandibular disproportion and illustrates the correction of each produced by bimaxillary surgical correction (bilateral sagittal set-back of the mandible and Le Fort 1 advancement of the maxilla), (**255**).

The role of orthodontic treatment

Orthodontic co-operation is essential to successful orthognathic surgery, especially in the growing child although adult treatment is often greatly helped also. The surgeon should understand the language of the orthodontist, and the principles of treatment planning. The days are past when it was enough for the orthodontist to plan and the surgeon to carry out operations to prescription. Today there is great scope in this field for innovative teamwork. Mutual respect for each other's contributions is a fundamental requirement.

Discussion will be limited here to an outline of the leading areas in which orthodontic treatment complements orthognathic surgery. The newer types of functional treatment during growth, for example the appliances proposed by Fränkel (**256** and **257**) offer some hope that orthodontic treatment may be able effectively to alter the skeletal base relationships of the jaws on selected patients treated during the actively growing period. Techniques of longterm extraskeletal traction (**258** and **259**) can certainly modify growth patterns. However, in general it remains true that patients referred for surgery are either those unsuitable for orthodontic treatment alone, or unwilling to undergo the lengthy periods of correction required. The skeletal base relationships should be considered as separate from the dentoalveolar component, although the two are fully interdependent. Skeletal base correction requires surgery; the dentoalveolar problem may be corrected either orthodontically or surgically. Individual teeth require orthodontic movement as a rule, although one-tooth osteotomies have an occasional place.

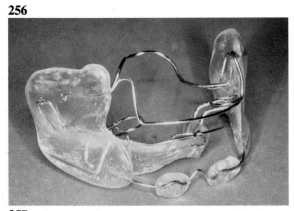

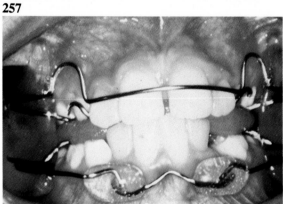

Assessment will have distinguished between malocclusion confined to the dentoalveolar segments and resulting in secondary aesthetic imbalance, and malocclusion secondary to skeletal base disproportion and probably complicated by compensatory tooth movement (for example, retroclination of lower incisors in Class 3 cases). As part of the treatment plan such secondary compensatory occlusal changes must be corrected, either by presurgical orthodontic treatment or postoperatively. In the latter case space must be built into the treatment plan to allow postoperative correction which may be by orthodontic treatment or by allowing the new muscle balance which accompanies the altered relationships between hard- and soft-tissues to restore normality.

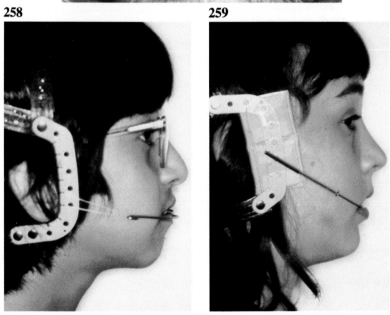

256 and 257   Fränkel orthodontic appliance.

258 and 259   Extraskeletal traction.

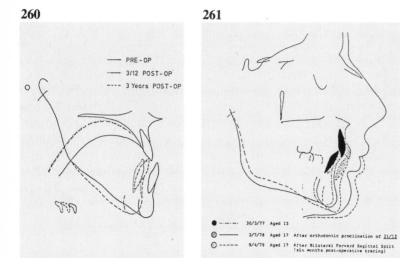

260 Incisor decompensation following bilateral body ostectomy.

261 Conversion of Class 2 Div 2 case to Class 2 Div 1 before mandibular advancement.

Figure **260** shows such a case where incisor retroclination has been recognised preoperatively but not treated, space being allowed for postoperative correction brought about under the altered influence of tongue and lip (case of bilateral body ostectomy). In many cases secondary tooth movements prevent the repositioning of the arches and must be corrected before or during surgery.

Figure **261** shows a typical and common example of this problem, the Angle Class 2 Div 2 case requiring preoperative orthodontic proclination of the upper incisors before mandibular advancement is possible. It is essential at an early stage in growing children to identify those who may require later surgery, and then to avoid compromise orthodontic treatment which may prejudice the surgery. Examples may be seen in the early extraction of upper premolars to reduce an overjet, later preventing full mandibular advancement and thus compromising the aesthetic result, with resultant bimaxillary retrusion; or in the retraction of upper incisors in Class 2 Div 1 cases to reduce overjet followed by later reversal of this move to advance the mandible.

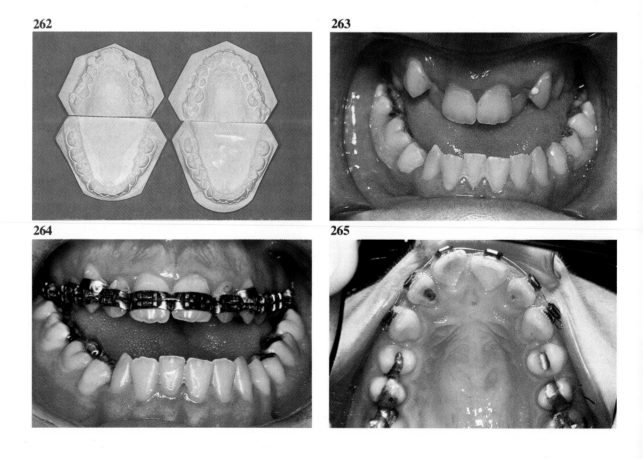

266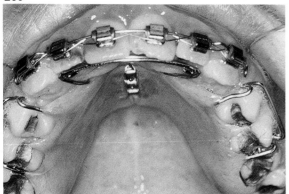

267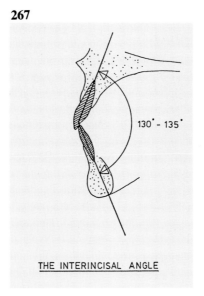

268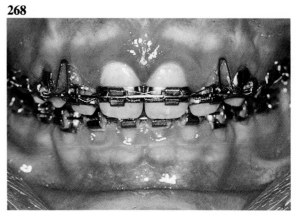

THE INTERINCISAL ANGLE

262 to 268   Preoperative orthodontics.

Preoperative orthodontics aims to correct compensatory tooth movements and arch malalignments, thus re-creating the primary malocclusion and allowing balanced surgical correction of the skeletal bases with acceptable restoration of interarch dental relationships.

The commonest applications are:

(a) Preoperative arch alignment to allow good interarch dental intercuspation (**262, 263** and **264**).

(b) Preoperative arch expansion (usually maxillary arch) or contraction, either by rapid maxillary expansion, especially in cleft palate cases, or routine expansion (also carried out in **262, 263** and **264**). The clinical result of this may be to worsen the occlusal and facial problem before surgery (**263** and **264**, the case shown in **262**, illustrate the increase in open bite which accompanies maxillary expansion before surgery). In non-cleft cases where the tongue is postured forwards allowing maxillary contraction to occur preoperative maxillary expansion becomes stable after mandibular set-back, where the tongue is returned to the upper palatal area.

(c) Alteration in the intercanine width is often necessary when the anterior segments cannot be fitted together or when narrowness of the anterior maxillary arch prevents mandibular advancement to the full extent necessary (**265** and **266**). This is unnecessary when anterior maxillary osteotomies are to be undertaken as the arch is easily widened (or narrowed) and moulded by operative midline splitting.

(d) Correction of incisor axial inclinations has already been discussed. The extent required is gauged by cephalometric analysis, and an interincisal angle of 130° to 135° is sought, although compromise results are common in this area. This angulation is felt by most orthodontists to represent a stable relationship, other things being equal (**267**).

(e) The creation of space between teeth at the sites of inter-dental osteotomies, while not essential, is useful where possible and reduces the chances of damage to teeth.

Where preoperative orthodontics involves the use of fixed appliances the same bands may be used for postoperative intermaxillary fixation, probably the most satisfactory of all methods where combined treatment is undertaken (**268**).

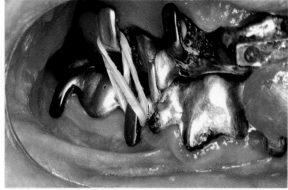

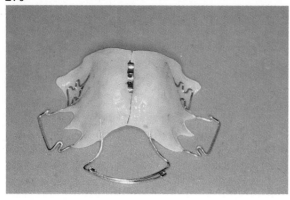

Postoperative orthodontics aims at finalisation of occlusal irregularities and retention of the results of surgery during the postoperative year. Slight overcorrection of intermaxillary relationships is often built into the treatment plan, and after the removal of IMF elastic traction to bring the arches into their ideal position is routine in some centres and has much to commend it (**269**).

If orthodontic appliances remain in place then the elastics can be applied to the bands on the teeth, usually at night-time only for six months. Otherwise cast cap splints can be left on for a further three months, but patients rarely tolerate this because of the cosmetic problem it produces. Removable appliances for night traction or removable functional appliances may be used. Whenever maxillary expansion or labial segmental surgery has been undertaken, a retention appliance is inserted immediately after fixation is removed and used for six months. An impression is taken at the time of splint removal and the appliance fitted the same day. Where incisor control is necessary a labial bow is incorporated in the appliance.

The postoperative phase may coincide with ongoing orthodontic treatment, and retention is then easily incorporated in this (**270**). All retention plates are worn continuously for 6 months, then at night for a further 3 months. In cleft palate cases retention is prolonged until a fixed bridge can be constructed across the cleft.

In general terms preoperative orthodontic treatment should be confined to that necessary to make surgery possible, leaving detailed finalisation of the occlusion until the postoperative phase. It is impossible to guarantee the exact position which the arches and individual dental segments will adopt after surgery. Most changes of significance will be complete within 6 months of the operation; there is much to be said for deferring further active orthodontic treatment until this period is over, unless the patient is still actively growing. For the same reason detailed spot grinding of teeth preoperatively is unwise, only gross cuspal interferences being dealt with before surgery. Postoperative spot grinding is beneficial and may be carried out after 3 months.

269 Postoperative elastic traction.

270 Postoperative retention appliance.

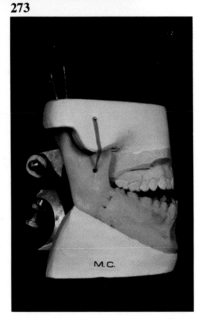

Model planning

The planning of occlusion requires the use of plaster models of the teeth (**271**) and sometimes of full mandibular or maxillo-mandibular models (**272** and **273**). During the first visit impressions of the teeth should be taken and a careful bite registration made. Models should be cast and trimmed ortho-dontically, so that the occlusal relationship can be seen instantly by setting the models down on the bench (**274**). Duplicates of these models are cast. At the second visit the accuracy of the bite registration and model trimming should be checked against the patient's occlusion, and maxillary and mandibular midlines noted on the models. This simple routine will avoid many time consuming errors.

At an early stage of assessment the general lines of possible correction become clear from simple inspection of the patient, the models and the radiographs. The object of *model planning* is twofold: (a) To determine the intended occlusion and arch form, and (b) To decide the exact amount and direction of movement of the arches or segments of the arches. Both must be undertaken at the same time as the photocephalometric study, or important factors will be overlooked.

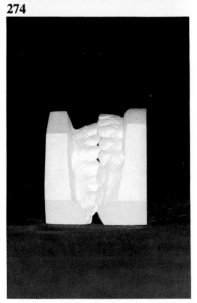

271 to 274   Models used in the planning of occlusion.

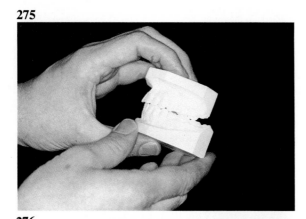

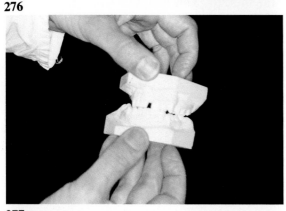

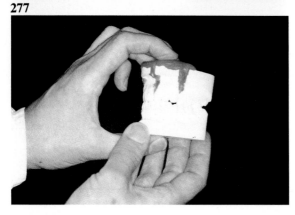

Determination of the intended occlusion and arch form is the first objective. Cases can be divided into two groups. Either the arches can be brought into a totally new relationship without breaking their continuity (**275**), or they cannot (**276**).

In the first case, if the new relationship is acceptable occlusally, there is no difficulty in relating this change to the profile plans and no further model planning is necessary. Operation will involve movement of the total arches in relation to one another, and will therefore be sited in the mandibular ramus, condyle or condylar neck, or in the maxilla above the dento-alveolar segment, or in a combination of these sites. The same result may be achievable after moderate spot grinding of the teeth to eliminate gross cuspal interference, or after simple orthodontic correction of the position of one or two teeth; both these possibilities can be tested on the model, orthodontic tooth movement being simulated by simple section with a fine saw. The process will be repeated with new models at the termination of such orthodontic treatment.

If the arches cannot be fitted together in this way, then it is necessary to consider the segmental movements required to produce the best occlusion. By inspection the segments involved can be determined; if two possibilities present each may be tried with a duplicate model. The model is sectioned and the movement required determined by trial and error (**277**). A number of complex articulators exist to make this task easier, but the movements can be achieved quite simply with the aid of some soft wax to secure the segments temporarily. Segments of the models may require to be cut away empirically to allow the trial movements to take place. Commonsense is needed to avoid movements which would be prevented by encroachment on dental roots adjacent to sectioned areas, and the radiographs should be consulted to verify root morphology, which may be marked on the models (see **283** and **284**). In this way the desired occlusion and arch form are planned in a gross manner. Next, these movements must be reduced to precisely measured dimensions and directions in the laboratory.

275 **Arches can be fitted together** without breaking their continuity.

276 **Arches cannot be fitted together.**

277 **Sectioning of model** to determine the movements required.

Determination of the exact amount and direction of arch or segment displacement is the second aim. Total arch repositioning without sectioning either arch is adequately planned on a plane line articulator having two positions for one of the models on the articulator arm (**278** and **279**). The based models are mounted on the articulator so that the occlusal plane is parallel to the bases, upper and lower. The midline of the face should be marked on the mounted models, and it is helpful to mark the interpupillary line (or a line parallel to it) and the alar to tragus line.

The displacement of the arch or arches will be guided by the photocephalometric planning, and in turn will itself lead to modification of that planning. This is why at least one posterior tooth and the most prominent incisor tooth are marked for each jaw on the profile plan. Rotational movements of one jaw (model) in relation to the other, which accompany the transition from the preoperative to the planned occlusion, will occur automatically if the teeth are fixed in IMF after osteotomy in the planned position.

The relationship of the whole dentoalveolar block to the rest of the facial skeleton is planned on the photocephalometric plan and brought about by translating that plan into effect at surgery according to the technique chosen. Thus, for example, the maxilla may be raised anteriorly by removal of a predetermined segment of supra-apical bone, and the mandible positioned in relation to the maxilla by preplanned IMF.

278　　　　　**279**

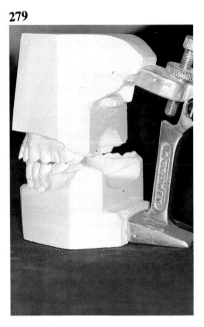

278 and 279　Two-position plane line articulator.

280

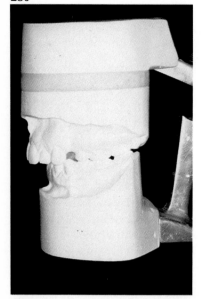

283

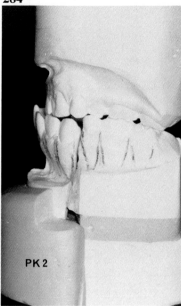

PK 1

284

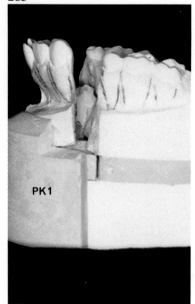

PK 2

281

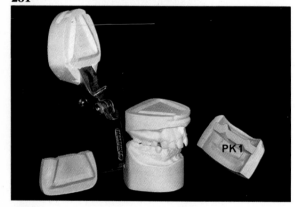

PK 1

285

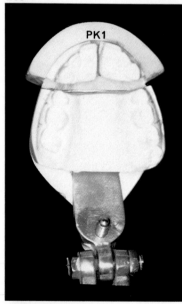

PK 1

282

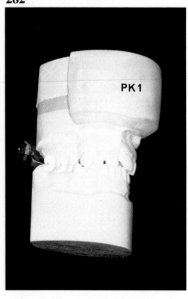

PK 1

280 to 286 Model planning for segmental surgery.

286

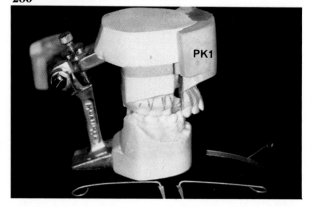

PK 1

Model planning for segmental surgery must be precise; the three-dimensional movements of the segments must be known and capable of exact reproduction at operation. The method followed is essentially that of Lockwood (1974) and is illustrated in a case of anterior maxillary ostectomy; the method is readily adaptable to any type of segmental surgery.

Figures **280, 281** and **282.** The models are articulated on a planeline articulator in the preoperative occlusion. The lower model is based directly onto the lower arm of the articulator, but a removable spacer is cast between the upper model and the plaster cap over the upper arm of the articulator. This spacer (green on the model, and about 19mm (¾in) thick) fits into localising grooves scored into the upper surface of the maxillary model base, and is itself localised to the articulator cap. The whole complex is trimmed at the sides and top as shown (**280**), but at this stage the spacer is intact.

When the site of proposed ostectomy is known, the spacer is sectioned a few millimetres posterior to the probable ostectomy site. Additional localising grooves are cut on the anterior surface of the premaxillary model segment(s) and the articulator cap, and the complex is reassembled without the anterior section of the spacer. An anterior localising key, the preplanning key PK1, is cast (**281** and **282**) so that when in place the various sections are firmly held in their preoperative relationship – even after the premaxilla has been separated by an 'ostectomy' on the model (**283**). It is convenient when working on the upper model to invert the complex (**283** to **284**).

Figures **283** and **284.** The preplanning key is removed and the maxillary model is sectioned, taking more plaster away posteriorly than necessary to allow free movement of the anterior segment(s) to achieve the desired occlusion. It is often helpful to have marked the position of the dental roots on the model beforehand, after careful inspection of both model and radiographs. No plaster may be removed where this would endanger the roots. With the preplanning key replaced (**283**), the amount of plaster removed is demonstrated, but this is not a necessary manoeuvre at this stage. The premaxillary segment is secured to the rest of the maxillary model and the whole complex reassembled without the preplanning key. A second key, the planning key PK2, is now cast to hold the anterior segment in its planned position, and any gaps in the alveolar or palatal parts of the model are eliminated by adding plaster to the posterior part of the model. Thus, with the planning key (PK2) in position, segmental movement is fully determined on the models (**284**).

Figures **285** and **286.** When the complex is reassembled with the preplanning key (PK1) holding the premaxillary segment(s) in the original position (**285** and **286**) the exact amount of bone to be removed from the alveolar and palatal areas is represented by the space between the anterior and posterior segments. This can be measured exactly, and appropriate templates prepared from malleable metal strips for use at operation after they have been sterilised (**286**).

Splints can now be constructed to position the segments with preplanned connecting bars attached via precise locking plates. Alternatively, occlusal wafers may be constructed to secure the fragments in the planned position at operation.

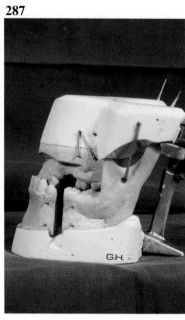

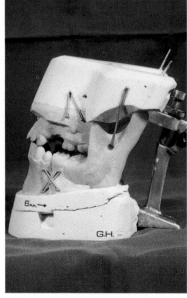

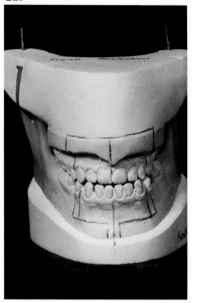

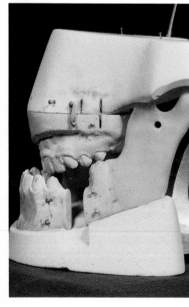

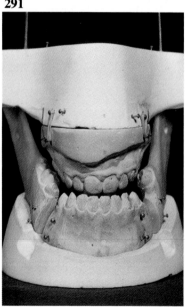

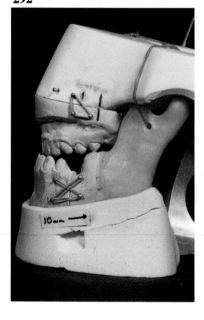

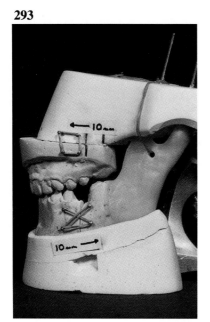 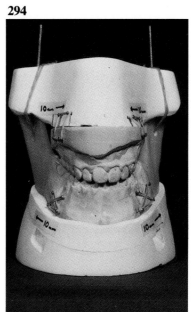 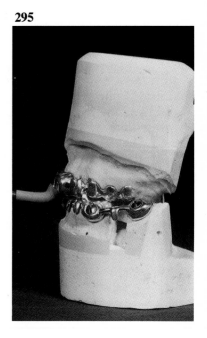

296

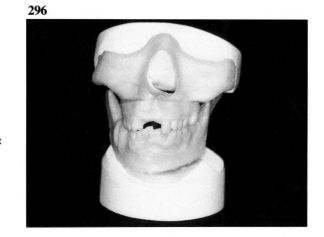

287 to 296   Full mandibular models: for bilateral body ostectomy of the mandible (**287** and **288**); for symphyseal ostectomy (**289**); for bimaxillary surgery (**290** to **295**); for a complex asymmetry after trauma (**296**).

Full mandibular models may be constructed in any situation where it is anticipated that complex three-dimensional movements, especially rotational movements, may interact unfavourably; or where it is necessary to incorporate precisely contoured onlays, whether bone grafts or alloplastic materials. With increasing experience the need for these models is reduced. They are time consuming and expensive to produce. However, there are some situations when their use may clarify the nature of tentative proposals for such complex surgery with great benefit. Examples are shown involving bilateral body ostectomy of the mandible (**287** and **288**), bimaxillary surgery (**290** to **294**, with the final occlusion established for splint construction **295**), and a complex asymmetry after trauma (**296**). (The last model was made by Mr B. Conroy, MBE.)

Summary of planning

The outcome of the assessment scheme outlined in this section is a definitive treatment plan. Little has been said about the need for full routine dental examination, but this is an obvious preliminary. The final treatment plan should therefore include: (a) All preliminary surgery including the extraction of teeth and removal of buried teeth or other pathological conditions treatable surgically; (b) Dental conservation and periodontal treatment; (c) Decisions on the type of surgery and its timing, and (d) Decisions on the presurgical and postsurgical orthodontic management, including the management of retention. The practical organisation of this assessment programme will take a minimum of three visits covering diagnosis, preliminary and final treatment planning. The following scheme expands that set out at the beginning of this section:

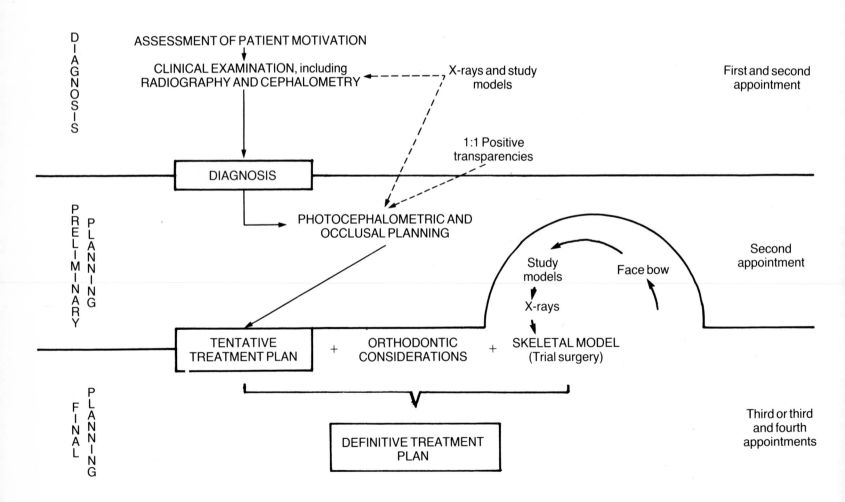

SECTION 3

Clinical presentation of facial disproportion

Abnormal skeletal anatomy can be classified in many different ways. It may be described simply in terms of mandibular and maxillary morphology, which may or may not be further complicated by associated abnormalities in other parts of the skull, especially the cranium. The pathogenesis of these complex anomalies has been discussed in Section 1.

A working classification is necessary for purposes of communication and also as a memory aid during clinical evaluation, but there is a constant danger of both over-simplification on the one hand and over-complication on the other. The many complex inherited,congenital and environmental factors which combine to modify normal growth and development inevitably result in a wide range of skeletal patterns. These may well confound rigid classification, and several abnormalities may coexist in the same patient, or secondary problems occur as a result of primary anomalies.

Classification in this section will therefore follow a simple morphological pattern designed to direct attention to leading features of facial skeletal abnormality, rather than attempting a framework within which every patient can be conveniently catalogued. Only by combining the information collated in all three relevant sections (ie Sections 1, 2 and 3) can a realistic evaluation of individual patients be made; and it will become apparent when this is done that no two patients are really identical, although several common clinical pictures are recognisable.

298

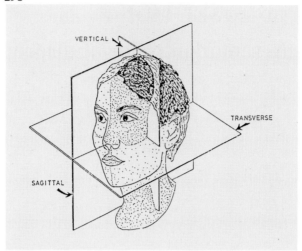

298 Facial planes.

Attention must be directed (**298**) to each of the three planes of facial orientation – *sagittal,* or anteroposterior, *vertical,* and *transverse.* Each of these planes must be considered at the three main levels of the face, Cranial (upper-third), Orbito-maxillary (mid-third) and Mandibular (lower-third), and the clinical markers of abnormality sought by applying the principles outlined in the previous section. The clinical examination of the full face, of the oblique and profile face, and the radiological and cephalometric evaluation will then determine the site and nature of the abnormalities to be corrected. It is, in the author's view, too simplistic to apply this routine absolutely rigidly (for example, mandibular excess divided into vertical excess, sagittal excess, and transverse excess) although the principle is helpful.

In this section the principal features of these abnormalities will therefore be illustrated, and in this exercise the continual overlap and interaction of the three planes at each of the facial levels will be constantly observable by the thoughtful reader. Certain common associations, or complex syndromes and anomalads (see also Section 1) emerge and can be described in terms of their common presentation; for treatment purposes they must also be considered in the analytical manner described above. In this category fall the craniostenotic syndromes, mandibulofacial dysostosis, facial microsomia and related anomalads, the Robin anomalad, and the many genetically programmed disturbances of endocrine, metabolic and other body systems. To define the site and nature of deficiency or excess is the first step towards formulating a treatment plan.

In broad principle the following classification will be followed:

1. **Symmetrical disproportion of the jaws**
   Mandibular enlargement
   Mandibular deficiency
   Maxillary enlargement
   Maxillary deficiency
   (Bimaxillary disproportion)

2. **Asymmetrical disproportion of the jaws**
   Unilateral mandibular enlargement
   Unilateral mandibular deficiency
   Unilateral maxillary abnormalities

3. **Cleft lip and palate syndrome**

Symmetrical disproportion of the jaws

Mandibular (lower-facial) enlargement

Progenia. This is simple protrusion of the chin itself, in a patient with normal mandibulomaxillary skeletal base relationships. Most commonly, however, it complicates other jaw disproportions both prenormal (**299** and **300**) and postnormal (**301** and **302**). (See **189** to **193,** and **829** to **831**.) Though often described in relation to excessive bony prominence of the chin button (pogonion in cephalometric terms), it is important to realise that the relative contributions of hard and soft tissues are unimportant; only the *total* chin thickness has any meaning in facial aesthetics. This is measured (see **189**) anterior to the line NB projected inferiorly on the skull tracing, and should approximate 16mm on a normal lateral skull film. The examples shown illustrate the way in which the prominence of the chin distorts the labiomental curve, and makes it impossible to restore good nose/chin relationships without intrinsic reduction of chin prominence, in addition to correction of any basic jaw disproportion.

299

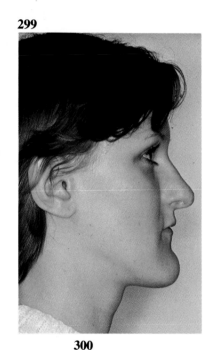

301

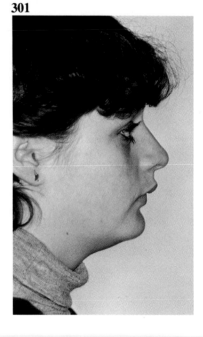

299 to 302   Progenia complicating mandibular protrusion or retrusion.

300

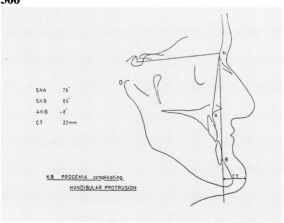

302

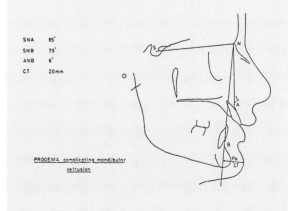

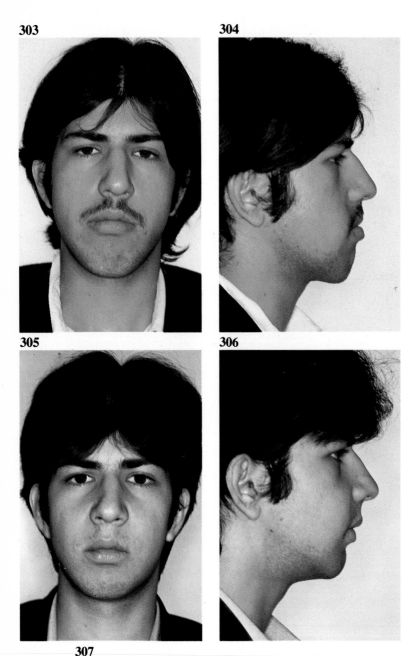

303

304

305

306

Vertical mandibular excess. Excessive bone in the vertical dimension is clinically significant in two mandibular sites – the anterior mandible and the ramus. The latter site is rarely a problem in symmetrical cases but is important in unilateral mandibular hemihypertrophy (**437** to **443**). Increased subapical bone in the anterior mandible is a very common problem, sometimes associated with over-eruption of the lower incisors in high angle cases with or without anterior open bite. Therefore it occurs most commonly as a part of the long face 'syndrome' in one of its many forms (**365** to **368**), and only rarely as an isolated feature. Anterior facial height is found to be increased, and on analysis the anterior lower dental height (**179**) is increased relative to other lateral film measurements (**307**).

The case illustrated (**303** and **304**) has associated maxillary problems, but the effect on facial aesthetics of the increased anterior subapical mandibular bone is clearly seen. There is disproportionate height in the lower face, and the chin appears too long and narrowed inferiorly. After correction (**305** and **306**), involving complex bimaxillary surgery in addition to the vertical correction of the anterior mandible, the restoration of balance is seen and the nature of the original problem more clearly demonstrated.

307

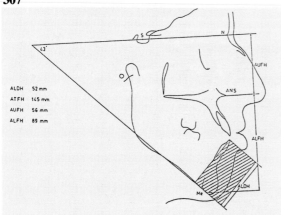

303 to 307   Vertical mandibular excess complicating long face 'syndrome'.

308

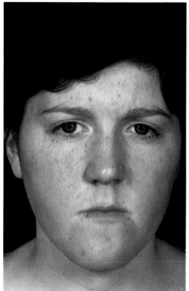

309

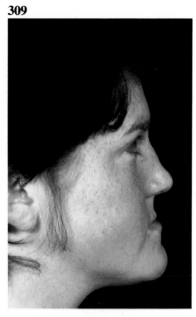

Sagittal mandibular excess. Terminology for this group is difficult, but the condition is easily recognised. Formerly called mandibular prognathism, or protrusion, the tendency today is to speak of sagittal mandibular excess.

The enlargement is not, however, always confined to the sagittal plane and may well also involve increase in both transverse and vertical dimensions. The characteristic feature is the proportionate involvement of the whole lower face, including the investing soft tissues, especially the pterygo-masseteric group. The appearance both clinically and radiologically is of a normally shaped but oversized lower jaw. Both the gonial angle and the SN:MP angle may lie within normal limits. There is no anterior open bite, indeed there may be an increased reverse overbite, but the incisor and molar teeth are in a prenormal relationship, often with posterior lateral crossbite. The condition is frequently associated with lower incisor retroclination, and there may be a false impression of mid-third recession. The case shown (**308** to **311**) is typical.

310

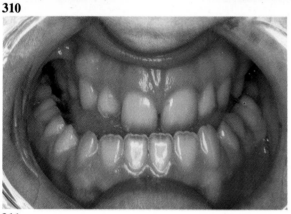

311

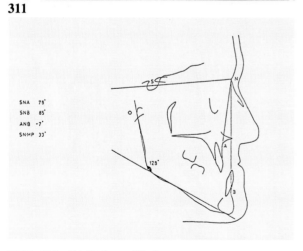

SNA 79°
SNB 85°
ANB -7°
SNMP 33°

308 to 311 Sagittal mandibular excess.

312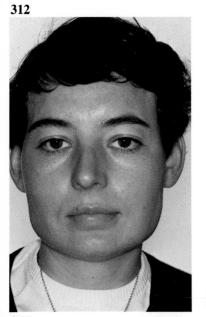

313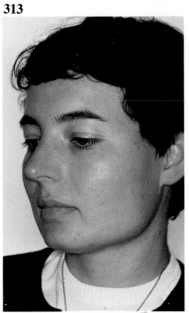

Bilateral masseteric hypertrophy. This is mainly enlargement in the transverse plane across the rami of the mandible. The skeletal abnormality is secondary to enlarged masseter muscles, although the internal pterygoids may also be enlarged.

The gonial angles are acute and there is overdevelopment of the angles of the mandible generally in the area of masseteric insertion (**312** and **313**). This is seen on the lateral or orthopantomographic view (**314**) as a heavy angle, and on the PA view (**132**) as a lateral flare of the bony angles. Clinically the prominence is exaggerated when the teeth are clenched together (**315**) activating the masseters, which can be seen and felt in excessive contraction. There is sometimes painful impairment of function, with headache, tension in the jaws, trismus and muscular pain in the affected region (Beckers, 1977). In many cases the complaint is of cosmetic deficit only.

314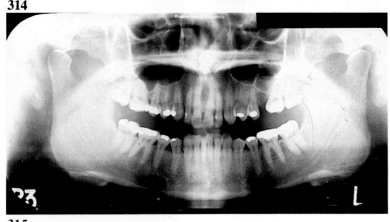

315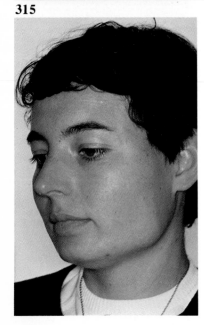

312 to 315   Bilateral masseteric hypertrophy.

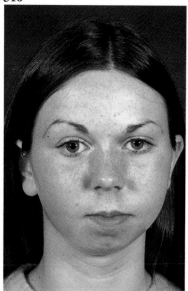

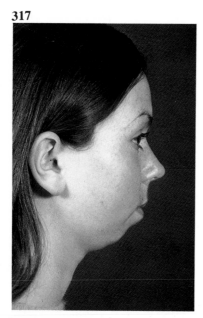

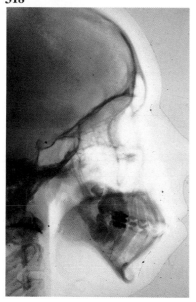

316 to 318   Severe microgenia.

Mandibular (lower-facial) deficiency

Microgenia and retrogenia. In profile, microgenia is simple retrusion of the chin with a normal maxillomandibular skeletal base relationship; like progenia it more usually complicates a prenormal or postnormal skeletal base relationship. Again, it is total chin thickness which matters, and a projection of chin much below 16mm anterior to the line NB projected inferiorly must be regarded as deficient.

The term retrogenia relates to the deficient chin in profile, while the term microgenia properly relates to the total chin area, but clearly both may describe the same patient. In view of the importance of chin to cranial base relationships, it is not surprising to note that definitions of retrogenia vary considerably. Some authorities relate chin position to a vertical line passing through soft-tissue nasion and lying at right angles to the Frankfort horizontal (or its clinical equivalent). Thus Gonzales-Ulloa and Stevens (1968) classify retrogenia on the extent of retraction from this meridian: first degree retrogenia is defined as retraction of less than 10mm, second degree retrogenia from 10mm to 20mm, and third degree retrogenia in excess of 20mm. Other analyses relate to natural head position lateral cephalometry rather than to 'tooth together' positions.

The problem with these classifications is that retrogenia is easily confused with retrognathia, but they do serve to emphasise the importance of relating the chin to the whole profile, and of observing the habitual posture of the particular patient's head. **316, 317** and **318** show a severe microgenic in profile and full face, and the lateral skull view for comparison. Here there is clearly associated mandibular retrusion but the anterior mandibular deficiency can be seen sagittally, transversely and vertically. This case is seen in profile before and after mandibular advancement and double sliding genioplasty in **847** and **848.**

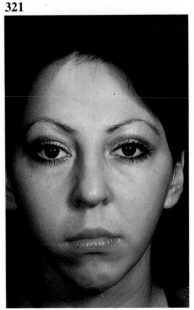

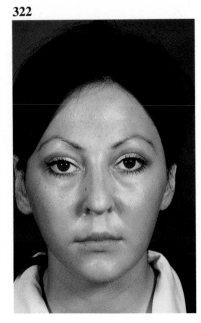

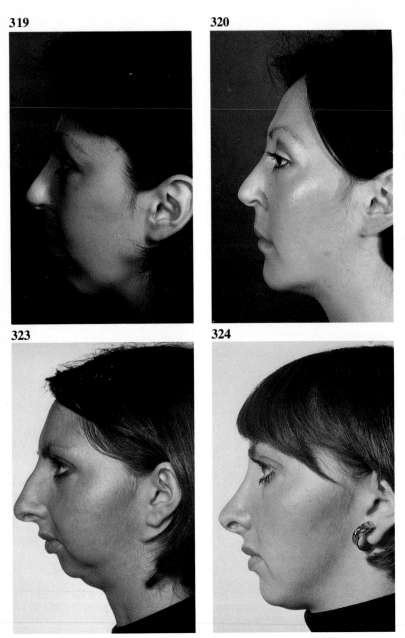

The case in **319** to **322**, shows a lesser degree of retrogenia and microgenia before and after mandibular advancement and horizontal augmentation genioplasty, to bring out the areas of anterior deficiency. Here the lateral or transverse defect has been observed and corrected.

323 shows a common association – nasal distortion with a dorsal hump, combined with mandibular deficiency and microgenia. Correction (**324**) required rhinoplasty (performed by P.K. Davis Esq, MS, FRCS), mandibular advancement and horizontal augmentation genioplasty. Thus the importance of recognising the underdeveloped chin as a separate entity is emphasised. Throughout this book the reader will find other examples. Note the microgenic faces seen in cases of unilateral mandibular deficiency later in this section.

319 to 322 **Retrogenia and microgenia (319** and **321)** corrected by mandibular advancement and horizontal augmentation genioplasty.

323 and 324 **Nasal distortion with a dorsal hump, combined with mandibular deficiency and microgenia,** corrected by rhinoplasty, mandibular advancement and horizontal augmentation genioplasty.

Sagittal mandibular deficiency. Mandibular skeletal hypoplasia presents in a wide range of clinical patterns extending from mild skeletal prenormality within the range of orthodontic improvement, if not total correction, to the extreme 'bird-face' deformities resulting from bilateral condylar hypoplasia or agenesis, **325** to **327** illustrating such a case.

The general features of *mild* mandibular deficiency are shown in **328** to **331**. This is a moderate but typical case of skeletal postnormality showing neither the characteristics of excessive posterior rotational growth (clockwise rotational growth, face directed to the right) nor of excessive anterior rotational growth (counter-clockwise rotation). It is a mean type of deficiency characterised by slight retrusion of the chin, most obvious in profile but not severe enough to distort the overall balance of the face in full face view. Vertical proportion of middle to lower face is normal and the face is neither square nor tapered at the mandibular angles.

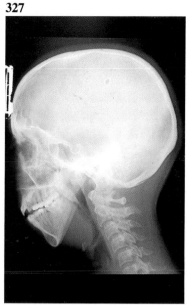

325

326

327

325 to 327   Extreme 'bird-face' deformity.

328 to 331   Mild mandibular deficiency.

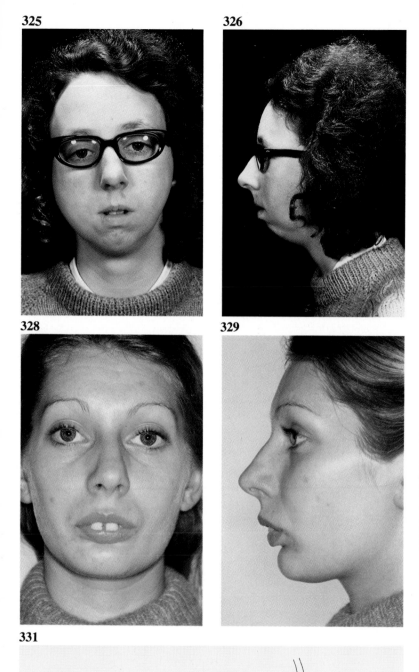

328

329

330

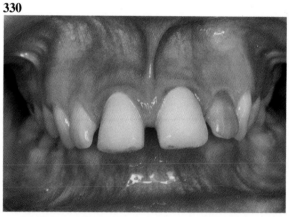

331

The proclination of the upper incisors resulting from the action of the lower lip beneath them has resulted in excessive incisor display with spacing between the centrals and the centrals and the laterals. This is a variable feature, depending not only on the degree of skeletal postnormality but also on the lip morphology and relationship to incisor length. There is a Class 2 division 1 incisor relationship with increased overbite and overjet, and a postnormal molar relationship. The naso-labial angle is normal, but the labiomental curve is increased in this case severely because of the influence of the maxillary incisors.

Cephalometrically this group tends to show good balance between ramus height and body length which may be only slightly small in relation to the other cephalometric figures, and vertical relationships are good. The degree of skeletal dispro-portion in the anteroposterior plane is indicated by the ANB difference, the cranial base is normally sloped or slightly tilted

99

up from sella to nasion in relation to normal angulation. Occlusally there is likely to be an increased curve of Spee, the maxillary arch is often contracted anteriorly with decreased intercanine distance, and there may be a crossbite in the molar regions.

Mandibular deficiency: low angle type

328 to **331** represents only the centre of a range of deficiency problems encountered in the mandible. It is misleading to think of these cases as anteroposterior problems only; more realistically they represent vertical, A-P and transverse growth abnormalities reflected throughout the face. Wolford *et al* (1978) have presented an excellent review of this spectrum of abnormality based on the examination of 1,945 Caucasian cephalograms subjected to critical computer analysis. From their results, amply borne out in clinical experience, it is necessary to consider mandibular deficiency as a spectrum ranging from the low angle type of case to the high angle case. Significant differences in treatment planning arise from the distinction.

332 to **338** show a typical 'low angle' type of mandibular deficiency (**332, 333** and **334**). Growth has occurred more horizontally than vertically, with resultant anterior rotational direction; the cranial base tends to be longer and flatter, with resultant figures for SNA higher than normal, the ANB difference being variable but inevitably with SNB greater for a given difference than in the high angle cases. The gonial angle and the SN:MP angle are both low, with a real tendency to greater ramus height and body length (another manifestation of anterior rotational growth patterns). The lower-facial height is reduced, while upper-facial height is not, and there is always a reduction therefore in total anterior facial height. There is often a deficiency in the subapical mandibular bone extending along the whole length of the body, although this is sometimes more evident anteriorly. Posterior facial height is increased in relation to the other types of mandibular deficiency (**335**). Occlusally (**334**) the arches are U-shaped with an increased overbite and overjet; the curve of Spee is increased. There may be premolar crowding.

332
333

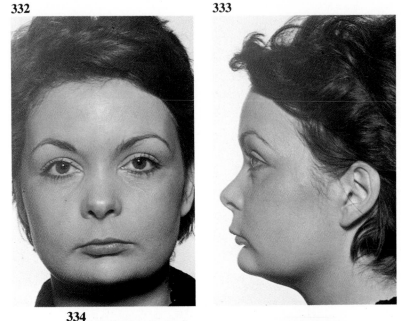

334

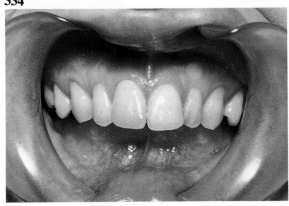

335

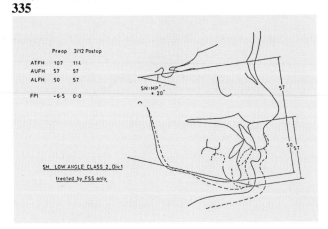

336

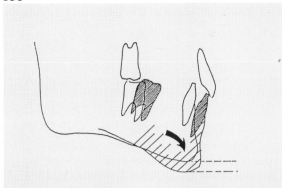

337   **338**

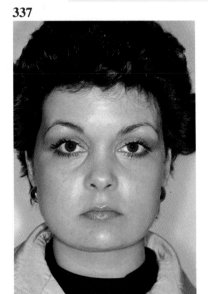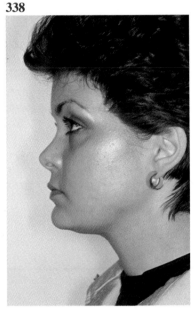

332 to 338 Low angle type of mandibular deficiency
(**332** to **334**) treated by mandibular advancement only
(**337** and **338**).

In full face view (**332**) the face is very square with obvious reduction of height in the lower-third. The upper and mid-face appear normal and well balanced, but the mouth is wide with the lips compressed together. In profile (**333**) the upper and mid-thirds again appear normal with good nasal projection and nasolabial angulation. The labiomental curve is deeply furrowed, the lack of lower anterior height is noted, and the mandibular plane is very flat. It is common for the chin contour to stand well forward to the lip in token of the decrease in subapical bone.

It is always important in this type of case to assess the maxillary height – where there is vertical maxillary deficiency, a large freeway space and mandibular overclosure associated with a low angle mandibular deficiency the case is one variety of 'short face syndrome' (see **374** to **378**). Advancement of the mandible in low angle cases produces the so-called clockwise rotation as a result of incisal guidance and therefore results in an increase in anterior lower-facial height (ALFH) with greater forward movement of the incisor tips than of the pogonion (**336**). This may leave an open bite laterally, which does not close readily by further eruption of the teeth, especially in the over 20s or in the presence of premolar crowding.

In this case (treated by the author some years ago) the increase in ALDH resulting from mandibular advancement (**337** and **338**), while significant, only corrected the preoperative FPI of –6.5 to 0. In other words there remained a 10% disproportion between AUFH and ALFH; this is the result of failing to give proper weight to the deficiency in the subapical mandibular bone height. Correction of this problem is either by total subapical osteotomy with bone grafting (**812** to **815**) or by vertical augmentation genioplasty (illustrated **832** to **838**). Comparison of the case illustrated here postoperatively (**337** and **338**) with the properly treated case (**1078** to **1084**), demonstrates the point at issue.

339

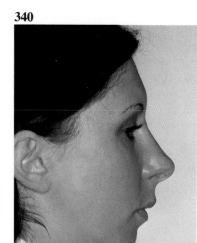

340

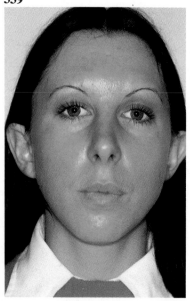

341

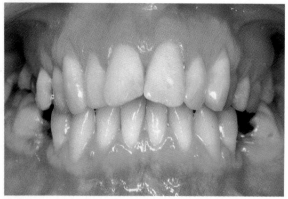

342

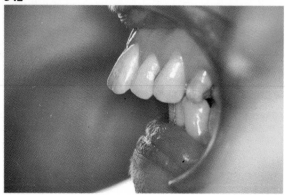

Mandibular deficiency: high angle type

Here growth is more vertical than horizontal, with a resultant posterior direction of rotational growth (clockwise rotation). The cranial base tends to be shorter than the low angle case with a greater slope; the result is to produce relatively low values for SNA and SNB regardless of the ANB difference, which is of course greater than normal in these skeletally postnormal cases. The gonial angle and SN:MP angle are both high with relative shortness of the mandibular ramus and the body. Posterior facial height is therefore short, but to lengthen it surgically would stretch the pterygomasseteric tissues and induce instability. Anterior upper-facial height is usually increased a little, but the lower-facial height is increased also anteriorly, making the face long and narrow with a pointed chin. There is minimal width at the mandibular angles. In keeping with the length of the face the alar flare is reduced and there is a 'pinched' look about the nasolabial region, with increased nasolabial angulation in profile. Chin thickness is usually reduced, and there may be excessive upper incisor display depending on the length of the upper lip and mid-face, and on the degree of overjet. Occlusally there is a Class 2 Div 1 malocclusion with a tendency to maxillary arch contraction and molar crossbite (**339** to **343**).

343

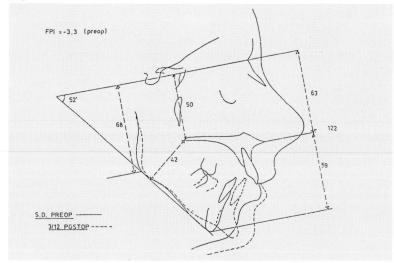

339 to 343 High angle type of mandibular deficiency.

344

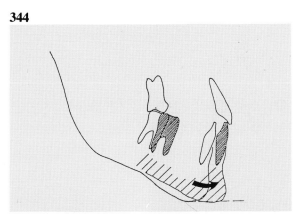

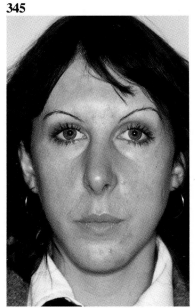 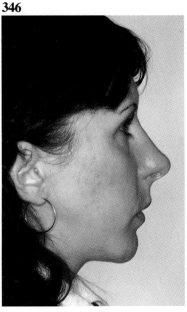

High angle cases may force a compromise on the surgeon. Ramus length cannot be increased and maxillary surgery may be rejected by the patient in the absence of noticeable mid-facial elongation. Counterclockwise surgical rotation (**344**) fortunately does not increase anterior lower-facial height, but advances the pogonion more than the incisor tips (compare with **336**). Despite this the patient usually requires a horizontal augmentation genioplasty, with possible vertical reduction, to correct chin thickness and improve the labiomental curvature.

Logically these cases are a variant of the long face problem (just as the low angle cases are variations of the short face problem), and vertical reduction of maxillary height with autorotation of the mandible combined with advancement is the indicated treatment. The previous case shown (**339** to **343**) was also operated on before these points were fully appreciated, and the compromise is seen in the result (**345** and **346**) following mandibular advancement by bilateral sagittal splitting and advancement genioplasty. The profile is greatly improved but in full face the vertical dysplasia remains in evidence.

Therefore, in summary, mandibular deficiency presents in a range of variation from the low angle case requiring advancement and increase in subapical bony height, with due regard to the possibility of maxillary vertical deficiency; average angle cases where mandibular advancement (with or without anterior maxillary surgery and genioplasty according to profile) is usually sufficient; and high angle cases requiring bimaxillary surgery with genioplasty, or the acceptance of aesthetic compromise in the full face view especially. Low angle cases are the most predictable and stable of these, while high angle cases present some of the least stable of orthognathic corrections.

344   High angle type: counterclockwise surgical rotation.

345 and 346   Case shown in **339** to **343** after mandibular advancement by bilateral sagittal splitting and advancement genioplasty.

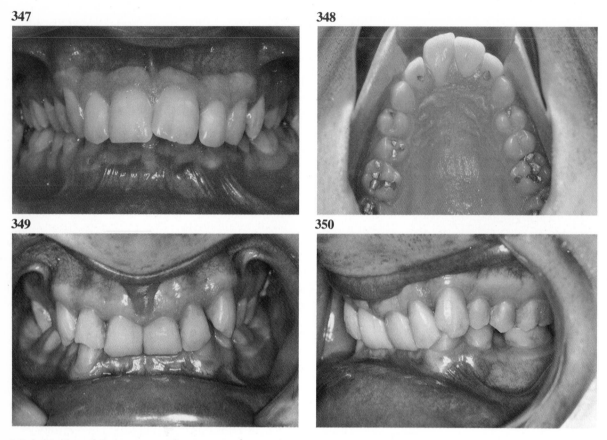

347 **348**

349 **350**

347 to 350 **Severe overbite** in Class 2 Div 1 malocclusions (**347** and **348**) and Class 2 Div 2 malocclusions (**349** and **350**).

Mandibular deficiency: variant patterns

Where the overbite is severe in Class 2 Div 1 malocclusions the lower incisors may bite into the palatal mucosa with significant trauma (**347** and **348**). In Class 2 Div 2 malocclusions this problem may be compounded by similar trauma to the lower labial mucosa from the upper incisors (**349** and **350**), the latter problem occurring most often in low angle mandibular deficiency cases.

Maxillary enlargement

Dentoalveolar protrusion. As in the mandible incisor proclination must be distinguished from alveolar protrusion, which can be assessed clinically and confirmed cephalometrically.

The cranial base is often sloping in cases of sagittal maxillary enlargement and therefore the absolute values for SNA may be very misleading; the extent of premaxillary or alveolar protrusion, as distinct from incisor angulation, is best judged clinically. The incisor, and sometimes the molar, relationships will be postnormal, usually with a Class 2 Div 1 incisor relationship although Div 2 may occur. There is usually an excessive ANB

difference, the nasolabial angle is too acute, and there is relative prominence of the para-alar region despite narrowing of the nose at the alar base (**351** and **352**). In the presence of competent lips the upper incisors may well be retroclined and the lowers proclined in compensation, but with lip incompetence the reverse occurs, as here (**353**). Incisor spacing or midline diastema may be present.

A partly artistic evaluation of the relative contributions of maxillary enlargement and mandibular deficiency to the skeletal base relationship is necessary. The effect of posturing the mandible forwards may be an immediate impression of bimaxillary protrusion, indicative of maxillary enlargement. However, the position is frequently complicated by: (a) Posterior maxillary vertical excess, or (b) Anterior maxillary vertical deficiency, either of which will lead to an upward slope of the palatal plane and possible open bite anteriorly. The former tends to be associated with high angle mandibular deficiency, as does (c) Total vertical maxillary enlargement. These complications make individual analysis of each case essential to distinguish the component parts of the problem.

Two cases are shown, the first (**351** to **354**), exhibits mild upper incisor proclination with midline spacing, tilting of the

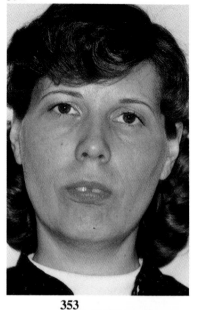
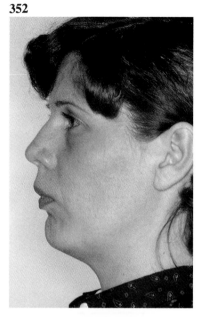

columella, and excessive upper incisor display. Correction by anterior maxillary ostectomy is indicated. The second case (**355** to **357**) is complicated by posterior vertical maxillary enlargement with shortness of the upper lip and secondary high angle mandibular deficiency and anterior open bite. This case requires much more extensive panfacial surgery. It represents a form of maxillary alveolar hyperplasia with vertical increase in the posterior alveolus (measureable cephalometrically), a high palatal vault, and narrowness of the maxillary arch.

This type of open bite case was first documented by Hall and West (1976). Without anterior open bite the effect of maxillary alveolar hyperplasia (MAH) is that of excessive growth of the alveolus in all directions, to a variable extent, with a flatter palate, variable overbite, deeper in Class 2 cases, and correctable by procedures including posterior maxillary ostectomy. This is discussed by West and Epker (1972). The term MAH is probably confusing, and the author prefers to regard these as cases of dentoalveolar maxillary enlargement involving one or all of the primary dimensions (A-P, vertical or transverse).

353

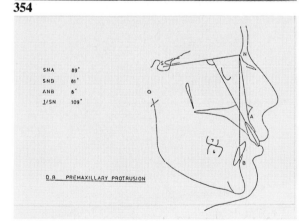

354

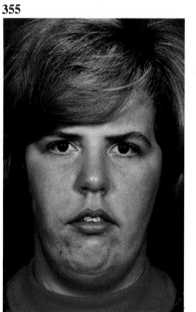
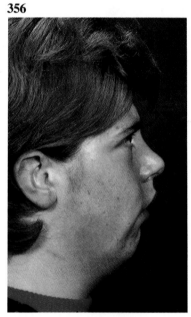

```
SNA     89°
SNB     81°
ANB      8°
1/SN   109°
```

D.A PREMAXILLARY PROTRUSION

351 to 354   Dentoalveolar protrusion showing mild upper incisor proclination with midline spacing, tilting of the columella and excessive upper incisor display.

355 to 357   Dentoalveolar protrusion complicated by posterior vertical maxillary enlargement with shortness of the upper lip and secondary high angle mandibular deficiency and anterior open bite.

355   **356**

357

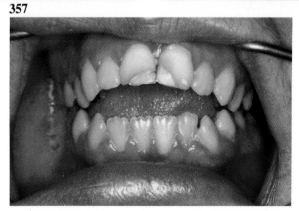

Panmaxillary enlargement

In no area is observation of the anteroposterior, transverse and vertical components of abnormality more important than in the maxillary basal bone. Enlargement in all three directions is usually pathological and may extend onto the alveolar process, as for example in Paget's Disease affecting the maxilla (**358** and **359**).

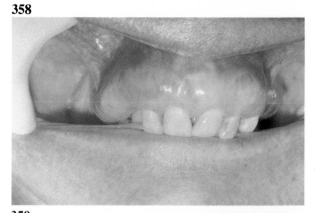

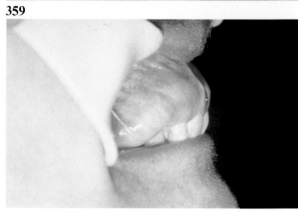

358 and 359 Panmaxillary enlargement caused by Paget's disease.

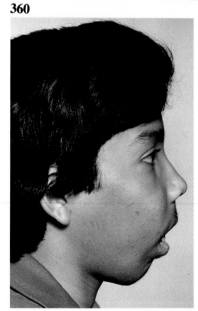

Increased transverse dimensions will carry the dentoalveolar segments away from each other laterally, and there may be spacing of the dentition, but this is rarely of other than occlusal significance, especially when combined with relative transverse mandibular deficiency, which combination may result in the lower dentition occluding entirely within the upper. Antero-posterior enlargement usually presents as dentoalveolar enlargement but on occasion cases are seen where the infraorbital bone is excessively prominent and nasal base projection too great, leading to one form of increased facial convexity (**360**). These cases are rare and cannot be fully corrected by total maxillary set-back with a segment removed from the region anterior to the pterygoid columns; unfortunately this can only be done at the dentoalveolar level and fails to correct the protrusion of the upper anterior face. The latter may be contoured, by removal of bone from the outer surfaces of the maxilla; osteotomy is usually impossible where pathological obliteration or partial obliteration of the maxillary sinuses has occurred.

Such a case is seen in **360** to **364** caused by bone thickening secondary to thalassemia major. Increase in the maxillary 'red marrow' in compensation for erythrocyte shortage accounts for the maxillary hyperplasia during childhood and adolescence, and makes surgical reduction during the growing phase a haemorrhagic procedure. Note the 'hair on end' appearance to the calvarium (**364**).

361

362

363

364

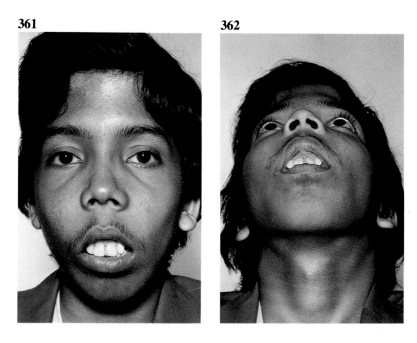

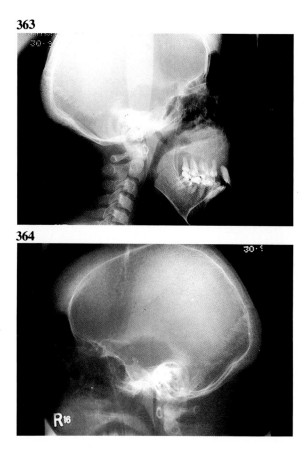

360 to 364 Panmaxillary enlargement in a patient with thalassemia major.

The long maxilla, vertical maxillary excess

The most important, and the most common, group of patients with maxillary enlargement are those presenting with vertical maxillary increase, called VME (vertical maxillary excess) in the USA. Again there is a wide spectrum of abnormality; already in this section we have seen the interaction of abnormalities in the different parts of the facial skeleton.

The so-called long face syndrome includes cases of high angle mandibular deficiency (**339** to **343** and **344** to **346**) and cases of dentoalveolar maxillary enlargement. In recent years the indications for total maxillary shortening have been extensively described by Schendel *et al* (1976), Bell *et al* (1977) and Bell and MacBride (1977). The case illustrated shows the typical features (**365** to **368**). There is increased anterior lower-facial height with or without anterior open bite. The alar flare is narrowed and the nasolabial area recessed. On smiling there is excessive upper incisor display, and the lower third of the face is generally elongated and narrowed. The mouth is reduced in width with thin vermilion exposure, although there may be lip incompetence. The nasolabial recession is more marked in profile, the chin may be retropositioned, or, if relatively prognathic, the labiomental curve will be flattened and displeasing, as in the case illustrated.

Cephalometrically there is an increased SN:MP angle, normal or reduced SNA and variability in the SNB. Always there is vertical maxillary excess, usually greater in the posterior maxilla, with increased anterior lower facial height. The ramus height is increased where there is no anterior open bite. Anterior dentoalveolar height is always increased, and may be reflected in excessive incisor display. Schendel regards the condition as one of increased maxillary height with greater ramus growth in those cases showing no anterior open bite, but normal ramus height in those developing anterior open bite. In both instances correction is limited by the requirement that ramus height cannot be increased surgically without the danger of unstable pterygomasseteric tension.

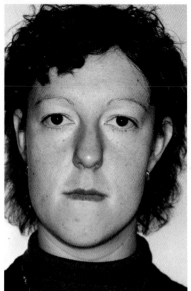

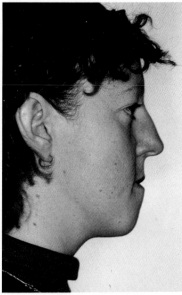

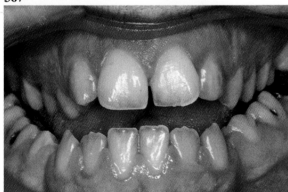

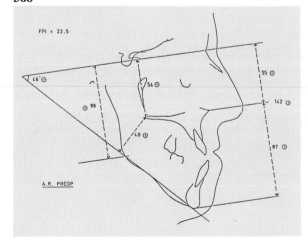

365 to 368 **Vertical maxillary excess** (long face syndrome).

Maxillary deficiency

This denotes inadequate bony development in the mid-third of the face at any level from the upper dentition to the orbits, and is usually taken in the wider context to include all mid-facial deficiency below the cranial level. While not strictly anatomical this has the advantage of including the whole range of mid-third hypoplasias. It is misleading to equate the levels of maxillary deficiency with the Le Fort fracture patterns familiar to the traumatologist; deficient development may affect very variable sites which do not correspond exactly with Le Fort's classification of fractures even though the lines of elective osteotomy have a general similarity to them.

As with the other regions discussed it is necessary to evaluate the vertical, anteroposterior and transverse planes deliberately and systematically. For general case description the maxillary deficiencies may be classified as: (a) Supra-apical maxillary hypoplasia; (b) Nasomaxillary hypoplasia, and (c) Total mid-facial hypoplasia, always allowing that there are many shades of intermediate overlap (369).

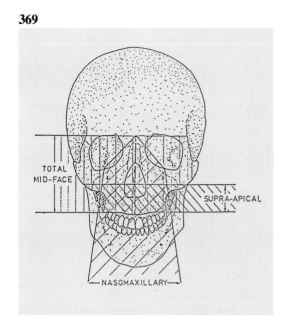

369

369 Maxillary hypoplasias: general areas.

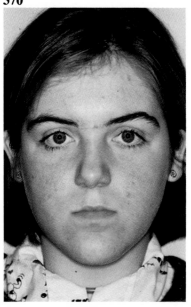

370

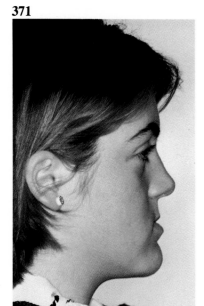

371

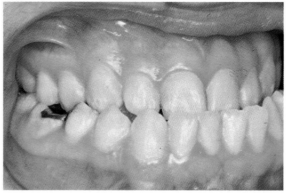

372

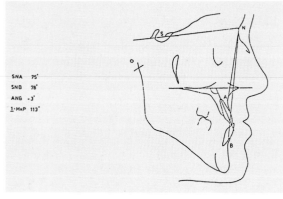

373

SNA 75°
SNB 78°
ANG -3°
1·MxP 113°

370 to 373 Supra-apical maxillary hypoplasia.

Supra-apical maxillary hypoplasia

This term denotes hypoplasia affecting more or less the region of the maxilla lying below a plane passing through the infra-orbital foramina anteriorly and the zygomatic buttresses laterally. It thus includes deficiency in the alar base regions and may be associated with recession of the anterior nasal spine, columella and nasal tip in relation to the rest of the facial skeleton. It is a common cause of maxillomandibular disproportion, and there may also be changes in the mandible.

The leading features are a prenormal occlusion, para-alar recession and sometimes molar crossbite (**370** to **373**). There may be lower incisor retroclination if there is unopposed lower labial pressure, and compensatory upper incisor proclination. A special type of case complicates cleft lip and palate patients with secondary maxillary hypoplasia (see pp. 286 and 287).

In this condition the main problem is anteroposterior and transverse, the latter more in the anterior than the posterior part of the maxilla. A special variant of the condition is vertical maxillary deficiency, described next.

Vertical maxillary deficiency, the short-face syndrome

Bell and his co-workers in Dallas have done much to define the characteristics of the so-called short face syndrome (Bell, 1977; Opdebeeck and Bell, 1978). Clinically (**374** to **377**) the face is broad and square, with reduced anterior facial height, especially when the teeth are in occlusion (**375**), and a low SN:MP angle. The nose is broad at the alar base, the alar flare is increased, the nasolabial angle is decreased, the lips are narrow with a broad oral commissure, and there is a deep reverse overbite. Depending on the degree of anteroposterior hypoplasia of the maxilla there may be an edge-to-edge or class 3 incisor relationship, made worse by mandibular overclosure in occlusion.

374   **375**   **376**

374 to 378   **Vertical maxillary deficiency** (short face syndrome).

377   **378**

The outstanding characteristic of all these cases is the inability of the patient to show the upper teeth because of the vertical shortening of the maxilla behind the lips and nose. There is always an increased freeway space, and the profile may look much more normal in the rest position of the mandible (**376**). In occlusion the mandible is overclosed and therefore appears more protrusive and with a more prominent chin than in fact is the case (**375**). Cephalometrically the reduced ALFH may or may not be associated with a reduced SN:MP angle. Opdebeeck and Bell (1978) found that ramus height is more significant in determining lower-facial height than is the SN:MP angle and they distinguish two groups of

patients. In the first group the FPI is little less than 10, the ramus height is increased markedly, and the SN:MP angle very low (one form of 'low angle' mandibular deficiency). Posterior dental height is increased or normal.

In the second group the FPI is very reduced (as here, **378**) the ramus is short (here it is long, although posterior total facial height is reduced a little), the SN:MP angle is normal or a little reduced (here a little low) but there is marked reduction in posterior dental height (reduced in this case). In the author's view the distinction between 'long ramus' and 'short ramus' cases is valid, but the maxillary features are very variable. In the presence of inadequate incisor display and an increased freeway space, maxillary elongation is the correct treatment.

379

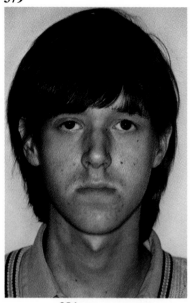

380

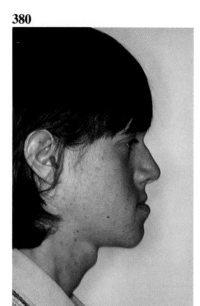

381

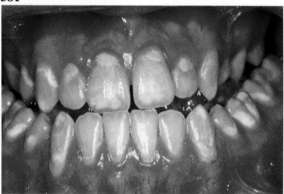

382

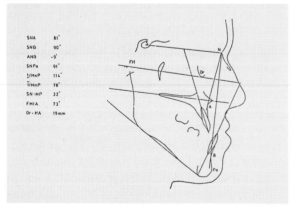

SNA	81°
SNB	90°
ANB	-9°
SNPo	91°
1/MxP	114°
ī/MnP	78°
SN·MP	32°
FMIA	73°
Or - NA	19mm

379 to 382   **Nasomaxillary hypoplasia** involving the dentoalveolar segment.

Nasomaxillary Hypoplasia

This condition has been described by Converse *et al* (1970) as 'foreshortening and hypoplasia of the nose and adjacent maxillary area', and these authors discuss the aetiology. A fuller discussion is given by Henderson (1980), and Henderson and Jackson (1973) classified the affected patients into four groups, which are illustrated in the following four cases.

Nasomaxillary hypoplasia: Group 1, Involving the dentoalveolar segment

This condition is characterised by recession of the nasal base producing a short nose, upturned or recessed at the tip (cf **379** to **382** with **112** to **115** which shows a more severe example of the same condition, having more serious nasal underdevelopment). The whole nasal skeleton is insufficiently projected forwards. The columella is usually short. There is hypoplasia of the medial (or medial and central) infraorbital rim and adjacent bone, leading to increased inferior scleral exposure. The dental occlusion is prenormal because of underdevelopment of the skeletal base. Cephalometrically the maxilla is retruded with relatively low values for SNA and negative facial convexity. The orbitale lies too far behind the NA line (in excess of 16mm, see Figure **246**). The maxillary plane may slope upwards anteriorly. The labial alveolar plate is likely to be thinned over the incisor roots, and the anterior nasal spine may be deficient. Anterior maxillary height is reduced, and this sometimes extends posteriorly, complicating the picture by vertical maxillary deficiency.

112

383

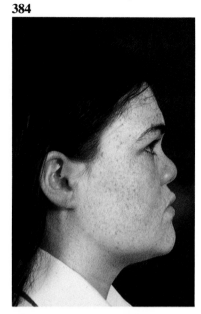

384

Nasomaxillary hypoplasia: Group 2, excluding the dentoalveolar segment (Binder's syndrome see Binder, 1962)

This is very similar to Group 1 except that the dentoalveolar segment is relatively normally related to the cranial base anteroposteriorly, but it is involved in anterior maxillary vertical deficiency. The maxillary plane is even more likely to be tilted upwards and the foreshortened nose sits on a deficient nasomaxillary base. The cranial base is often short and there may be marked cranial base sloping.

These two groups represent different degrees of a basically similar condition, but the relatively normal AP dental relationship makes management difficult in Group 2. Both require Le Fort 2 maxillary advancement to control and stabilise the forward correction of the nasal area, but in Group 2 it will be necessary subsequently to set back the dentoalveolar segment to its original position, usually some 6 to 9 months after the major maxillary correction when consolidation has occurred.

385

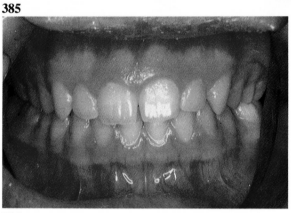

386

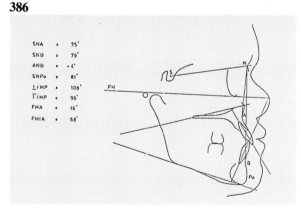

SNA	=	75°
SNB	=	79°
ANB	=	-4°
SNPo	=	81°
1/MP	=	108°
1̄/MP	=	96°
FMA	=	16°
FMIA	=	68°

383 to 386   Nasomaxillary hypoplasia not involving the dentoalveolar segment (Binder's syndrome).

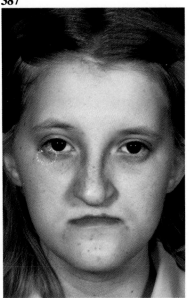

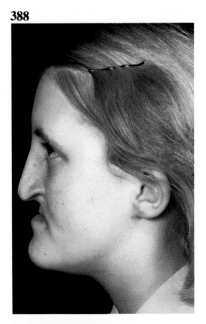

Nasomaxillary hypoplasia: Group 3, Cleft palate syndrome

Among secondary cleft palate deformities, particularly those which have undergone extensive maxillary and palatal surgery in infancy, there is a significant number of cases exhibiting underdevelopment of the maxilla up to and including the nasomaxillary and medial orbital areas. This is an important group and yields the commonest indication for Le Fort 2 maxillary advancement. The case shown in **387** to **390** is typical, showing, in addition to the dentoalveolar collapse and clefting, recession of the nasal base and hypoplasia of the adjacent maxillary area. The nose is often well developed, but may be small and will show the full range of characteristic nasal deformities of the secondary cleft palate nose. The features are shown, and the problem will be taken up again in the discussion of cleft palate syndrome cases (pp. 298 to 302). Vertical maxillary deficiency is an almost constant feature of all cleft palate cases.

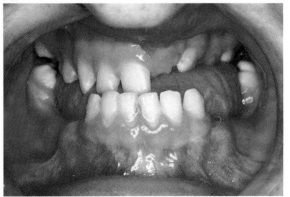

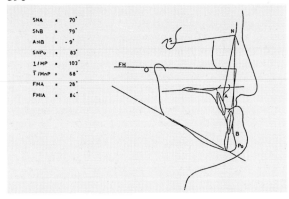

387 to 390   **Nasomaxillary hypoplasia** complicating cleft palate.

Nasomaxillary hypoplasia: Group 4, Panfacial problems

Nasomaxillary hypoplasia, like all maxillary deformities, may complicate other facial dysharmonies, but there is common involvement of this area in two situations worth noting separately. The first is illustrated here and has been seen a number of times, although it is difficult to recognise a common aetiology. Mandibular asymmetry in association with nasomaxillary hypoplasia shows mild asymmetric mandibular enlargement magnified by the maxillary defect. The case shown in **391** to **395** illustrates rather more lateral infraorbital involvement than the other cases shown, although this may occur throughout the groups and is indicative of the need for wider correction along the lateral infraorbital rim. The other association is with mild symmetrical mandibular enlargement, giving rise to a forward slope of the face, the sloping face syndrome (Henderson and Jackson, 1973) (**396** and **397**).

391 **392** **393**

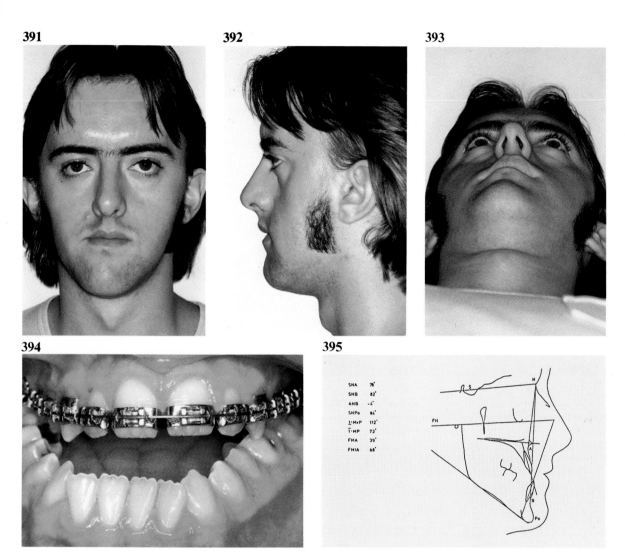

391 to 395 Nasomaxillary hypoplasia complicating mandibular asymmetry.

394 **395**

SNA	78°
SNB	82°
ANB	-4°
SNPo	84°
1·MxP	112°
1·MP	73°
FMA	39°
FMIA	68°

396

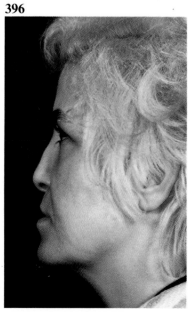

397

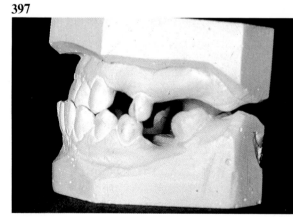

396 and 397 Nasomaxillary hypoplasia in association with mild mandibular enlargement (sloping face syndrome).

115

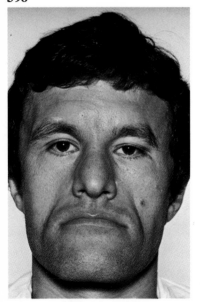

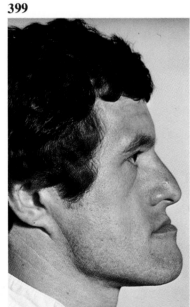

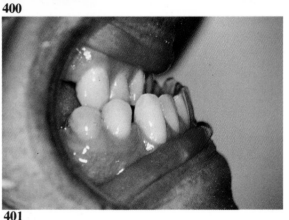

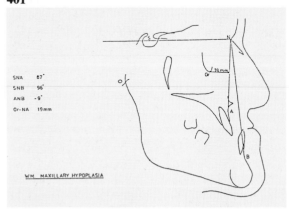

SNA	87°
SNB	96°
ANB	-9°
Or-NA	19mm

WM MAXILLARY HYPOPLASIA

398 to 401 **Lateral maxillary deficiency** with strong nasal projection.

Lateral maxillary deficiency

There is an intermediate group of cases exhibiting mid-facial deficiency which includes the dentoalveolar segment (antero-posteriorly and transversely, sometimes vertically) and the medial and lateral infraorbital regions extending onto the malar prominences, but sparing the nasal base. These cases (**398** to **401**) show strong nasal projection, and are best treated by the Küfner procedure (Küfner, 1971) (p. 256) or by Le Fort 1 advancement supplemented by infraorbital and malar proplast augmentation.

Total mid-facial hypoplasia

Maxillary deficiency affecting the whole mid-face, including the orbital walls and zygomatic regions may occur without cranial malformations, but the commonest presentation involves one of the craniostenotic syndromes. This leads into an area beyond the scope of this volume, as the whole assessment, diagnosis and management of these cases has developed into a complete and rapidly advancing subject, that of craniofacial surgery. There are, however, areas of overlap with orthognathic surgery in the management of the mid-face deficiencies and this area is covered here and in Section 4. It cannot be too strongly emphasised that a trained team is necessary for both the evaluation and treatment of most of these cases.

A case of post-traumatic mid-face retrusion with elongation of the face and transformation of the orbits into ellipsoid cavities of increased volume is shown in **402** and **403**. Such a case is indicative of the need for subcranial correction at the Le Fort 3 level. Many facial deformities of congenital origin raise the question of Le Fort 3 correction, usually on account of malar hypoplasia. It should be remembered that the operative morbidity of Le Fort 3 surgery is much greater than that of Le Fort 2 or 1 surgery.

The case shown in **404** to **406** was referred with a secondary cleft palate deformity and treatment planning led to the suggestion that here Le Fort 3 correction was necessary to restore lateral orbital support and malar projection. This was the author's advice to the patient who refused any surgery involving the orbits. Correction at the Le Fort 1 level was therefore combined with lower labial set-back to improve labiomental contour (**407** to **409**, before occlusal rehabilitation). The result is interesting and illustrates how little residual defect remains, although the lack of infraorbital and malar contour is obvious. The patient is well pleased and it is arguable that an acceptable result with minimal risk would have been obtainable by Le Fort 2 advancement, perhaps with lateral extension or proplast malar augmentation. On the whole the Le Fort 3 operation is best reserved for craniostenotic problems and some post-traumatic cases, but exceptions occasionally arise.

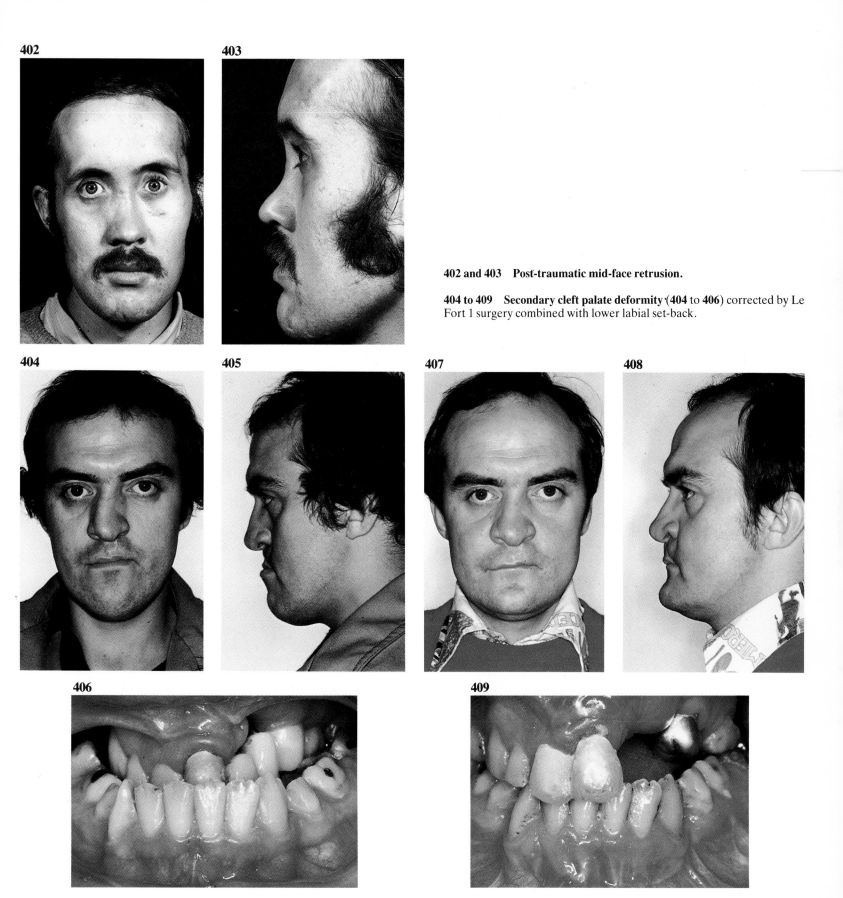

402 and 403   Post-traumatic mid-face retrusion.

404 to 409   Secondary cleft palate deformity (**404** to **406**) corrected by Le Fort 1 surgery combined with lower labial set-back.

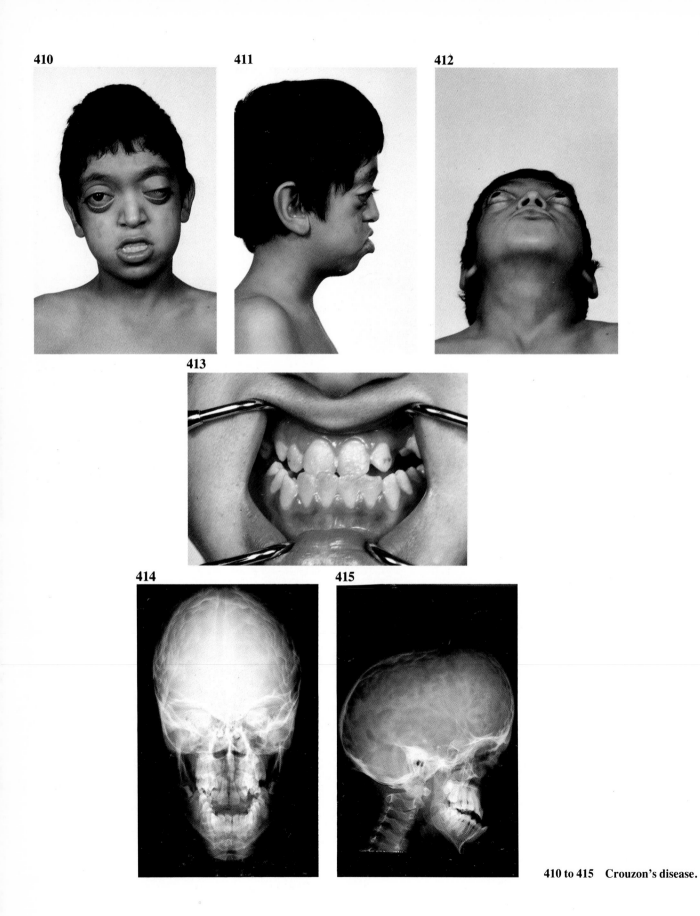

410 to 415 Crouzon's disease.

118

Crouzon's disease

In this craniostenotic syndrome the maxillary deficiency involves the whole maxilla and the orbital and zygomatic areas share in the underdevelopment. Typically, as here, the cranial base is sloping to an extreme degree, with backward facing displacement of the cranial base. There is severe maxillary underdevelopment with gross shortage of bone in the antero-posterior dimension at the dentoalveolar level. Commonly the maxillary incisors are proclined in dental compensation. Even if these are aligned orthodontically, correction of the whole mid-face by advancement in one block from orbit to dentition may still be insufficient to restore orbital depth. In these circumstances a combination of Le Fort 1 and Le Fort 3 procedures allows differential repositioning of the upper and lower components. Where there is reasonably good vertical growth in the maxilla anteriorly, this can be accomplished in one stage, but where there is a loss of vertical height a second stage Le Fort 1 with vertical augmentation correcting the overadvancement of the dentition at the Le Fort 3 stage is the most satisfactory procedure.

Other features of Crouzon's disease are seen here (**410** to **415**) (the pathogenesis has been discussed in Section 1). Coronal synostosis gives the characteristic appearance to the forehead and cranial vault, although the forehead is not projected from the cranium during growth, and in many cases will require augmentation or frontal bone advancement, via a transcranial approach. The orbits are very shallow antero-posteriorly with marked exophthalmos (see also **244** and **245**).

The maxillary retrusion is gross, evidenced by lack of lateral and inferior orbital support, recession of the nasal base and nasal profile (especially at the bridge), marked para-alar hollowing, and often an acute nasolabial angle (as here) caused by the combined effect of incisor proclination and maxillary retrusion. Growth appears to be anteriorly rotational, with the mandible relatively prognathic and sometimes really so; narrowness of the ramus may compensate for this to some extent. Vertically the anterior upper-facial height tends to be reduced and the posterior increased, but the severe cranial base slope makes a nonsense of using normal cephalometric values for comparison. In fact the cephalogram is of little use in planning correction of these cases, although serial cephalometry during growth yields valuable information.

Occlusally the maxillary dentition is often crowded and contracted and oral hygiene may be a problem with these children unless careful instruction in the prevention of dental disease is given during the formative years. Prolonged orthodontic treatment is frequently required, and presents a greater problem than usual as these cases tend to be sent long distances for surgical management, away from easy orthodontic liaison. Ocular hypertelorism, with or without orbital dystopia also complicates many cases, although on occasion hypotelorism occurs. A wide range of variation is observed and the reader is referred to texts of craniofacial surgery for details of cranial assessment (vital in all cases, even those apparently requiring only mid-facial advancement at the sub-cranial Le Fort 3 level).

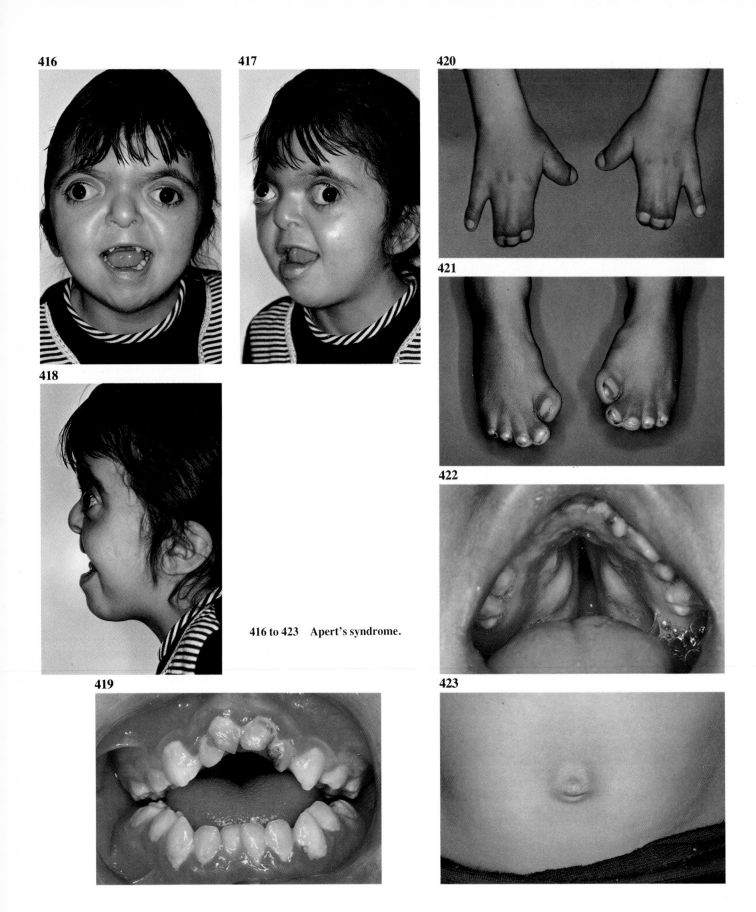

416 to 423   Apert's syndrome.

Apert's syndrome

The features of this syndrome are very similar facially and cranially (**416** to **418**) although there is a much greater tendency to anterior open bite (**419**) because of anterior maxillary vertical deficiency. The syndrome is recognised by associated congenital anomalies, especially syndactyly in the hands (**420**), feet (**421**), and palatal arching, often with clefting of the palate (**422**). This patient also shows exomphalos (**423**). Many other complex combinations of abnormality occur and the reader is referred to standard texts of facial syndromology (Gorlin and Pindborg, 1964; Goodman and Gorlin, 1977) for detailed descriptions.

Asymmetrical disproportion of the jaws

This defies logical classification. It may be based on morphology (eg mid-third, orbital, lower-third) or on aetiology (eg developmental, acquired, etc). All attempts to harmonise the variations in one classification fail, and the pattern of description will be based on the simple morphological distribution described on page 19. An expanded version of this is of value, and in the following morphological classification the congenital and developmental groups are in italics. Most groups may produce secondary changes.

A. Lower facial enlargement

1. *Asymmetrical mandibular enlargement*
   With anterior open bite
   Without anterior open bite

2. *Unilateral condylar hyperplasia*

3. *Unilateral mandibular hemihypertrophy*
   (Cases intermediate between 2 and 3 are described)

4. New growth. Tumours and dysplasias which include both hard and soft tissues. These may involve the mid-face and upper-face also. Osteomata, osteochondromata (especially of the condyle), lymphangiomata, plexiform neurofibromata, etc.

5. *Asymmetrical masseteric hypertrophy*

6. *Hemifacial, and hemibody hypertrophies (very rare)*

B. Lower facial deficiencies

1. Acquired unilateral mandibular hypoplasia
   Traumatic, infective and inflammatory, irradiation
   May produce ankylosis

2. *Congenital unilateral mandibular hypoplasia*
   Condylar aplasia

   Condylar hypoplasia
   Facial microsomia (may be bilateral, but never symmetrically)
   (metabolic, ? congenital, ? acquired)

3. *Hemifacial, and hemibody hypoplasia (very rare)*

C. Mid-third asymmetries

1. *Cleft lip and cleft palate syndromes*

2. Localised maxillary pathology – irradiation, fibrous dysplasia, lymphangiomata, plexiform neurofibroma, etc. May involve lower- and upper-face also. Some may be congenital.

3. Secondary maxillary asymmetries – usually secondary to mandibular anomalies during growth. *Congenital, developmental* or acquired.

4. Hemifacial atrophy (Romberg's syndrome). Aetiology uncertain.

5. *Hemifacial hypoplasia, or hemifacial hypertrophy (rare)*

D. Upper facial asymmetry

1. *Cranial asymmetries*, plagiocephaly, etc.

2. Acquired cranial asymmetries, as fibrous dysplasia, etc.

3. *Orbital dystopias*

E. Facial clefts

Tessier clefts 1, 2, 3, 4, 5, 9, 10, 11, 12 and 13 (see Tessier, 1979).

Asymmetrical lower facial enlargement

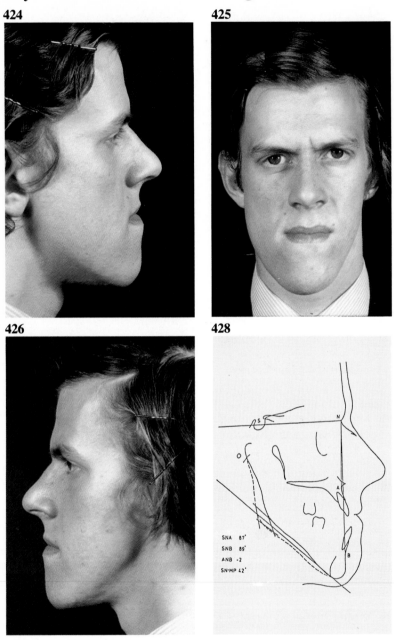

424 to 428 Asymmetrical mandibular protrusion with anterior open bite.

Asymmetrical mandibular protrusion with anterior open bite

The case shown in **424** to **428** is typical. While argument proceeds as to whether this type of case is an eccentric bilateral mandibular protrusion because of bilateral condylar hyperplasia of unequal drive, the presentation is of mandibular protrusion with deviation of the chin to one side, high SN:MP angulation and anterior open bite. It is an asymmetrical form of long face, and correction demands attention to the several areas of abnormality, both mandibular and maxillary, in the anteroposterior and vertical dimensions principally.

Asymmetrical mandibular protrusion without anterior open bite

Again this type of case may represent unequal condylar excess, but there is clear evidence of mandibular protrusion, chin deviation and Class 3 incisor and molar relationships. However, in the case shown in **429** to **432** there is no anterior open bite although there may be mild supra-apical maxillary hypoplasia.

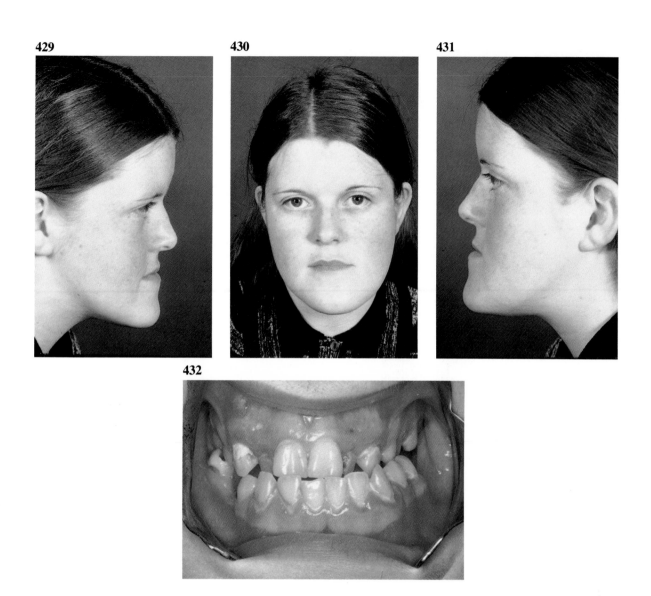

429 to 432 Asymmetrical mandibular protrusion
without anterior open bite.

433

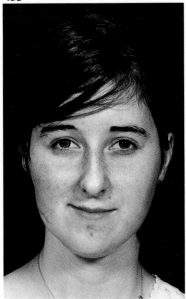

434

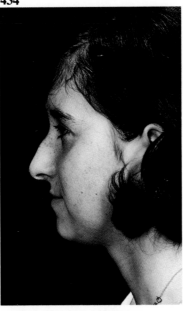

Unilateral condylar hyperplasia (433 to 436)

In this condition there is elongation of the affected condylar neck and subcondylar region generally, with deviation of the chin towards the normal side. There may be mild mandibular protrusion, but this is rarely very noticeable. The lip line slopes down towards the affected side. On the unaffected side there may be a lateral crossbite, and sometimes the occlusal plane slopes upwards to this side, reflecting (as does the lip line) secondary over-eruption of the maxillary teeth on the affected side to maintain occlusal contact.

In severe cases a lateral open bite occasionally develops on the affected side. The displacement of the lower midline is greater at the lower border, or anatomical mid-chin, than at the incisor midline, so that the incisor apices are carried to the non-affected side more than the crowns, giving an appearance of apical drift in a stream of basal bone growth. The condition usually presents in early adolescence with increasing deformity until growth of the mandible is complete, usually by the end of the second decade. These appearances are most easily seen in PA views of the mandible (**436**), although orthopantomography may help to compare the length of the condylar necks.

435

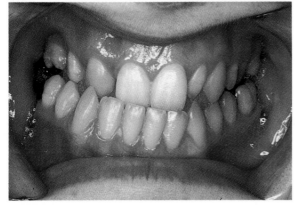

436

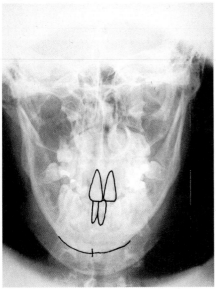

433 to 436   Unilateral condylar hyperplasia.

437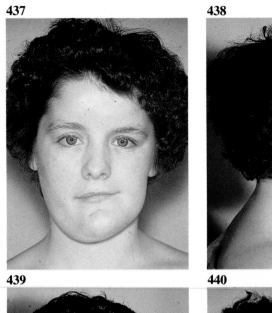

438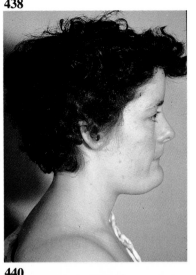

Mandibular hemihypertrophy (437 to 443)

In this condition one side of the face appears enlarged with the lower border lying at a lower level on the affected side, showing marked convexity, or bowing, when viewed laterally. There is little or no displacement of the chin, although the form of the soft tissues of the chin may appear slightly distorted towards the unaffected side. The lip line slopes downwards to the affected side. The incisor midline is not deflected to the abnormal side in most cases and there is often an open bite on the affected side laterally. The maxillary cheek teeth tend to over-erupt to attempt closure of this lateral open bite with resultant downward slope of the maxillary plane towards the abnormal side and increased vertical maxillary height unilaterally. Radiographically there is enlargement of the whole mandible, condyle, ramus and body, on the affected side, with displacement of the inferior alveolar canal towards the lower border.

439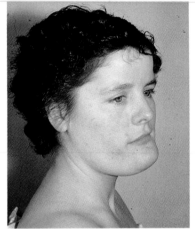

440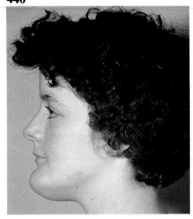

441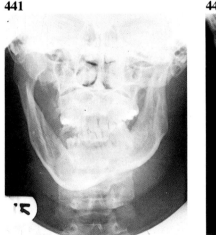

442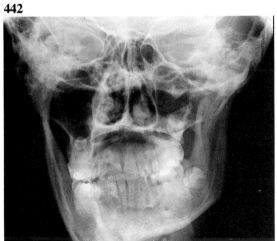

443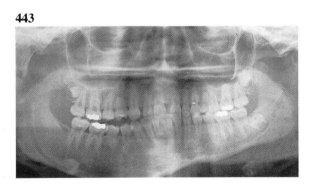

437 to 443 Mandibular hemihypertrophy (442 and 443 show a separate case – see also p. 318).

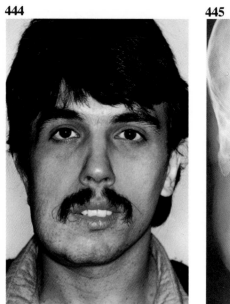

444

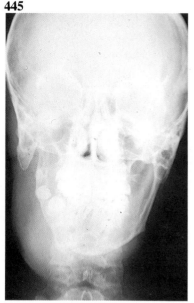

445

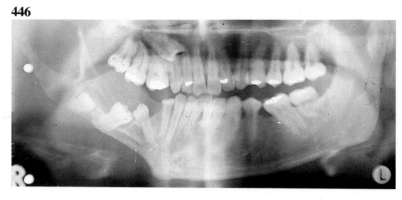

446

444 to 446 **Plexiform neurofibroma** involving the lower half of the right side of the face.

447 to 455 **Plexiform neurofibroma** with extensive involvement of the soft tissues of the right side of the face.

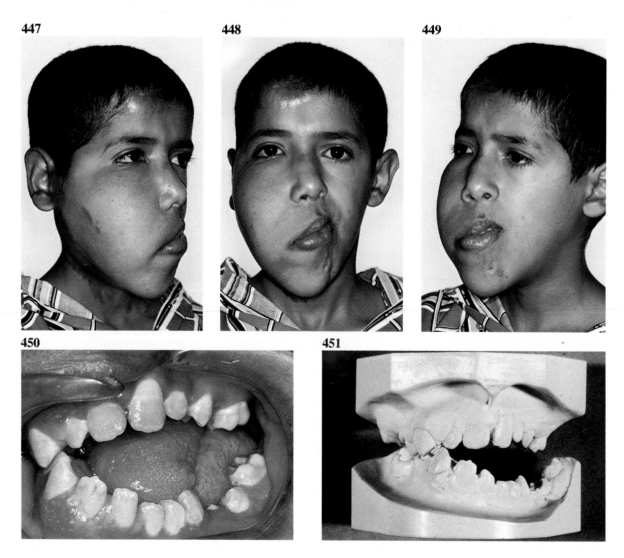

447

448

449

450

451

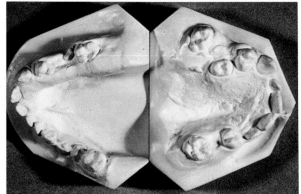

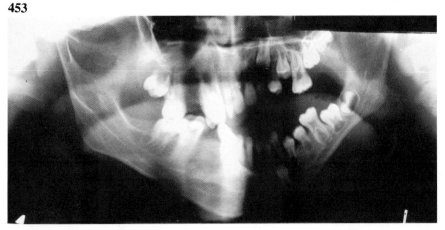

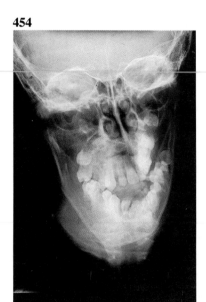

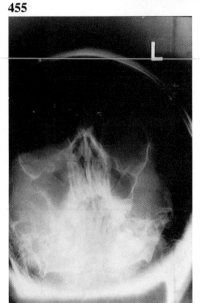

Pathological causes of lower facial asymmetry

Lower-facial asymmetry caused by *new growth, bone dysplasia, or similar pathological processes* presents in a wide variety of ways, but it is worth remembering that several of these conditions develop slowly over a long period and present confusing pictures of deformity unless recognised for what they are. Some affect the middle and upper facial tissues also, either separately or together.

Two examples of plexiform neurofibroma are illustrated here, the first (**444** to **446**) confined to the lower-third of the face while the second (**447** to **455**) affects the whole of the face producing a false impression of congenital hemihypertrophy (note however that the teeth are not enlarged in neurofibroma).

Von Recklinghausen's neurofibromatosis is a developmental abnormality inherited as an autosomal dominant. It is characterised by multiple subcutaneous neurofibromata, *café au lait* cutaneous pigmentation, and sometimes mental retardation and epilepsy. The condition starts in infancy, is progressive,

and facially may affect the trigeminal and facial nerves leading to a dense intertwining mass of neurofibromatous tissue with secondary maxillary and mandibular deformity. An incidence of between 1:2000 to 1:3000 of the population is quoted, and some 4% to 7% of cases involve the orofacial tissues (Pindborg and Hjørting-Hansen, 1974). Some one-third of cases also have skeletal involvement (Heard, 1962). A useful discussion of the maxillofacial changes is given by Müller and Slootweg (1981) who discuss the possible mechanisms of skeletal involvement, which may be resorptive or hyperplastic.

The first case shown (**444** to **446**) illustrates an expansive plexiform neurofibroma involving the lower half of the right side of the face, especially the submandibular region. There is associated rightsided mandibular hypoplasia with deepening of the sigmoid notch, condylar hypoplasia and elongation of both condylar neck and coronoid process. Dental eruption is inhibited on the affected side of the mandible (**446**). There is associated *café au lait* pigmentation of the skin and one tibia shows gross overgrowth. Müller and Slootweg ascribe sigmoid notch deepening to pressure atrophy secondary to localised neurofibroma of the inferior alveolar nerve, histologically proven in two of their cases.

The second case (**447** to **455**) shows much more extensive involvement of the soft tissues of the right side of the face including the parotid and submandibular regions, with extensive infiltration of the tissues of the lips and malar regions. The right side of the tongue and palate are affected (**450, 452**) with vertical maxillary hyperplasia on the same side and an anterior and lateral open bite to the left side (**451, 452**). There is some maxillary and mandibular enlargement on the right and also hypoplasia of the left mandible with some evidence of sigmoid notch atrophy (**453**). The latter may be again caused by localised involvement of the inferior dental nerve, but the general leftsided mandibular hypoplasia may be a result of lateral displacement of the enlarged tongue during development. The ear is set low and flat against the skull (**448**), a characteristic deformity, with vertical enlargement. The complex asymmetry which results from these anomalies requires extensive panfacial reconstruction combining skeletal and soft tissue correction.

456

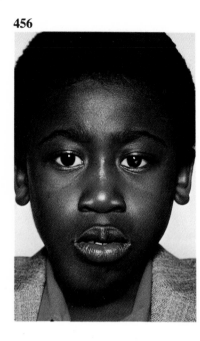

457

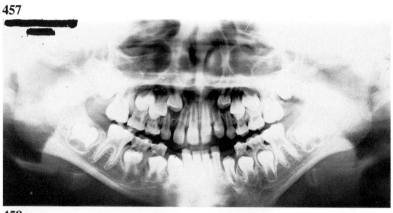

458

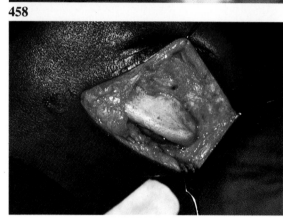

456 to 458   **Mandibular hypertrophy** associated with a haemolymphangioma in the overlying soft tissues.

459 to 462   **Fibrous dysplasia** causing asymmetrical enlargement of the mandible with involvement of the malar region and orbital displacement.

463 to 468   **Osteochondroma – two cases.**

461

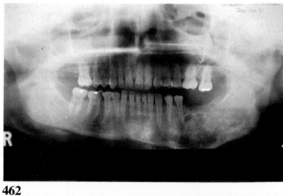

459

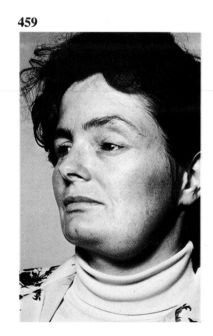

460

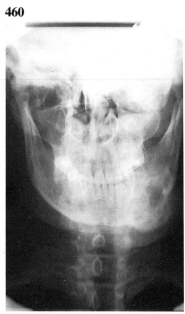

462

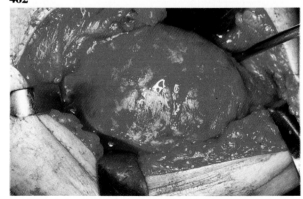

463

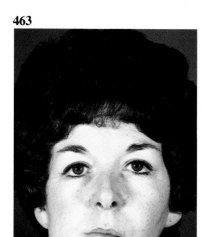

466

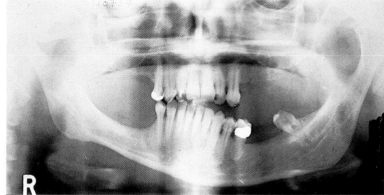

467

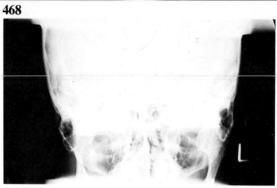

468

464

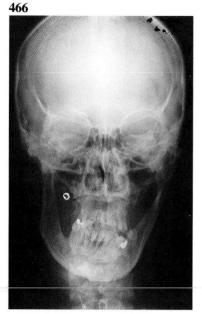

465

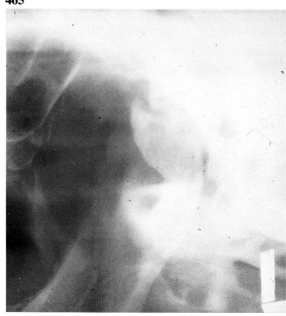

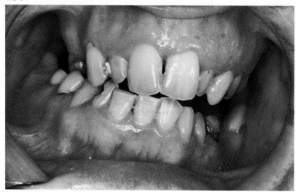

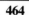

There is some evidence that increased vascularity will stimulate local hyperplasia of bone, several conditions occurring during the growing period and associated with locally enhanced blood flow being related to adjacent areas of bony excess not otherwise involved in the primary pathology.

The boy shown in **456** to **458** has a localised area of mandibular hypertrophy to the right of the mandibular symphysis in direct relationship to a longstanding haemolymphangioma in the overlying soft tissues (previously resected). The area is seen at operation (**458**) and is difficult to explain on any other basis.

Fibrous dysplasia is one cause of slowly progressive, painless, asymmetrical enlargement of the mandible (**459** to **462**). This usually requires serial recontouring during the active phase or there will be secondary distortions which prove more difficult to correct. Diagnosis is usually clear from the history and radiographic appearance, together with normal blood chemistry and positive biopsy confirmation. This case also involves the malar region with orbital displacement.

Osteochondroma or osteoma of the mandibular condyle produces a picture at first easily confused with condylar hyperplasia (**463, 464**). The mandible deviates with development of lateral open bite on the affected side and the diagnosis is apparent when the enlarged condyle is seen radiographically (**465**). Condylectomy not only restores symmetry (see **1264** to **1270**) but allows histological examination of the tumour mass. Presentation tends to occur at a later stage of life than with condylar hyperplasia or hemihypertrophy.

Further radiographic views of this condition are shown in **466** to **468**, although the case is different.

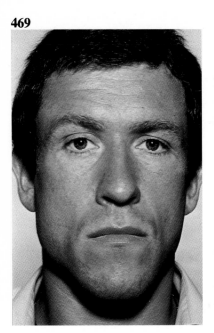

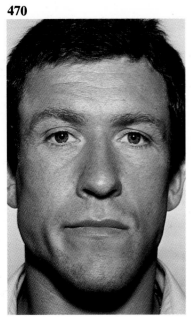

469 to 470   Asymmetrical masseteric hypertrophy.

Asymmetrical masseteric hypertrophy (469 and 470)

This condition is identical to the bilateral variety (**312** to **315**) except that one side is much more developed than the other. The masseter becomes much more prominent on clenching the teeth (**470**) and the mandibular changes are similar to those in bilateral masseteric hypertrophy, with enlargement of the mandibular angle and lateral flaring. Both sides are usually more prominent than normal and the condition, while asymmetric, is nearly always bilateral.

Asymmetrical lower-facial deficiency

This requires the surgeon to distinguish between cases of acquired and congenital or developmental origin. The major problems of treatment planning depend on the degree of abnormality in the investing soft tissues, largely although not exclusively related to the aetiology. The reader is referred to Section 1 for a discussion of the pathogenesis of the facial microsomias, which form a significant proportion of the patients in this group although exhibiting the wide variation of involvement which might be expected from the causal mechanism postulated by Poswillo (1973).

The extent of involvement of the various tissues (bone and periosteum, muscle, skin and fascia) which together determine the functional matrix within which growth occurs is a prime objective of assessment. In some cases of acquired origin, for example after severe facial burns or ablative surgery with or without radiotherapy in infancy, the soft tissues may well be significantly deficient, affecting both growth and the timing of surgical correction. For the most part it is the congenital and developmental conditions, especially the microsomias, which present with soft tissue deficiencies. An excellent review of the literature to 1975 is given by Towers (1975).

Acquired unilateral mandibular deficiency

Deficient development of the mandible may follow early trauma, infection, or pressure from contiguous soft tissue tumours (see also **444** to **455**). Intracapsular fractures of the mandibular condyle, especially crush fractures, may lead to ankylosis with failure of growth, or to simple growth retardation. Infection may spread from dental crypt infections, osteomyelitis of the ramus or middle-ear infections; blood-borne organisms settling in the joint are much rarer.

471 to **476** illustrate a typical case of unilateral mandibular hypoplasia caused by infection during the first decade of life (thought to be at 7 or 8 years of age). Osteomyelitis of the right ramus led to sequestration and surgical sequestrectomy, and the subsequent failure of mandibular growth illustrates the three dimensional distortion of the facial skeleton. The chin is deviated to the affected side with a small and distorted ramus, abnormal condylar shape, and mild mandibular retrusion in profile, the chin being more retruded than the alveolar region. The normal tongue and labiobuccal musculature encourages a much more normal occlusion than would be expected from the basal bone distortion, resulting in much greater distortion at the lower border than at the occlusal level (**474** and **476**). The 'twist' thus induced results in a flattening of the contralateral side, sometimes misleading the observer into thinking that the problem is overdevelopment of that side. Secondary maxillary vertical hypoplasia on the affected side will sometimes incline the occlusal plane upwards towards the affected side.

471 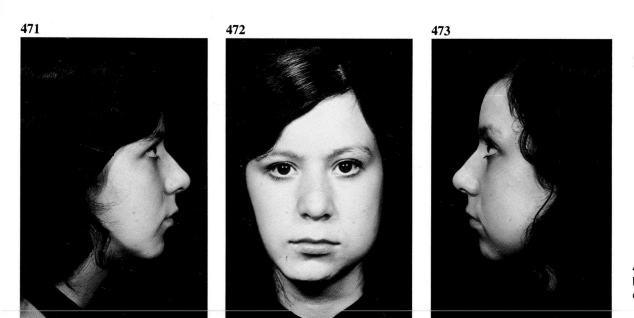 **472** **473**

471 to 476 Unilateral mandibular hypoplasia caused by infection in childhood.

474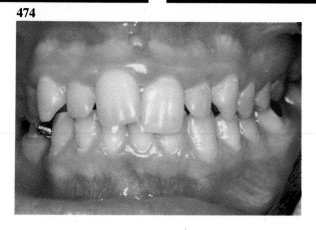

475 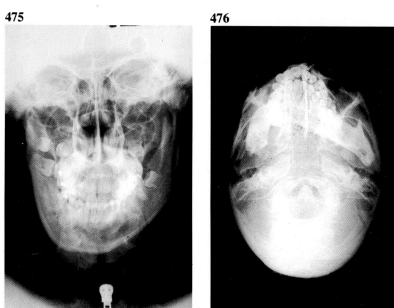 **476**

477

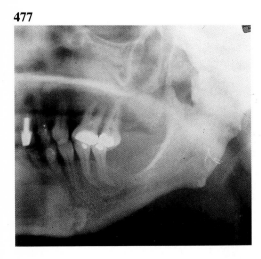

478

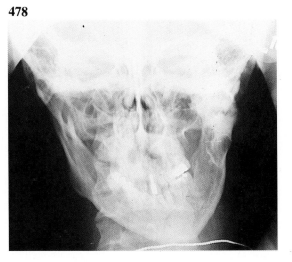

477 and 478 Ankylosis resulting from trauma to the condylar area in infancy.

479 to 482 Ankylosis with asymmetry, lack of forward and vertical mandibular growth, and severe occlusal disruption.

479

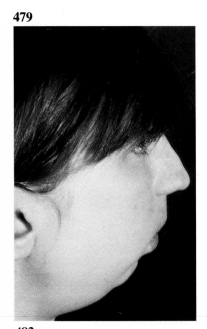

480

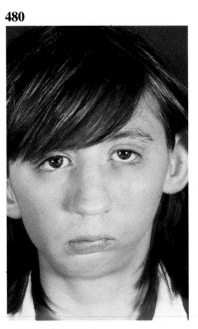

481

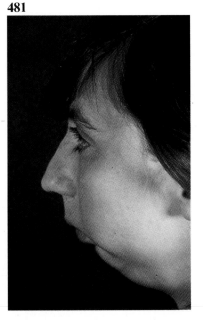

482

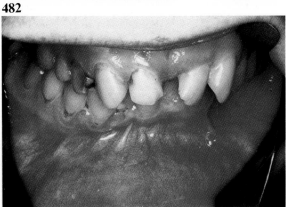

When trauma to the condylar area occurs during infancy the resulting ankylosis may cause severe disability and growth inhibition. The radiographs in **477** and **478** are typical, and resection of the affected area (previously performed twice in this patient) is usually followed by recurrence of bony ankylosis, with vast masses of bone on the lingual side as well as the region of the articulation itself. The case shown in **479** to **482**, affected more on the right than the left, demonstrates characteristic deformity, with asymmetry, lack of forward and vertical mandibular growth, and rather more severe occlusal disruption, associated with ankylosis and generalised somatic underdevelopment.

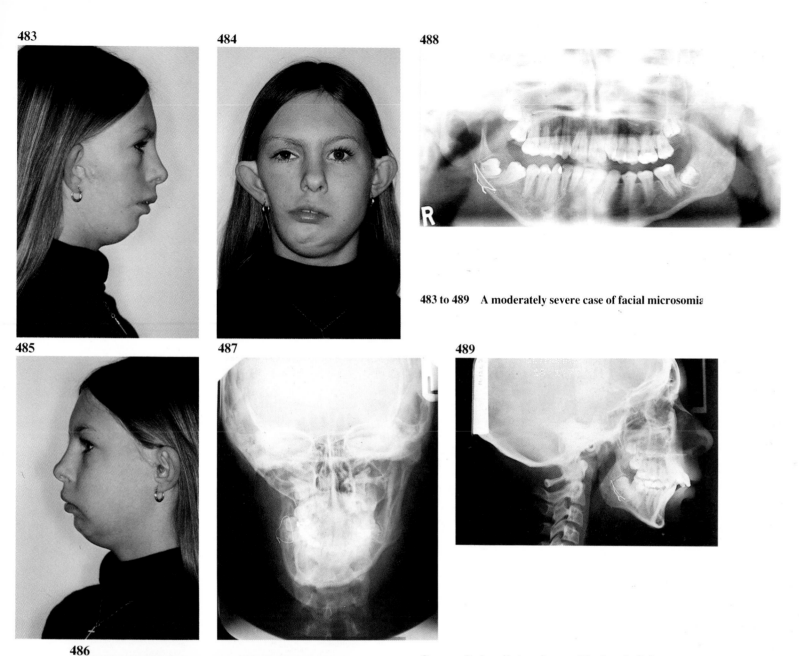

483   **484**   **488**

485   **487**   **489**

486

483 to 489   A moderately severe case of facial microsomia

Congenital unilateral mandibular deficiency

Facial microsomia

The stigmata of this condition are underdevelopment of the affected side of the mandible, mainly the condyle and ramus, together with deficient muscles of mastication, temporal bone, vertebrae and ocular abnormalities. Deformities of the external ear and accessory auricles are most often the first noticed indication. There may be macrostomia and facial nerve involvement.

The actual presentation of an individual case may range over the whole spectrum with great variability. **483** to **489** show a case with a moderately severe presentation, and also show that both sides of the face may be affected, although always to

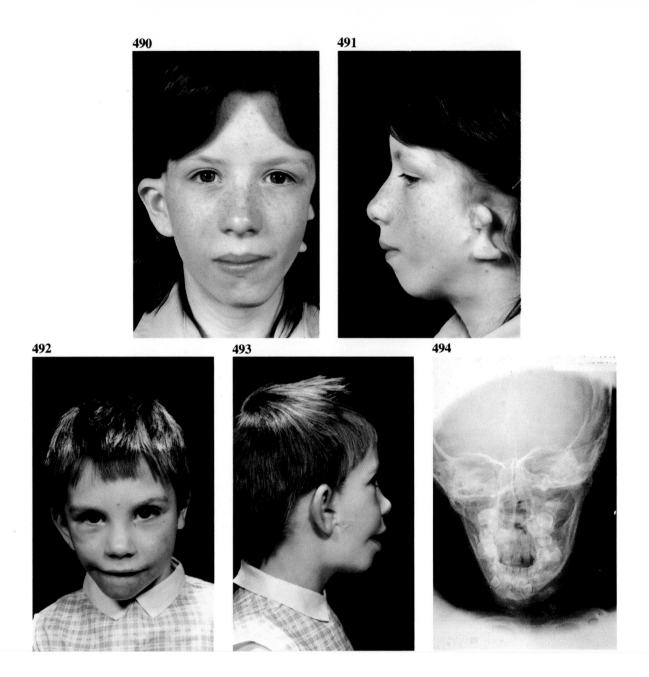

a different degree, thus consistently producing asymmetry. The low position of the external ear can be seen, especially on the right, which is the more severely affected side. Both ears protrude laterally and hearing is reduced on the left. Complete atresia of the external auricle is sometimes found. The mandibular hypoplasia is evident with characteristic contour on the right. On the left side there is relatively little masseteric involvement and the antegonial notch can be seen. On the right side there is gross shortage of soft tissue including the masseter, and there is no notch. An early attempt at bone grafting the ramus (see the wire) has completely resorbed, which would be expected from the shortage of soft tissues. Some temporalis function has stimulated coronoid growth. Again, this case illustrates the upward slope of the maxillary occlusion with secondary inhibition of vertical maxillary growth on the affected side, and typical secondary malar flattening.

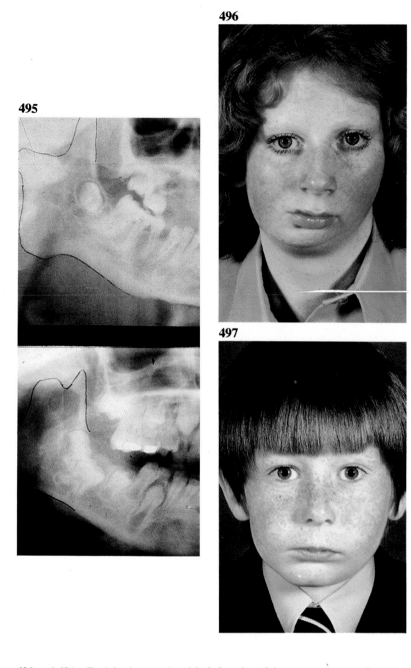

496

495

497

Facial microsomia shows a wide degree of variation. Sometimes (**490, 491**) the leading problem is the external ear with hearing defects, while the mandibular and soft tissue problems of the rest of the face are quite minimal. In other cases (**492** to **494**) mandibular deficiency, macrostomia and external auricular defects all contribute to the problem about equally. The degree of antegonial notching and concomitant muscle deficiency may not be apparent on superficial examination but can be detected on palpation, electromyography and radiological examination (**495,** see also page 46; **496** relates to the upper radiograph and **497** to the lower). Muscle activity can often be deduced from specific development of muscular processes. For example, marked coronoid development indicates temporalis activity. See Section 1 for a fuller discussion of the variations of facial microsomia, related there to pathogenesis.

490 and 491   Facial microsomia with deformity of the external ear and hearing defect.

492 to 494   Facial microsomia with mandibular deficiency, macrostomia and external auricular defects.

495 to 497   Detection of antegonial notching by radiological examination.

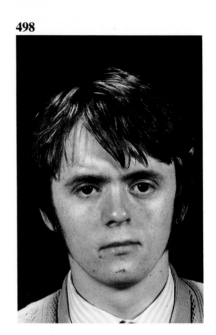

498

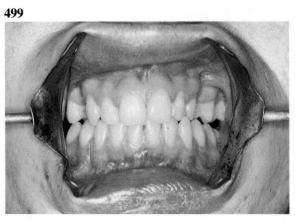

499

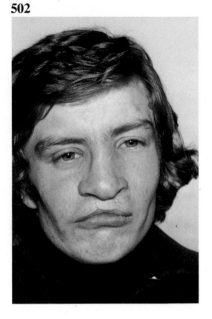

502

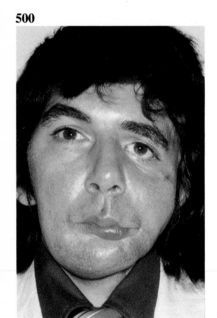

500

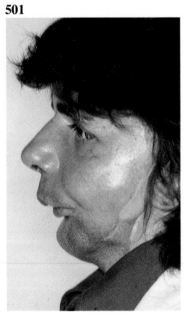

501

498 and 499 **Localised maxillary asymmetry** caused by irradiation for a skin lesion over the left maxilla.

500 and 501 **Underdevelopment of the face** resulting from extensive treatment of a tumour in infancy.

502 **Torticollis** causing secondary underdevelopment of mandible and maxilla.

503 to 506 **Fibrous dysplasia** affecting the maxilla and zygoma.

507 **Severe asymmetry** caused by facial trauma.

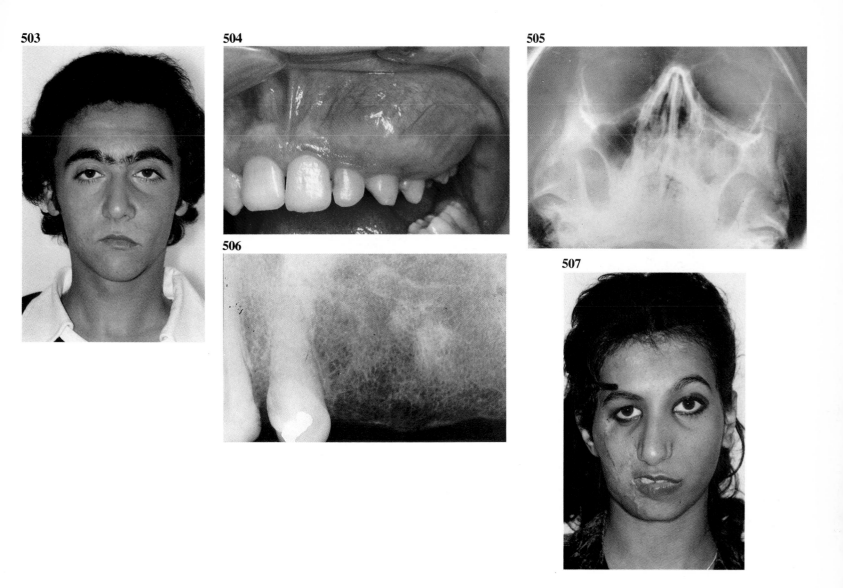

503 504 505 506 507

Mid-third asymmetries

These may present from a variety of causes and classification is unhelpful. Many facial asymmetries, for example the microsomias, involve the middle and even the upper-face as part of the basic failure of development, and the same applies to neoplastic malformations and osteodystrophies. The most common maxillary asymmetry occurs in the cleft lip and cleft palate syndrome, described in Section 5. Localised pathology, irradiation or surgery during growth will produce localised maxillary deformity. (See also **447** to **455** and **459** to **462**.)

Localised maxillary asymmetries may occur as a result of irradiation during development (**498, 499**) in this case for a skin lesion over the left maxilla. Proplast augmentation is the treatment of choice, if any is needed at all. Tumour oblation in infancy followed by extensive surgery for reconstruction, recurrence and irradiation, accounts for the underdevelopment of the face in **500** and **501,** which involves the vertical position of the orbit as well as the maxillomandibular region. Torticollis (**502**) will produce secondary underdevelopment of mandible and maxilla. Fibrous dysplasia (**503** to **506**) commonly affects the maxilla and zygoma with increasing swelling, which may displace the orbital floor superiorly unless serially reduced during the active phase. Severe facial trauma (**507**) may inhibit development of the maxillary and malar regions resulting in severe asymmetries which are difficult to correct.

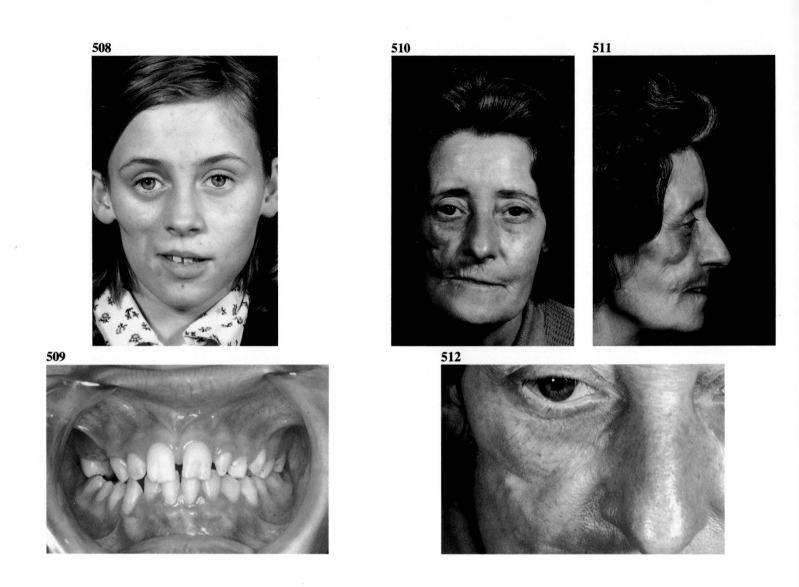

508 to 512 Progressive hemifacial atrophy.

Progressive hemifacial atrophy may involve the whole of one side of the face (and in rare instances of the body), but most commonly the mid-face is most affected as in **508** to **512**. Both congenital and progressive developmental groups are described, but the aetiology is obscure. There is slow atrophy of the affected area of the face, with wasting of subcutaneous fat, usually starting in the second decade (Gorlin and Pindborg, 1964) and slowly spreading to involve the surrounding tissues, including bone and cartilage. The tongue may be involved in cases affecting the whole of one side of the face.

The younger patient shown (**508** and **509**) shows a more usual presentation, already advanced by early adolescence and showing signs of involvement of the lip and infraorbital tissues.

There is loss of bone above the canine and premolar teeth (**509**). After progressing for some years the condition remains stable throughout life, although second progressions have been observed. In the established condition (**510** and **511**) the deformity is ageing and severe; on close inspection the skin is atrophic and papyraceous (**512**), sometimes with increased local pigment. There may be associated neurological abnormalities, and the full 'Romberg's syndrome' is usually associated with a *coup de sabre* deformity of the midline or paramedian region of the face. There is difficulty in distinguishing the condition from some cases of scleroderma on clinical grounds alone. A full description is given by Gorlin and Pindborg (1964).

513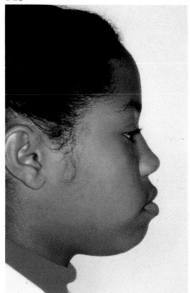

514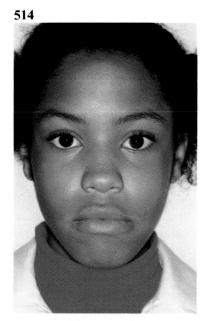

515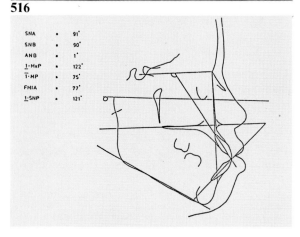

516

SNA	•	91°
SNB	•	90°
ANB	•	1°
1̲·MxP	•	122°
1̅·MP	•	75°
FMIA	•	77°
1̲·SNP	•	121°

513 to 516   Bimaxillary alveolar protrusion.

Special clinical groups

There is a multiplicity of syndromes involving the face about which whole reference books of considerable size have been written, and to which the reader is referred for comprehensive discussion of their clinical presentation and variability (see for example, Goodman and Gorlin, 1977, and Gorlin and Pindborg, 1964). All these present, within the structure of the facial complex, abnormalities which can be related to the descriptions given above – they derive their group identification more from the aetiology and the clinical associations than from special facial skeletal morphological characteristics. Nevertheless, it is proposed to present a few of these groups for special consideration in view of the particular problems of management they pose.

Bimaxillary alveolar protrusion is characterised by gross proclination of both maxillary and mandibular anterior teeth, usually with real protrusion of the alveolar bone over the skeletal bases of both jaws. The condition is racially normal in black races and those of oriental origin. In these races the lips are often thick and full, and lip seal is maintained without strain. In Caucasian races there is lip incompetence at rest. The appearance of thickened and everted lips gives rise to aesthetic demands for treatment; and it is quite common for expatriates living in European or American cultures to seek conformity to Western ideals of normality.

The case shown in **513** to **516** is typical. The patient presents both maxillary and mandibular protrusion with relative advancement of the alveolar bone relative to the cranial base and the mandibular base respectively. The ANB difference is within normal limits, but both upper and lower incisors are grossly proclined. The nasolabial angle is too acute and the labiomental curve flattened, sloping backwards to a deficient chin in terms of horizontal projection. The occlusion is usually good with well-aligned arches, although a tendency to Class 3 dental relationships may occur (**515**); sometimes the upper anteriors are more prominent than the lowers with an increased overjet. The lips are thickened in appearance although less in section.

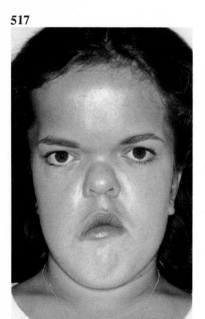

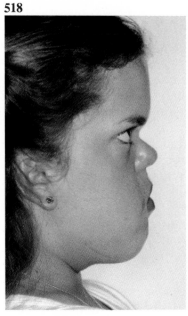

519

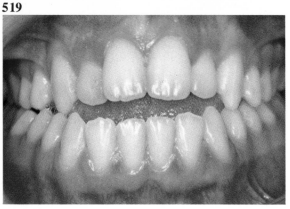

Achondroplasia (short-limbed dwarfism) is characterised by a special form of severe nasomaxillary hypoplasia. Apart from the general features (dwarfed body with lumbar lordosis, abdominal protuberance, short limbs, prominent buttocks and an enlarged cranium) the facies are immediately recognisable. The gross deficiency in the mid-face is associated with a short nasal dorsum, very recessed nasal bridge, and small button-like nose in full face view (**517**). The enlarged cranium combines with the recession of the nasal bridge to produce a deeply depressed appearance to the frontonasal area generally. The short nose makes the upper lip appear long, with an upturned nasal tip and columella exaggerating the nasolabial angulation (**518**). The maxillary arch is usually contracted and crowded anteriorly, a reflection of the lack of maxillary development (**519**).

Cephalometrically the orbitale lies too far behind the NA line, and the other features described are clearly depicted (**520**). The problem of treatment really turns mainly on whether or not the patient will benefit from compromised Le Fort 2 correction with rhinoplasty when the other features of dwarfism cannot be camouflaged. Very few cases present for treatment, and there appears to be greater acceptance of the condition by those afflicted than is the case with other facial syndromes. On balance, it is doubtful whether the patient is best served by major facial reconstruction.

517 to 520   Nasomaxillary hypoplasia associated with achondroplasia (short-limbed dwarfism).

520

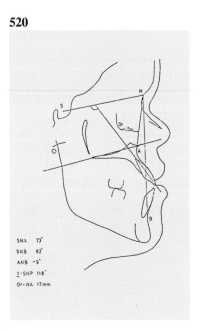

SNA   73°
SNB   82°
ANB   −9°
1·SNP 118°
Or-NA 17mm

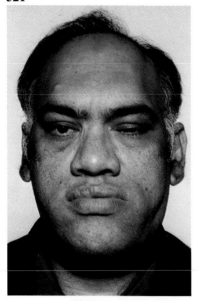

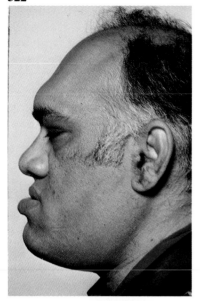

Acromegaly is caused by increased secretion of growth hormone from an adenomatous or hyperplastic anterior pituitary gland. There is an insidious onset, usually in late adolescence, with enlargement of the head and face, including the tongue, and of the hands and feet. Facially (**521** and **522**) the tissues thicken and coarsen, with enlargement of the nose, lips, supraorbital ridges and cheek bones. The mandible is increased in bulk in all dimensions, with spacing of the anterior teeth which also become proclined (**523**). The mandibular angles become squarer, and the frontal sinuses enlarge markedly. The sella turcica is expanded by the pituitary enlargement. These features are seen clearly on the lateral radiograph (**524**) which demonstrates also the real mandibular prognathism, and the increase in the calvarium. The condition must be recognised and treated before any attempt is made to correct the mandibular excess. Surgery is likely to be complicated by haemorrhage of a severe degree and by airway obstruction. Very careful postoperative monitoring is essential.

523

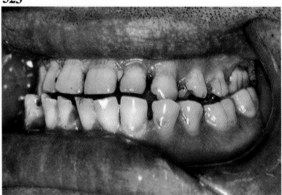

524

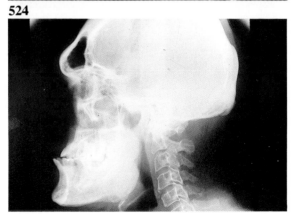

521 to 524   Acromegaly: facial effects.

525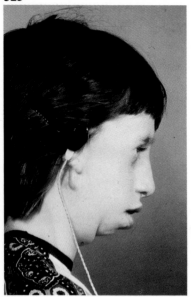

526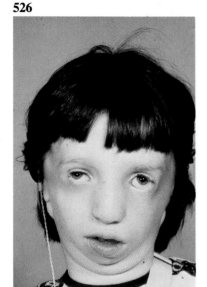

Treacher Collins syndrome is discussed in Section 1. The facial appearance is characteristic with an antimongoloid slope to the palpebral fissures, hypoplastic or absent malar bones, malformed external ears and frequently ossicular defects or meatal atresia, with resultant conductive deafness (note the hearing aid on the right side, **525**). The temporal bones may be hypoplastic although the rest of the calvarium is usually normal. The glabellar angle is flat with apparent enlargement of the nose by contrast with the deficient malar regions. The orbits appear to be deficient inferiorly with three-dimensional lateral rotation. There may be colobomata in the outer thirds of the lower eyelids. The mandible is deficient, with marked antegonial notching (see **135** and **136,** the radiographs of the patient shown here). The chin is recessive. The gonial angle is increased.

There is sometimes an extension of hair-bearing skin extending down onto the cheek regions. There is frequently macrostomia of one or both sides, crowding of the dental arches and cleft palate. The essential feature is that the deformities are symmetrical, and the reasons for this are discussed in Section 1.

525 to 528   Treacher Collins syndrome.

527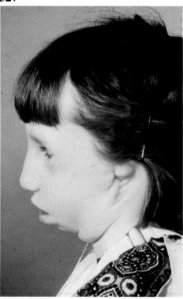

528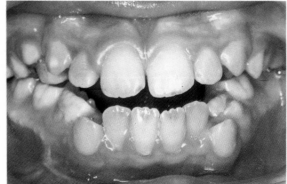

SECTION 4

Treatment methods and techniques

Part 1

Surgical access to the facial skeleton

General principles

Access to the facial skeleton is required for all facial osteotomies. In elective surgery performed to improve facial appearance, it is of prime importance to maintain the normal function and viability of the tissues and to get cosmetically pleasing results when healing is complete. These considerations limit the methods of surgical access. Incisions should be placed intraorally wherever possible, or failing this, within the hairline, along tension lines or within the conjunctivae.

Occasionally intranasal incisions allow limited supplementary access. Many osteotomies can be performed from within the mouth, but others are more safely and accurately performed through extraoral incisions offering a better view of important structures and greater operative flexibility. One incision will often give access to adjacent parts of the facial skeleton, though in many procedures a combination of selected incisions is required. When this is done careful regard must be paid to possible prejudice of blood supply to a particular segment. The main principles to be followed may be summarised thus:

(1) *Adequate exposure.* This must be sufficient to allow bony cuts to be made with any required separation of soft tissues from bone, but does not necessarily mean that the full extent of the osteotomy must be directly seen. Several areas can be cut 'by feel' provided the soft tissues can be protected adequately with suitable tissue retractors. The importance of properly designed retractors for this work cannot be over-emphasised.

(2) *Good postoperative cosmesis* by careful placement of incision lines and attention to suturing technique, including the technique of suture removal.

(3) *Good postoperative function.* Scars can interfere with function by developing contractures. Intraorally this may present difficulties in the construction of dentures if incision lines cross the margins of the denture periphery. Badly designed incisions around the teeth result in poor gingival reattachment with resultant periodontal disease. Extraorally scars may limit the movements of the eyelids with both cosmetic and functional implications.

(4) *Preservation of essential structures*, especially motor and sensory nerves is important. Disruption of the branches of the fifth or seventh cranial nerves will produce unacceptable motor weakness or sensory loss, sometimes completely destroying the surgical result. Less essential structures may well be sacrificed.

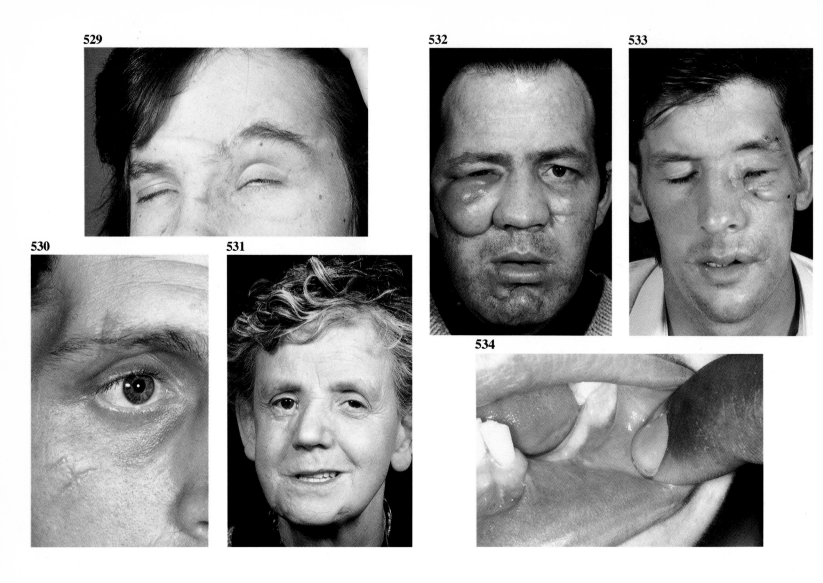

529 to 534 Traumatic scarring, causing disturbed appearance and function.

(5) *Maintenance of adequate nutrition and waste elimination* for all skeletal elements and soft tissue pedicles or flaps. Most important is the maintenance of an adequate blood supply; this will be discussed in detail in relation to individual incision lines and exposures. It is desirable also to avoid severing lymphatic and venous channels over areas wide enough to obstruct drainage pathways unnecessarily, or oedema may develop in the postoperative period.

Traumatic scarring illustrates the results of misplaced incision lines. **529** shows the difference in healing between various lines of laceration in the medial nasal and supraorbital regions, and also the disturbance of motor function of the left eyelid as a result of damage to seventh nerve filaments. **530** again illustrates the obvious scarring which results when an otherwise inconspicuous scar turns across the RSTLs (see page 156), and the same effect on the zygomatic prominence. **531** illustrates the ectropion which results from scar contraction involving the lower right eyelid, and **532** shows the result of impeded lymphatic drainage on the right side.

A less extended incision on the left has not had the same result (3 months after injury).

Figure **533** shows the obvious nature of an incision crossing a natural facial boundary line (the left upper lip) as well as the effect of asymmetrical disturbance of the tissues around the eye. Finally **534** shows the result of traumatic damage to the vestibular sulcus, with obvious problems for prosthetic rehabilitation.

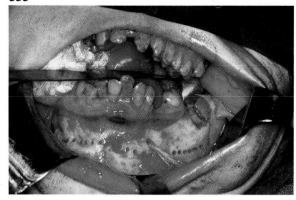

535

535   Full intraoral exposure of the mandible.

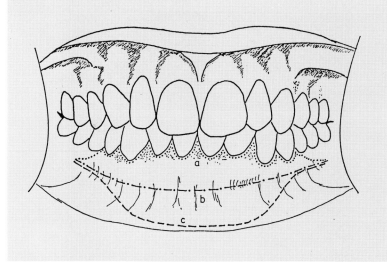

536

536   Symphyseal exposure.

Intraoral access

The mandible. Access to the mandible from within the mouth will be considered in two parts, (a) Access to the anterior mandible, and (b) Access to the body, angle and ramus. In practice the whole mandible can be exposed intraorally at one time by joining the anterior and posterior incisions, and in this way the lateral, anterior and inferior (ie lower border) surfaces are available for surgery at one time (**535**). (See also **542**.)

Exposure of the anterior mandible is necessary for genioplasty, for all subapical anterior osteotomies including symphyseal ostectomy, anterior mandibuloplasty, and lower labial segmental procedures. The structures to be preserved are the two mental nerves and their terminal (labial and buccal) branches. Three possible incisions are shown (**536**), all directed towards degloving the anterior mandible to a greater or lesser extent. The labial incision (c) is recommended for all procedures which will increase the bulk of the anterior mandible, such as advancement genioplasty with simultaneous increase in vertical height.

The standard mucogingival incision (b) is adequate for most purposes, and is simpler. It bleeds much less and is therefore less likely to produce postoperative swelling of the lip. However, it does frequently undergo some postoperative breakdown with healing by secondary granulation, which does not seem to matter but may give rise to discomfort and food trapping.

The gingival margin incision (a) is not recommended. It makes for too tense a soft tissue flap, and requires mucoperiosteal release at the corners to give anything like adequate exposure. Gingival recession may follow its use, particularly if there is any tension during closure; and it is contra-indicated if IMF is to be used as the flap must be closed before the teeth are brought together.

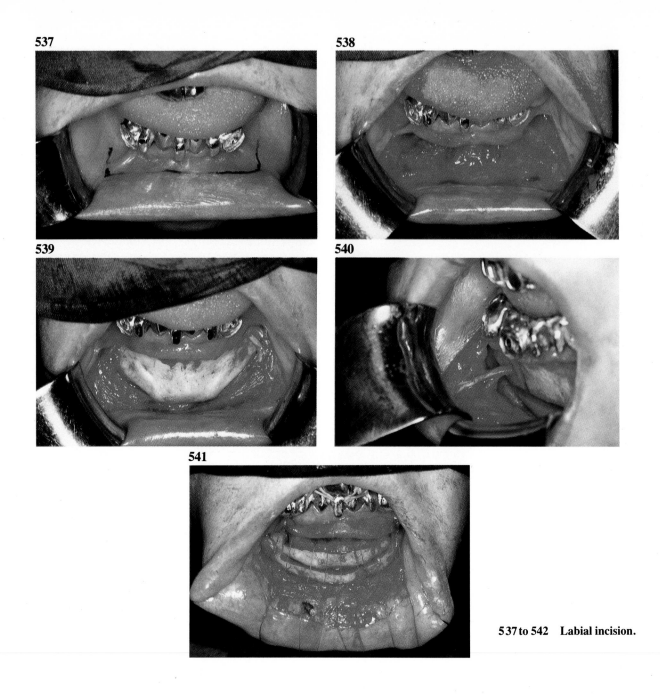

537 to 542   Labial incision.

The labial incision is carried onto the lip for its full width, sweeping upwards to the alveolus in the premolar region on each side (**537**). If radiographs indicate that the mental foramina are further back than usual the incision is also carried back to the first molar region. Only the mucosa is incised and this is dissected away from the underlying muscle layer (**538**). Care must be taken not to damage the labial branches of the mental nerves on the lip where they lie just submucosally. The muscle layer is next divided with a scalpel carried directly onto the alveolus over the apices of the incisor and canine teeth, but not distally to this until the mental nerves have been identified

and dissected to the mental foramina at their emergence. The muscle is thus divided at a different level to the mucosa, allowing closure in two displaced layers over the area of maximal tension.

During this second, deeper incision the periosteum is divided and the incision is carried distally above the mental foramina. The periosteum over the symphysis and around the mental nerves is raised with a rugine to the extent indicated by the procedure to be undertaken. This will include the whole symphysis onto its posterior surface for some genioplasties, for symphyseal ostectomy or anterior mandibuloplasty (**539**). Less

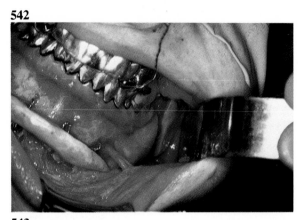

542

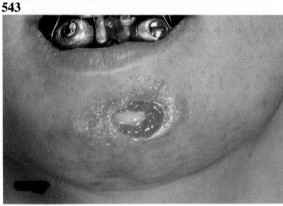

543

543 Chin ulceration caused by pressure bandage.

cannot be stretched. Also the adequacy of detachment of the integument over a wide area should be checked; often a small bridge of periosteum is still attached to the lower border.

The widest detachment is needed when a combined forward sagittal split and advancement genioplasty has been undertaken (**542**), and the anterior and posterior dissections joined together, reducing integumental tension markedly. Never apply a pressure bandage over the chin especially when a genioplasty has brought reciprocal pressure to bear on the tissue surface of the flap. **543** illustrates a pressure ulcer brought about in this way, no doubt aggravated by occult maceration of the skin following wetting of the bandage during feeding and washing.

Access to the lingual aspect of the anterior mandible to remove a segment of bone for segmental set-back is unnecessary. The forefinger is placed against the lingual plate, supporting the mucoperiosteum while the cut is made with a bur (**544**). This will allow the sensation of the moving bur to be transmitted to the finger through the soft tissue during cutting, at the same time helping to avoid unnecessary elevation of periosteum from bone in an area where the bone is dependent on its soft tissue pedicle for its blood supply. With practice this can be done sufficiently delicately not to divide the periosteum under the bur point at all. Where no tooth or bone is to be removed it may be necessary to insert a Howarth's raspatory between the periosteum and bone immediately behind the osteotomy site to allow access from above for a cortical vertical cut. Detachment should be confined to the area of the cut and the proximal part of the mandible, maintaining maximum attachment to the anterior segment.

Exposure of mandibular body, angle and ramus

Access to the mandibular body, angle and ramus via intra-oral exposure is by simple subperiosteal dissection, but a number of practical points arise (**545**). The incision should be started on the buccal aspect of the third molar and carried

exposure is needed for labial segmental surgery alone. Where the chin is to be advanced to any extent then the tissues should be raised from the mandible back towards the ramus and the related lower border. If full degloving is to be performed the mental nerves should be dissected free of the tense epineural tubes which invest them, out into the soft tissue of the lip and cheek (**540**). This allows easier retraction without tension and reduces the chances of accidental severance during manipulation of the lip and perimental tissues. A small, sharp-pointed pair of scissors is used for the dissection of the epineurium.

When the mucogingival access is used the incision is similar except that there is only one cut directly to bone and two layers cannot be developed. Closure is by 4/0 interrupted catgut in the muscle layer and 3/0 horizontal mattress silk in the mucosa. All sutures should be inserted in each layer before any are tied in that layer, otherwise the tissues will be fragmented by traction on tied sutures during placement of successive ones (**541**). Sometimes closure is difficult and this always indicates tension due to the skeletal changes. The periosteum must be incised so that the anterior soft tissue is not in periosteal continuity with the posterior – remember that periosteum

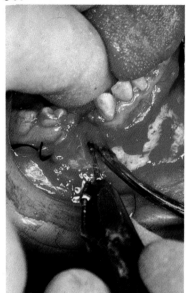

544

544 The removal of a segment of bone for segmental set-back.

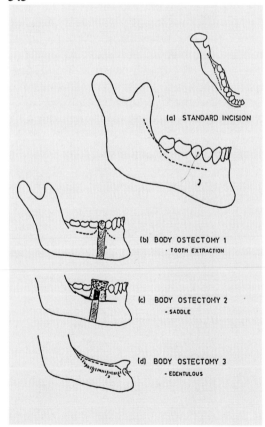

545

(a) STANDARD INCISION

(b) BODY OSTECTOMY 1
- TOOTH EXTRACTION

(c) BODY OSTECTOMY 2
- SADDLE

(d) BODY OSTECTOMY 3
- EDENTULOUS

545 Incision for access to the mandibular body, angle and ramus.

forwards along the buccal aspect of the jaw as far as required by the case, cutting down directly to bone just above the mucogingival reflection (a). A small mucosal cuff is left to facilitate suturing during closure, but the incision line must be kept high enough to be clear of possible future denture flanges. In the region of a body ostectomy the incision should be made to pass upwards to include the gingival margin of a tooth to be extracted (or which has been removed preoperatively) (b), or alternatively to a saddle area at the ostectomy site (c). This allows tailored coverage of the area of future bone grafting at the ostectomy site.

The buccal flap so formed may be sutured to the cheek or tongue during surgery until closure, when it can be trimmed to shape. If the mandible is edentulous (d) in the region being exposed, then the incision should be made parallel to the crest of the ridge but about 2mm below it to preserve good weight-bearing mucoperiosteum over the ridge while keeping clear of the potential denture periphery. With a suitable hooked retractor below the lower border excellent access to the lateral and inferior aspects of the mandibular body is obtained (**546**).

The incision should follow the line for third molar removal in the retromolar area, except that the distal part may be carried upwards and backwards over the external oblique ridge if the angle or ramus are to be exposed (**547**). The manner of doing this is important if the buccal pad of fat is to be avoided. The forefinger of the left hand (assuming the operator is right-handed) is placed over the external oblique ridge, palpating it and drawing the soft tissues laterally, stretching them over the ridge. The incision is carried up the ridge, initially through to bone but after about 1cm through mucosa only. The soft tissues being under tension then reveal the underlying buccinator fibres and these are divided, arresting haemorrhage from the small artery in this region by diathermy if necessary. This clears the field for later dissection and the incision is continued onto bone along the anterior surface of the coronoid process to about 1cm below its tip. This exposes the anterior fibres of the temporalis muscle which are detached with a sharp periosteal elevator.

The *mucosal* incision rarely requires to be extended far; upward retraction with a ramus retractor displays a wide field once the tissues have been reflected from the medial and lateral aspects of the ramus (**549**). However, too high an incision brings the buccal fat into the incision as does too lateral an incision. Subperiosteal dissection is started laterally with a large, fan-shaped dissector and carried to the lower border as far as the anterior edge of masseter, the attachment of which may give some resistance. A rigid channel retractor with a good hook to get underneath the lower border is used to strip the latter back to the angle and posterior edge, while freeing the periosteum with the dissector over the whole lateral surface of the ramus, except the condylar process. Again some resistance may be felt at the angle itself.

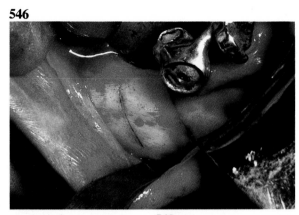

546

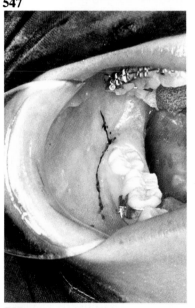

547

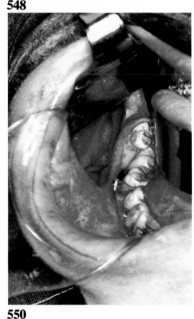

548

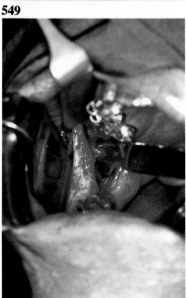

549

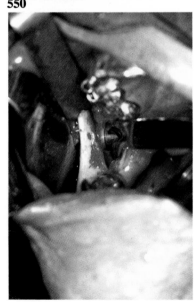

550

In underdeveloped mandibles the flare of the external oblique ridge may be relatively prominent with the angle recessed behind it. The tissues must be stretched out laterally with force to see the full extent of the angle and detach the muscle from it. A Ward's third-molar retractor, inserted back to front, is ideal for this purpose (**548**). If the ramus is to be exposed the medial tissues are dissected from it, feeling for the position of the lingula after the internal ridge has been freed. An assistant must forceably retract the tissues up the ramus with a ramus retractor. Once the lingula is seen or perhaps felt, then the level of entry of the inferior alveolar nerve and vessels is known, and the tissues may be stripped from the mandibular sulcus above and behind to the posterior border, at the base of the condylar process.

The sigmoid notch is identified and distinguished from the posterior border (especially in narrow rami). It is possible to expose the condyle from this approach but it is not an ideal access. With a long-channel retractor in place medially, above the lingula, a ramus retractor on the coronoid process and the third molar retractor laterally, good exposure of the whole ramus is obtained (**549**). The medial prominence of the internal oblique ridge may be reduced with a pear-shaped acrylic trimmer if it obstructs vision (for example in sagittal splitting), but the experienced operator will rarely find it necessary (**550**). There is no advantage in placing two retractors, buccally and medially, to meet around the posterior border; the practice is likely to cause pressure on the facial nerve against the mastoid process, with resulting paresis. It is difficult to detach the medial pterygoid muscle under direct vision in many cases because the flare of the mandible prevents direct access, but this can be overcome after the ramus is split (see page 175).

During body ostectomy, or other procedures confined to the body or anterior parts of the mandible, the lingual dissection must be kept to a minimum to preserve the blood supply from the lingual aspect. The gingival attachment may be divided with a curved No. 11 blade for one tooth on either side of an osteotomy line to allow the placement of a slim retractor. It is never necessary to expose more widely. Generally, mandibular exposure should be wide on the buccal and labial aspects to give necessary surgical access, but minimal lingually to preserve blood supply. This is also important on both aspects of the condylar process during sagittal splitting, or avascular necrosis of the proximal fragment may occur. The genial tubercles also mediate important nutrient afferents.

546 to 550 Incision for access to the mandibular angle and ramus.

The Maxilla

In exposing the maxilla intraorally the essential consideration is to maintain an adequate blood supply to those segments which are to be mobilised. The biological basis of low level maxillary mobilisation has been investigated in depth by Bell and his colleagues (Bell, 1969 and 1973). Their work comprised carefully controlled studies of vascularisation and revascularisation, and of bone healing, after a variety of maxillary osteotomies performed on adult Rhesus monkeys used as experimental analogues. With microangiographic and histological techniques they demonstrated minimal early transient vascular ischaemia, minimal bony necrosis, and early bony union after total (Le Fort 1), anterior, and posterior maxillary osteotomies. Other workers have used blood flow as an indicator of postoperative changes (as Nelson *et al*, 1978). The results are confirmed by the now substantial clinical experience of many surgeons that similar principles apply to human maxillary surgery, despite early doubts as to the comparability of the monkey experiments.

The arterial supply to the maxilla is traditionally seen in terms of several named arteries derived from the internal maxillary artery, always with the knowledge that extensive collateral channels are present between adjacent areas in the head and neck generally. However, in designing access incisions for this type of maxillary surgery it is more appropriate to think in terms of *pedicle supply* to the segments after mobilisation. The collateral circulation within the maxilla and its soft tissue investment forms a complex network of supply to both bone and teeth comprising labial, buccal, and palatal afferents, apical, intra-alveolar and pulpal vessels, and palatal, periodontal and gingival plexuses – all intercommunicating and not irreversibly committed to the *in vivo* centrifugal pattern of flow after disturbance of the intramedullary haemodynamic balance which occurs as a result of osteotomy. Perhaps the most important pedicle supply is that derived from the palate, but even this is not dependent upon preservation of the greater palatine arteries.

The blood supply to the lower maxilla is to be thought of as palatal or vestibular (551). The preservation of a broadly based, well attached palatal or vestibular mucogingival pedicle on at least one side of any segment to be mobilised should be adequate to ensure the viability of that segment; if both vestibular and palatal pedicles are provided this is even better, but it is not necessary and in many cases will compromise the surgery. If the base of a pedicle happens to coincide with a known axial arterial supply (for example, the greater palatine vessels at the base of a palatal pedicle) so much the better, but it has been demonstrated that this is not essential (Bell *et al*, 1975). If an incision is designed so that it would, if raised for minor surgical access to the underlying bone, give a soft tissue flap with a good blood supply, broad at the base, then it is likely to be true that an underlying bony segment would be well supplied if mobilised while still attached to that flap.

Intraoral access to the maxilla may therefore be gained in many alternative ways. Ideally, from the point of view of maximum blood supply with minimal interference with normal haemodynamics a series of vertical vestibular incisions (554) offers the best access. However, from the surgical point of view this would preclude the use of downfracturing methods of maxillary mobilisation – methods which have revolutionised maxillary surgery in the last decade. So, from the surgeon's viewpoint the best incision is the horseshoe vestibular incision (552) made high in the sulcus from first molar to first molar. The divided horizontal and vertical incisions, of which one variant is shown (553) are all safe and can be used to facilitate access where specific maxillary contours are difficult to cut or dissect by tunnelling techniques. When the palate is to be reflected, access must be gained by vestibular tunnels, as the blood supply will depend on the vestibular pedicles alone (555). The cleft palate patient presents special problems which will be discussed in Section 5.

The following general guidelines are offered:

(1) Never detach both palatal and vestibular pedicles from a dentoalveolar segment at the same time if that segment is to be mobilised.

(2) Palatal pedicles are better than vestibular pedicles. They are more firmly attached and may have a superior blood supply.

(3) Vestibular pedicles, being less firmly attached to bone, are more vulnerable to injudicious retraction than are palatal pedicles. If reliance is to be placed on them, their boundary incisions should be placed first, any necessary 'tunnelling' completed, and all osteotomy cuts from the vestibular aspect of the maxilla made *before* elevation of the palatal mucoperiosteum. In this way potential compromise of the vestibular blood supply can be anticipated before it is too late. This is most likely to occur in cleft palate cases where it is proposed to close the fistula at the same time as maxillary advancement, which is entirely dependent on good vestibular supply. If this should fail, then a two-stage procedure can easily be substituted.

(4) Aim to detach no more of the soft tissue from the segment itself than is strictly necessary for the required bony surgery to be completed.

(5) The area at greatest risk of ischaemia is the canine area (from the vestibular supply). This is a good area to maintain an intact vestibular pedicle if the palate has to be raised locally, especially when combinations of anterior and posterior segmental surgery are undertaken simultaneously. Vertical incisions are therefore best placed either mesially or distally to this area, and horizontal incisions away from it. This does not apply when the palatal mucosa is maintained intact, and it is a good reason for performing such combinations from above on the downfractured maxilla.

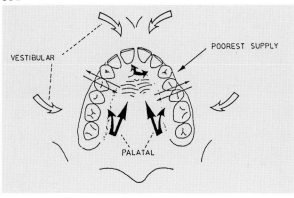

551   Maxillary blood supply.

(6) No reliance should be placed on ill-defined sources of blood supply from the nasal, medial antral or posteroantral areas.

552   Horseshoe incision.

553   Divided vestibular incisions.

554   Multiple vertical vestibular incisions.

555   Palatal and vestibular incisions.

Three groups of low level maxillary osteotomy are undertaken.

(a) *Anterior maxillary ostectomy*, or *osteotomy*, displacing the premaxillary segment, usually from canine to canine (but sometimes further forwards or backwards), in a backward, upward, downward or rotational manner. Rarely the segment may be brought forwards.

(b) *Posterior maxillary ostectomy* or *osteotomy*, mobilising the posterior alveolar segments, unilaterally or bilaterally, usually repositioning them upwards or transversely.

(c) *Total maxillary osteotomy* at the Le Fort 1 level, displacement being forwards, upwards, downwards or rotational. There are several variations of this procedure. High level maxillary osteotomies above the Le Fort 1 level are performed through combinations of intraoral and extraoral incisions; the principles applicable to intraoral exposure are similar to those governing low level access and will not therefore be described separately.

Exposure of the maxilla for total maxillary osteotomy where the palate is not to be cut across from below should be by the horseshoe incision (**552** and **556**). Dissection around the lateral, anterior, and posterolateral walls of the antra is by simple periosteal elevation from the incision line upwards. The mucosa overlying the alveolus below the incision should *not* be detached, but upper exposure should display the emergence of the infraorbital nerves, the zygomatic buttress up onto the temporal process of the zygoma, the anterior nasal spine and lower margin of the pyriform aperture of the nose. The incision should be kept high in the sulcus particularly posteriorly, to end above the first molar.

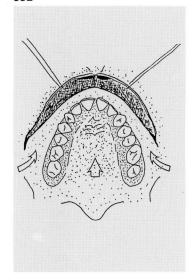

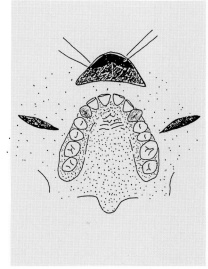

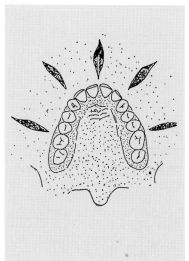

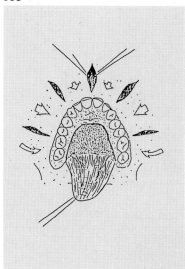

A substantial blood supply sweeps in to the alveolar region under the posterior part of this incision, and the high placement allows easier access to the pterygoid region where the pterygoid plates meet the posterior maxilla. Do not detach the tissues further than the entrance to the upper part of the pterygomaxillary fissure or brisk bleeding may result. After definition of the pyriform aperture, the nasal floor is elevated with a sharp dissector, carefully sweeping round from the floor to the lateral wall below the inferior turbinates, then back to the septum last. The angle between septum and floor is most likely to give difficulty, especially on the right side where the nasopalatine artery passes into the incisive canal most often. 557 to 558 show the divided vestibular approach by tunnelling below vestibular flaps.

556

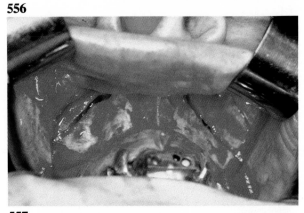

557

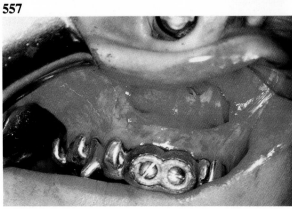

558

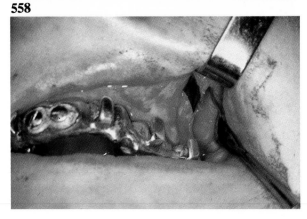

556 **Maxillary exposure: horseshoe incision.**

557 and 558 **Maxillary exposure:** divided vestibular approach by tunnelling below vestibular flaps.

Exposure of the anterior maxilla alone is necessary for the various forms of anterior maxillary osteotomy and ostectomy designed to reposition the premaxillary segment and to widen or narrow it transversely. For this segmental surgery the main consideration is again preservation of the blood supply to the segment or segments which are to be moved.

There are three accepted approaches, the Wassmund (described in 1927), the Wunderer (1963) and the Cupar (1954, 1955, also more recently popularised by Epker, 1969). Of these the Wassmund is the safest, relying on maintained labial and palatal pedicles to the anterior segment, the osteotomies being carried out under mucosal tunnels from midline and premolar vertical vestibular incisions on the lateral aspect of the premaxilla, and from palatal tunnels developed from the premolar region to the midline, using incisions around the palatal aspect of the necks of the first premolars and a midline incision in the palate (**559**).

The Wunderer technique (**560**), relies on the labial vestibular pedicle together with some blood supply from the incisive canal, two vertical premolar vestibular incisions being combined with a transpalatal incision allowing reflection of the palate posteriorly. In this technique the premaxilla is eventually fractured anteriorly to rest on its labial pedicle alone.

The last technique, the downfractured method, relies entirely on the palatal pedicle, which is adequate for the anterior maxilla just as the full palate is adequate for the whole maxilla (**561**).

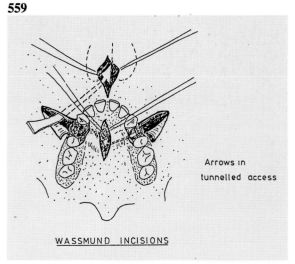

559

Arrows in tunnelled access

WASSMUND INCISIONS

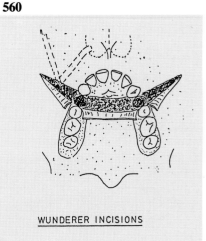

560

WUNDERER INCISIONS

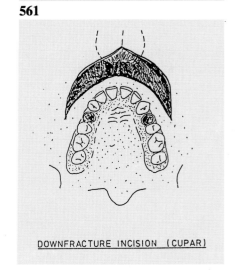

561

DOWNFRACTURE INCISION (CUPAR)

559 to 561   Incisions for access to the anterior maxilla.

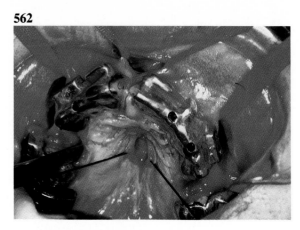

562 Wassmund approach.

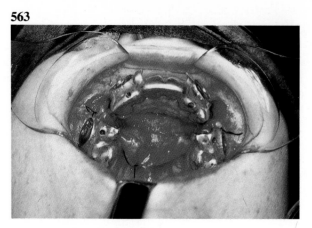

563 Wunderer approach.

The surgical technique of the Wassmund approach (**562**) requires that two buccal flaps are developed opposite the tooth or interdental space which is to be the site of osteotomy. It is best to make a vertical incision just anterior to the osteotomy site and reflect a small flap distally. The anterior mucoperiosteum need not be raised from bone over the dental roots at all; it is important in all these anterior segmental procedures to elevate mucoperiosteum as little as possible from the segment itself. The anterior surface of the premaxilla can then be exposed by elevation of the soft tissues under the flap above the canine and incisor region, meeting up with the dissection made from a midline vertical incision. The pyriform aperture of the nose is identified and defined. On the palatal aspect a midline incision does not prejudice the blood supply and tunnels can be developed subperiosteally from the premolar region (or other osteotomy site) to the centre of the palate.

Advantages. Excellent blood supply to premaxillary segment(s). Midline ostectomy easy. Heals well.

Disadvantages. Time-consuming, especially in the palatal vault. Poor if it is intended to elevate the premaxilla because it gives poor access to the superior nasal surface of the premaxilla, and to the turbinates and nasal septum after osteotomy.

The Wunderer approach (**563**) is identical to the Wassmund on the buccal and labial aspects, but a transpalatal incision is made from the mesial aspect of the osteotomy site, across the palate in an arc with its convexity forwards, keeping palatal to the incisive papilla. The anterior palatal mucoperiosteum is not elevated at all, but the posterior part is flapped back to allow access under direct vision to the transpalatal osteotomy. This technique is ideal when the premaxilla is to be elevated.

Advantages. Good visualisation of the osteotomy sites. Excellent when the premaxilla is to be raised, because it gives good access (after forward displacement of the premaxilla on a labial pedicle) to the nasal crest of the maxilla, the nasal septum and the floor of the nose. Good access labially and palatally when no teeth to be extracted.

Disadvantages. The poorest blood supply to the anterior segment, vulnerable to injudicious traction on the segment. Can be difficult to divide the nasal septum. Occasionally gives rise to oronasal fistula. More difficult to split the premaxilla in the midline.

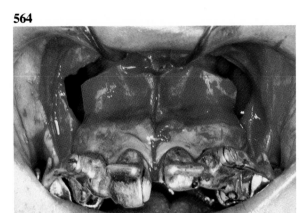

564 Premaxillary downfracture technique.

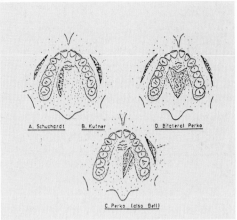

565 Incisions for access to the posterior maxilla.

The downfracture technique, shown with ostectomy cuts completed to indicate access through to the deep aspect of the premaxilla (**564**), mirrors the total maxillary downfracture except that it is only carried back to the osteotomy site. The 'horseshoe' incision is therefore carried around the anterior maxilla from osteotomy site to osteotomy site, and the mucosa tunnelled to the gingival margin, or incised vertically, at the site of the cuts. After removal of the planned bone segments buccally, the cuts are carried across the palate through the ostectomy sites and the premaxilla hinged downwards on the palatal pedicle. The procedure is best when lateral bone is to be removed, and poorest when only an interdental cut is to be made.

Advantages. Good access. Good blood supply. Easy midline ostectomy. Excellent visualisation superiorly, and therefore good for elevating the premaxilla. Mainly indicated for upwards movement when a tooth is to be removed allowing also backward displacement.

Disadvantages. Can be technically difficult to complete transpalatal cut. Avoid when no tooth has to be removed.

Exposure of the posterior maxilla alone (**565**) is required for posterior segmental osteotomies designed to raise, lower, or move transversely or more rarely anteriorly the molar or molar/premolar segments. The simplest approach was that of Küfner (1970) (B), who made only a horizontal incision above the apices of the involved teeth, gaining access to the palatal aspect transantrally. Schuchardt (1959) (A), made a corresponding incision palatally to make the palatal cut under direct vision; while Perko (1972) and later Bell (1975), made a hockey-stick incision along the midline of the palate as far forwards as the incisive papilla and then carried it out laterally just anterior to the proposed osteotomy site (C). When bilateral incisions were needed this turned into one Y-shaped palatal incision (D). The horizontal Küfner incision is common to all these techniques for access to the buccal aspect of the posterior maxilla. The indications, advantages and disadvantages will be discussed in Part 2 of this section, pages 270 to 271.

Extraoral access

Skin incisions on the face should be designed to provide adequate access to bone with minimal scarring. The healing of a skin incision has two phases macroscopically, initially a healing phase by primary intention, and the subsequent long-term stabilisation which involves both structural changes (conversion to scar tissue) and colour changes (from early red to white). The long-term result is more important than the short-term healing, and this means eversion of the skin edges during suturing and the placement of incisions along lines of maximum skin tension. The former allows scar contraction to flatten the final scar on the skin (rather than indenting it), while the latter minimises any tendency for the scar to widen, at the same time reducing the effects of keloid formation if that should occur.

The historically interesting lines of skin tension associated with Langer, 1861 (work recently largely translated and published in English by Professor T. Gibson, 1978), was based on the study of puncture wounds inflicted on the skin of cadavers after rigor mortis had set in. In the light of modern biomechanical research (Gibson and Kenedi, 1967) these lines are regarded as fallacious and misleading; according to these authors 'Langer's lines are an interesting phenomenon which is still to be fully explained'.

A more rational concept is that introduced by Borges and Alexander (1962), who refer to 'relaxed skin tension lines RSTL' and present detailed studies of their distribution over the face as well as elsewhere. According to their definition 'skin tension is the force that causes widening of scars; the force that makes a linear incision gape more widely if it is transverse to it than when it is aligned to it'. RSTL are determined by the tenting effect of underlying hard tissues, and must be distinguished from wrinkle-lines which result from muscular activity, including that of the muscles of facial expression; the two do not always correspond. Despite this, in the face and neck the muscles of expression are of primary importance; McGregor (1975) regards the lines of election for facial incisions to be at right angles to the direction of the resultant pull of the muscles of facial expression, which with ageing become set into a pattern of wrinkles. If an incision can be placed in such a wrinkle-line so much the better, if not it should lie parallel to one so that it may appear to be another wrinkle.

When in doubt about the relaxed lines of skin tension in a particular area the best technique is simply to relax the skin by muscle contraction (for example, ask the patient to furrow the forehead), or by passive manipulation (for example, by pinching the skin which leads to lateral extension of the folds and furrows in the same direction on each side). There are several areas around the eyes and forehead where RSTL and wrinkle-lines do not correspond. The recommendations made for access incisions in this text are based on the principles outlined above and on clinical experience. There are factors outside the surgeon's control, infection for example, which will modify the result; but a bad scar will always be worse if the incision which caused it was ill designed.

Facial incisions may be placed within the hairline or the eyebrow, or disguised by contiguity with natural boundaries between different facial areas. Surgical technique is most important. Except in the hairline or eyebrow, the scalpel blade should always be held at right angles to the skin surface to avoid bevelling, and the margins should be slightly undermined in the immediate subdermal layer to avoid damage to the branches of the facial nerve. In the hair or eyebrow the incision may slope slightly to parallel the hair follicles by inclining the blade after inspection of the direction of hair growth. Tissues should be handled gently, with delicate instruments; atraumatic needles and fine silk (or better, monofilament) should be used on the finer skin around the eyes, mid-face, and lips. Any subcutaneous catgut sutures should be placed with the knots buried deeply.

For a full discussion of the whole subject of suturing, and postoperative care of suture lines the reader is referred to McGregor (1975).

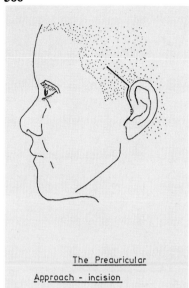

The Preauricular

Approach - incision

566 to 568 Preauricular access to the mandibular condyle.

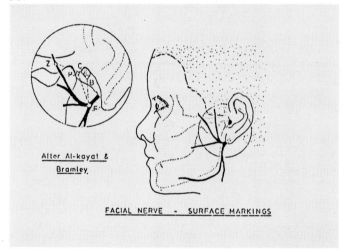

After Al-kayat & Bramley

FACIAL NERVE - SURFACE MARKINGS

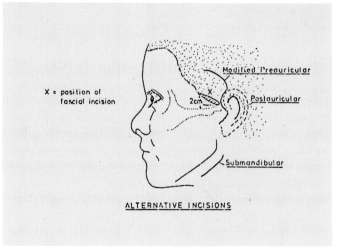

X = position of fascial incision

Modified Preauricular

Postauricular

2cm

Submandibular

ALTERNATIVE INCISIONS

Access to the mandibular condyle

This may be gained in a variety of ways, preauricular, endaural, postauricular, and submandibular. Intraoral access is of little value in orthognathic surgery, although oblique subcondylar osteotomies can be performed via this route (exposure as for the ramus, but dissection carried superiorly to display the condylar neck). Of these alternatives the author prefers the preauricular approach (Rowe, 1972) (**566**), which provides the best access with control of haemorrhage in an area liberally supplied with blood vessels. It reduces to a minimum the risk of damage to the facial nerve, always at risk in the region of the condylar neck. **567** shows the surface markings of the facial nerve, the main superficial structure to be preserved. It is probably damaged more often by heavy traction on the soft tissues than by direct trauma. The endaural route (Davidson, 1956) provides poor access and carries a danger of stenosis of the external auditory canal. The latter criticism also applies to the transmeatal postauricular approach (Axhausen, 1931), although reasonable access may be gained by a supra-meatal postauricular approach. For the submandibular approach see pages 160 to 163.

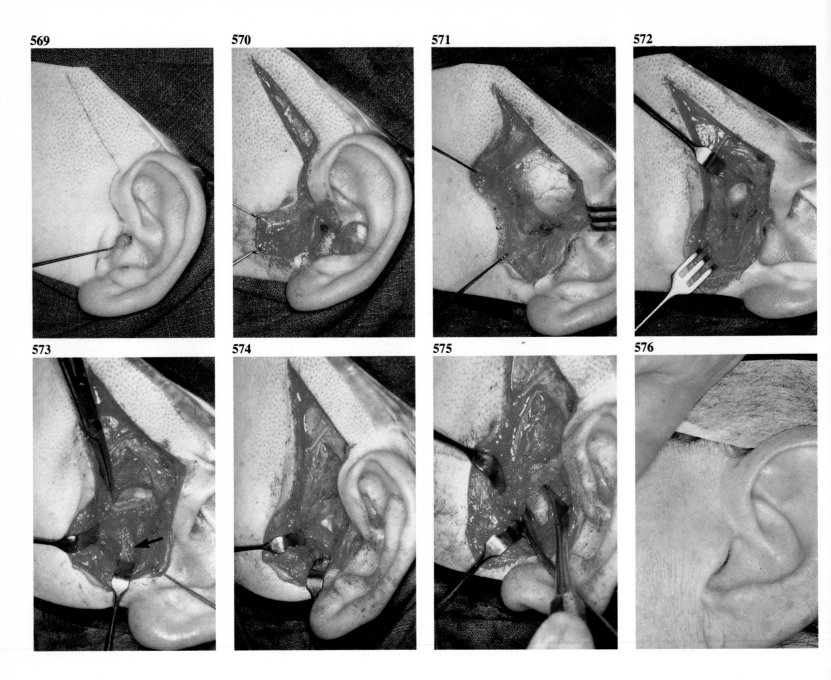

569 to 576 **The preauricular approach to the condyle:** surgical technique.

The preauricular approach to the condyle is marked out after the temporal hair has been shaved (**569**). The incision is carried obliquely downwards and backwards through the hair at about 45° to the zygomatic arch, curved down in front of the helix in a skin crease or elicited RSTL (pinching the helix and the skin together), and round onto the posterior surface of the tragus running about 1 mm to 2 mm behind the tragal crest. If a high condylectomy is to be performed the incision is stopped on the tragus; if a full condylectomy is intended the incision is brought out again just below the tragus onto the face, anterior to the lobe.

The incision (**570**) is deepened into the subcutaneous tissue in the temporal region and to expose the tragal cartilage in the ear. Once the avascular area immediately anterior to the cartilage has been identified (close up to the cartilage itself), a pair of McIndoe's scissors are passed deep down this plane posterior to the condyle itself, opened and withdrawn.

The temporal fascia is identified and exposed (**571**), and followed down until it passes over the zygomatic root, which can be palpated, located in the picture just below the cautery mark. The bridge of tissue separating the temporal and the pretragal parts of the dissection is now divided; branches of the superficial temporal artery and associated veins will be encountered, divided and coagulated or tied. During this stage the main superficial temporal vessels, the glenoid lobe of the parotid gland and the associated soft tissues are anterior to the plane of dissection.

Next the zygomatic root is exposed (**572**), incising through the temporalis fascia, sometimes through a few strands of temporalis muscle which bleed, directly onto bone. The post-glenoid tubercle is identified and marks the most posterior part of the subperiosteal dissection, which is carried forwards to display the origin of the zygomatic arch (**573**). Provided the dissection is kept below the periosteum the arch can be exposed for about half its length from this approach. If it is desired to obtain better zygomatic exposure, the approach must be extended superiorly and carried out through a longer incision of the temporalis fascia (see bifrontal flap, pages 169 and 170). Working from the zygomatic root above, the tissues are next reflected forwards from the temporomandibular ligament and the capsule of the temporomandibular joint. This is easier if an assistant moves the jaw through the towels, when the condyle will be felt to move under a palpating finger. The temporomandibular ligament can be seen (arrowed).

The capsule is opened with an inverted L incision (**574**), the posterior limb of which passes vertically up the back of the condyle. The condyle is then visible, and can be displayed by intracapsular dissection. A Howarth's elevator can be placed anteriorly and another posteriorly (**575**). Dissection may be carried down the condylar neck as necessary; if a very large condyle is encountered an additional incision may be necessary below the lobe of the ear (and below the facial nerve). The safest way to accomplish this is via a combined submandibular and preauricular approach.

The excellent cosmetic result obtained by this approach is illustrated in **576** (the case shown in the operative sequence, 3 months postoperatively). The author closes the temporal part of the incision with 3/0 silk, the prehelical part with 5/0 monofilament, and the tragal part with 6/0 monofilament, removing the latter two suture lines early (3rd or 4th day) and placing steristrips over the prehelical part of the incision for a few days. Drains are usually unnecessary because haemostasis should be obtained before closure. If a continual ooze is encountered, a vacuum drain is used and brought through the skin below and behind the lobe of the ear, above the line of the facial nerve. A light pressure dressing is applied over a cotton roll placed on the pretragal skin and a wool pack in the meatus.

567 shows in brief the important findings of Al-Kayat and Bramley (1979) who studied in detail the surgical anatomy of the facial nerve in its extracranial course. They emphasised that the temporal fascia divides inferiorly, about 2 cm above the malar arch into two layers, the superficial of which is attached to the lateral aspect of the malar periosteum, and the deeper to the medial aspect. The gap contains fat, and the zygomatic branch of the superficial temporal artery, plus the zygomatico-temporal branch of the maxillary nerve. At the malar arch level the periosteum blends firmly with the outer of these two layers together with the superficial fascia, within which run the temporal and zygomatic branches of the facial nerve. The temporal branches run superiorly in the looser superficial fascia over the temporal fascia. The bifurcation of the facial nerve (Point F) is located by reference to the lowest concavity of the bony external auditory canal (Point B) and the lowest point at the postglenoid tubercle (Point P), the variation in BF being from 1.5 cm to 2.8 cm, and the distance PF from 2.4 cm to 3.5 cm in a posteroinferior direction.

The temporofacial division of the nerve and the most posterior filaments of the temporal branch always lie anterior to a line drawn from F to P. These workers measured the distance from the most anterior concavity of the bony external auditory canal, Point C, to the point on the lateral surface of the malar arch midway between its upper and lower borders, where the most posterior twig of the temporal branch crosses it, Point Z. This distance ranges from 0.8 cm to 3.5 cm, and is therefore very variable. It follows that the nerve cannot be regarded as safe if an incision is made directly onto the zygomatic arch more than 0.8 cm in front of the point C.

From these observations a modified preauricular approach (**568**), uses a curved incision in the hairline, and does not separate the superficial fascia from the temporalis fascia as far as the zygomatic arch. Instead the lateral layer of the temporalis fascia is divided with an oblique (45°) incision starting at the root of the arch to gain access to the space between the lateral and medial divisions referred to above (**568**). Thus the zygomatic periosteum is safely divided from within this space (and therefore over the superior aspect of the arch), in the confidence that the facial nerve branches remain inside the reflected soft tissue flap. For wide exposure this is undoubtedly a safer approach and allows better visibility as the tense fascia is divided before the flap is reflected.

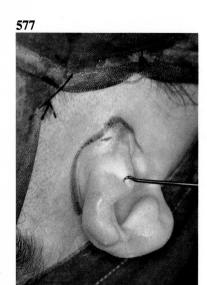

577

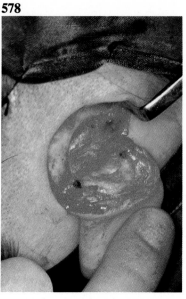

578

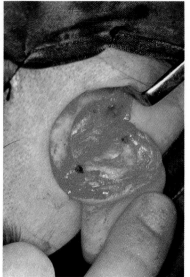

580 to 582   The submandibular approach to the mandible.

580

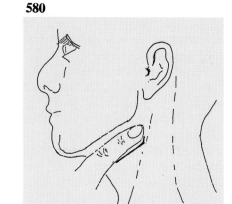

POSITION OF SUBMANDIBULAR

INCISION

579

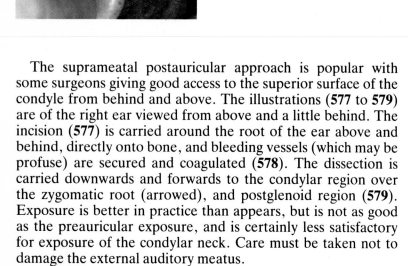

577 to 579   The suprameatal postauricular approach to the condyle.

The submandibular approach to the mandible

This is important because it provides the access for all major surgery of the mandibular body or ramus when intraoral exposure is inadequate. It also gives access to the condyle and coronoid process. Curiously the incision is ascribed to Risdon (1934) who made only a passing allusion to it (**580**). The main technical difficulty is in avoidance of the lower (mandibular and cervical) branches of the facial nerve which curves upwards and forwards at a variable level and with a variable degree of reticulation through the operative area (**581** and **582**).

The following tissues are divided from skin to mandible. (1) Skin; (2) Subcutaneous fat and superficial fascia; (3) The platysma muscle; (4) Deep cervical fascia; (5) A layer of loose connective tissue in which lie the facial artery and the anterior facial vein, plus the facial nerve (lying on the deep surface of the deep cervical fascia posteriorly, penetrating the fascia more anteriorly to reach the muscles of facial expression), and sometimes the anterior branch of the posterior facial vein; (6) Periosteum along the lower border of the mandible, with the attached masseter muscle posteriorly.

The suprameatal postauricular approach is popular with some surgeons giving good access to the superior surface of the condyle from behind and above. The illustrations (**577** to **579**) are of the right ear viewed from above and a little behind. The incision (**577**) is carried around the root of the ear above and behind, directly onto bone, and bleeding vessels (which may be profuse) are secured and coagulated (**578**). The dissection is carried downwards and forwards to the condylar region over the zygomatic root (arrowed), and postglenoid region (**579**). Exposure is better in practice than appears, but is not as good as the preauricular exposure, and is certainly less satisfactory for exposure of the condylar neck. Care must be taken not to damage the external auditory meatus.

581

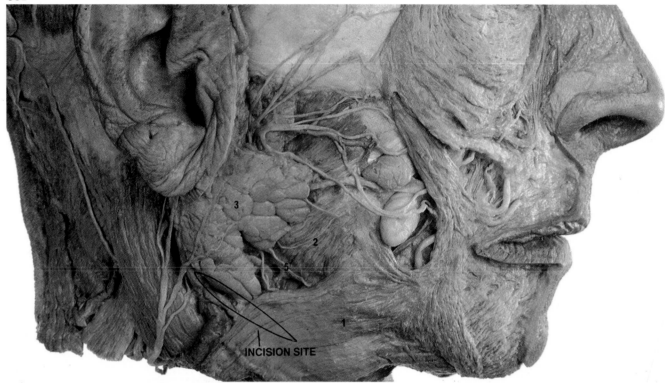

INCISION SITE

582

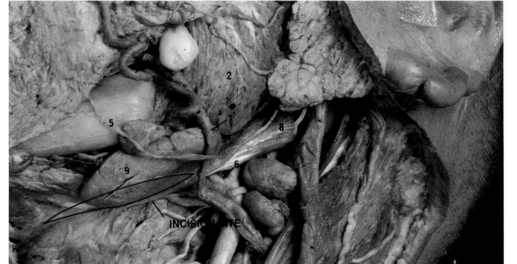

INCISION SITE

Key
1 Platysma
2 Masseter
3 Parotid Gland
4 Cervical Branch of Facial Nerve
5 Marginal Mandibular Branch of Facial Nerve
6 Facial Artery
7 Facial Vein
8 Posterior Belly of Digastric
9 Submandibular Gland

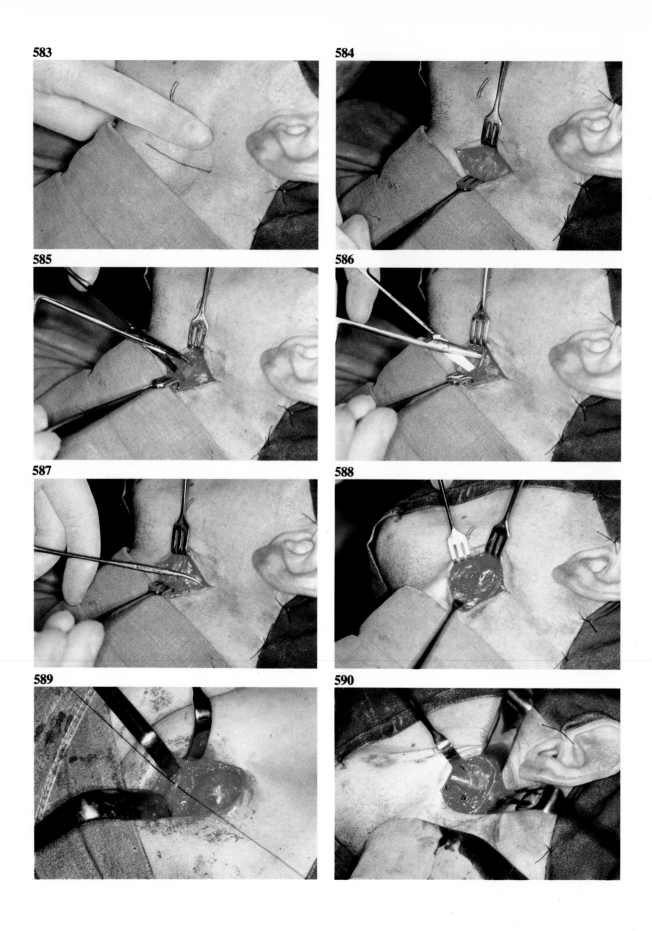

591

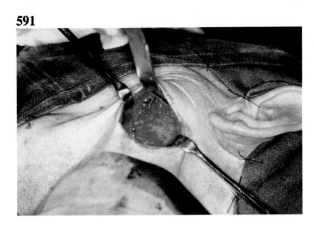

583 to 591   The submandibular approach: surgical technique.

The incision should be about 5 cm in length, placed in one of the skin creases running parallel with the lower border of the mandible, about 1½ fingers' breadth from the mandible (**580** and **583**). The exact placement will depend on whether the ramus or the body is to be exposed; if possible it should be placed posterior to the facial vessels (palpable over the anterior margin of the masseter), for access to the ramus, condyle, or coronoid process. For access to the body it will have to be placed more anteriorly, and the vessels will have to be divided. The posterior end of the incision may be curved slightly upwards around the angle for posterior access, but never near the lobe of the ear (see surface marking of facial nerve, **567**). After division of the skin, subcutaneous fat and superficial fascia, the platysma muscle is defined and exposed in the incision area (**584**).

The fibres of the muscle are separated along its long axis with blunt scissors (**585**), which are then passed deep to the platysma separating it from the deep cervical fascia underneath (**586**). It is helpful if neuromuscular blocking agents have not been used by the anaesthetist because the presence of seventh nerve fibres can be excluded by simple clip pressure along the line of proposed platysma division (**587**).

Alternatively, direct incision can be used with a nerve stimulator to hand. The platysma is divided along the line of the skin incision and the deep cervical fascia displayed (**588**). The fascia is exposed and incised with care, identifying the facial vessels where appropriate and dividing them between black silk ligatures (for easy identification). The facial nerve (cervical branch) will often be identified lying in close relation to the artery, over, anterior or posterior to it. Its course is very variable, and some caution is advised in applying data taken from cadaver studies, which are subject to postmortem distortions of the *in vivo* relations. If identified (eg. **589**) (and it is desirable to identify the nerve if possible), it should be retracted upwards with the superior flap, which also contains the lower pole of the parotid gland in its posterior part.

The lower border of the mandible and the attached masseter (**590**) is next identified and an incision carried down to bone. The periosteum is reflected from the ramus or body as required (**591**).

The preauricular approach and the submandibular approach may be usefully combined to give excellent access to the whole of the ramus and condyle when either incision is inadequate in itself. This most commonly arises in connection with temporomandibular joint ankylosis, but may be necessary in the correction of unilateral mandibular hypoplasia or enlargement involving the condylar and ramal regions of the mandible at the same time.

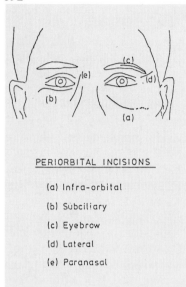

PERIORBITAL INCISIONS

(a) Infra-orbital

(b) Subciliary

(c) Eyebrow

(d) Lateral

(e) Paranasal

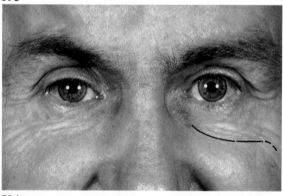

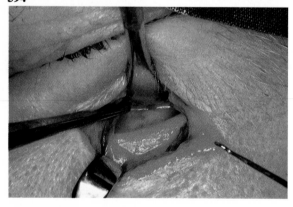

592 Periorbital access.

593 and 594 Infraorbital incision.

Periorbital access

Many corrective procedures of the maxilla, zygomatic regions and orbits require surgical access around the orbital tissues to the orbital walls, floor or roof; periorbital incisions also give access to the nasal root and the supraorbital regions, and sometimes are useful for access along the medial ends of the zygomatic arches. For most osteotomies involving the bone above the midorbital level the bifrontal flap is recommended (pp. 169 and 170), because it gives bilateral exposure and symmetry is easier to maintain or achieve.

The *infraorbital incision* (**592**(a)) is probably the most commonly used access, but it is not the best cosmetically. For the less experienced in orbital surgery it is perhaps the incision of choice; it should slope down laterally rather more obliquely than the crease lines because this is one of the areas where facial expression produces wrinkle-lines not quite in the same places as the RSTLs. If the incision is extended laterally (**593**, dotted line), the direction should be changed as shown, in the interests of improved lymphatic drainage and thus of reduced postoperative oedema. This lateral part is likely to be less satisfactory cosmetically and is better avoided.

The skin and subcutaneous tissue are incised, and the orbicularis oculi exposed; the muscle is divided by blunt dissection parallel with its fibre direction and at a different level to the skin incision (higher level as a rule) so that closure may be effected in two stepped layers. The periosteum is divided over the anterior aspect of the inferior orbital rim, and the orbital floor is exposed subperiosteally (**594**), together with the adjacent area of the anterior maxilla, identifying and preserving the emergent infraorbital nerve. Closure is in layers, 4/0 buried catgut in the muscle layer and 5/0 monofilament to skin.

The *subciliary incision,* **592**(b) (also called the blepharoplasty incision), is cosmetically excellent, gives good access to the orbital floor, the lateral orbital wall and rim, the lower medial orbital wall, and the medial half of the zygoma with the upper part of the anterior maxilla. The skin only is incised along the line shown (**595**) about 2mm below the eyelashes and to the extent illustrated. It is dissected by blunt scissors, undermining away from the underlying orbicularis oculi muscle (**596**) to a level coincident with the orbital rim; at this level the muscle layer is incised, the periosteum identified along the whole orbital rim, and then this also is incised onto the anterior maxillary surface.

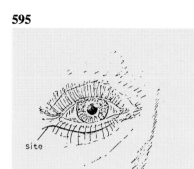

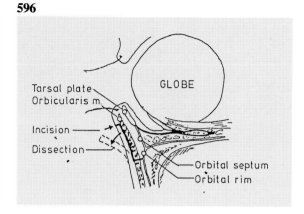

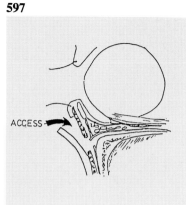

595 to 597   Subciliary incision.

Care must be taken to keep the periosteal incision below the tarsal plate which is displaced beneath a retractor towards the globe during this stage. The orbital floor is next exposed subperiosteally (**597**) to the extent required by the procedure undertaken. The anterior maxilla, zygoma and orbital rims can also be exposed by subperiosteal dissection. Closure is best with a single subcuticular suture (6/0 monofilament), the ends being left free to be withdrawn on the 5th postoperative day. Care must be taken with approximation of the lateral angle of the incision, and a separate suture placed here is worthwhile. Too high an incision, or careless closure, may result in troublesome ectropion.

The *eyebrow incision* (**598** and **599**) is the simplest to perform, incising the skin within the eyebrow and following the curve of the hair, before splitting the muscle parallel with the fibre direction and finally incising the periosteum over the lateral and superior angle of the orbital rim. The lateral part of the orbital roof and the lateral orbital wall is well exposed, but for wider exposure the bifrontal flap should be used. The illustrations are from a traumatic case and show the exposure of a zygomatico-frontal fracture line.

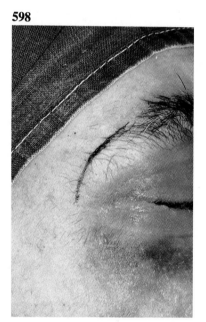
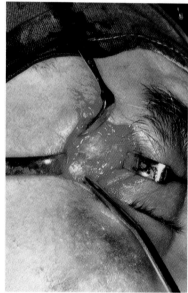

598 and 599   Eyebrow incision.

600 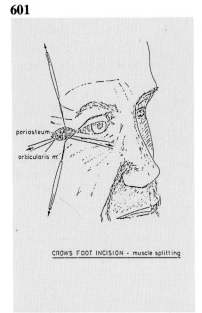 **601** **602**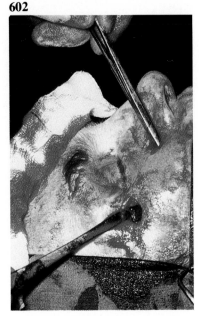

600 to 602   Lateral (crow's foot) incision.

603

603 and 604   Paranasal incision. Lachrymal duct (outlined), and tubercle (arrowed).

604

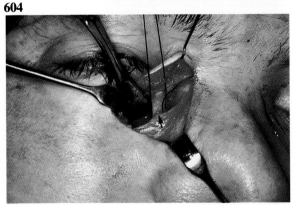

The *lateral (crow's foot) incision* uses the wrinkle-lines that sometimes develop radially from the lateral margin of the orbit (**600**). The muscle layer is split at right angles to the skin incision (**601**). The approach has little part to play in exposure for osteotomy cuts, but is useful (especially in older patients) for the placement of frontal suspension wires following maxillary mobilisation involving also the malar complexes, and for positioning proplast (**602**) or onlaying bone grafts.

The *paranasal incision* is an important access used in the Le Fort 2 osteotomy. The incision is carried through skin in the position shown (**603**), and the muscle layer defined. The external nasal artery is divided on the anterior aspect of the muscle, and the latter is split along the line of its fibres to define the angle between the nasal bone medially and the frontal process of the maxilla laterally. The periosteum is incised along this groove and down onto the anterior maxillary surface. Sharp subperiosteal dissection delivers the periosteum laterally until the anterior lachrymal crest is exposed.

This is followed in a lateral direction until a small thickening of the inferior orbital rim, the lachrymal tubercle, is seen and then further laterally until the infraorbital nerve is defined. The tubercle always overlies the lachrymal duct, which is likely to be in an anomalous position in deformities of this region. Once the duct has been exposed the orbital floor is raised on its lateral aspect, while the lachrymal groove is exposed medially to it. On the lateral margin of the groove the posterior lachrymal crest is dissected out, curving laterally into the orbit and always very thin. The dissection can then be completed behind the lachrymal duct (**604**). The nasal bones, pyriform aperture, glabellar region and anterior maxilla can all be freed subperiosteally and exposed to the dissection from this incision, and the other side can be reached across the nasal bridge when bilateral incisions have been performed.

605

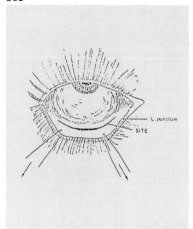

606

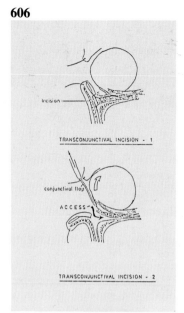

TRANSCONJUNCTIVAL INCISION - 1

TRANSCONJUNCTIVAL INCISION - 2

607

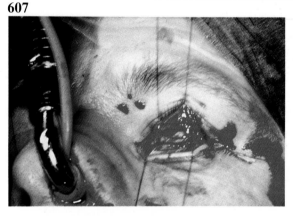

605 to 607 Transconjunctival incision.

The *transconjunctival incision* has been popularised by Tessier (1973) and offers access to the orbital floor, medial and lateral walls, together with some access to the anterior maxilla. It is least satisfactory for the latter, however, and is most useful for simple cuts across the orbital floor connecting medial and lateral osteotomies made via a bifrontal flap. The lower eyelid and conjunctival fornix are retracted with two fixation sutures, medial and lateral (**605**). The conjunctiva is incised after injecting a small amount of 1 in 200,000 noradrenaline solution. The incision runs parallel to the lower border of the tarsal plate about 2 mm below its lower border where the conjunctiva and the orbital septum are closely adherent (**606**). This incision should not start more medially than the lachrymal punctum, and extends laterally for the full length of the eyelid. By blunt dissection the periosteum is exposed along the whole length of the incision and incised, preferably over the orbital rim along the anterior maxillary margin (**606**). Tightness of the lower lid may make this difficult, in which case the incision should be made onto the rim. Subperiosteal dissection then exposes the orbital floor, etc. During the deeper dissection the superior conjunctival flap is retracted over the cornea with fixation sutures to protect the globe (**607**), and the lid is retracted forwards with a large Desmarre's retractor, or with fixation sutures, as in **607**. Closure is by continuous 6/0 monofilament, the knot remaining on the skin.

The technique requires to 'be learnt' because there is a strange sensation beneath the conjunctiva during incision, with an impression of 'bogginess' which misleads the inexperienced into thinking that the knife is not cutting. The tarsal plate must be carefully avoided during downward dissection to the orbital rim, which is palpated ahead of the scalpel. It is possible to leave the conjunctival incision without suture, but if this is done the periosteal layer must be closed carefully with absorbable sutures.

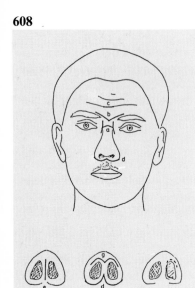

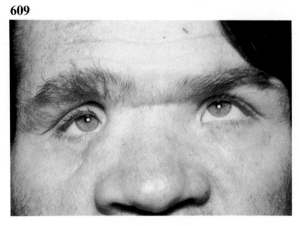

608 **Paranasal and intranasal incisions** for simultaneous maxillary osteotomy and corrective rhinoplasty.

609 **Depressed scar** following a transverse nasal incision.

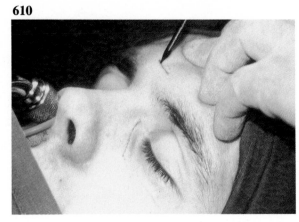

610 **Glabellar 'wrinkle' incisions.**

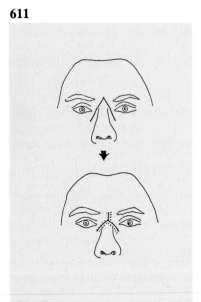

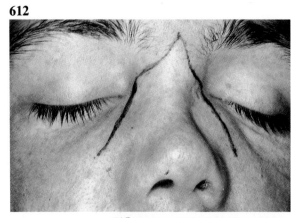

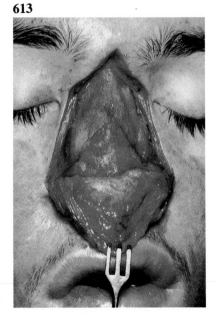

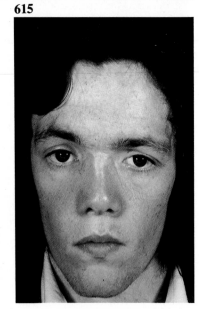

611 to 615 The V-Y incision.

168

Other *paranasal* and *intranasal incisions* of many types have been described and the reader is referred to standard texts on rhinoplasty for a full discussion of the different approaches to the cartilaginous and bony nasal skeleton. However, there are many cases which require both facial osteotomies and corrective rhinoplasty, particularly in the cleft palate group. Several incisions may be used to combine access for simultaneous maxillary osteotomy and first-stage rhinoplasty, and the most useful paranasal and intranasal incisions are illustrated here (**608**).

The H-incision (a) allows access to the nasal bridge and is tempting during Le Fort 2 osteotomy for tailoring the nasal bridge area. Particularly where the nasal skin is tight, the incision provides access to the bridge and the nasal septum; but it is when the skin is tight that the results are likely to be poor because the scar is stretched at its weakest point; indeed skin breakdown can occur. It is a poor incision and longterm scarring is often bad. A case is illustrated (**609**) showing a depressed scar following a transverse nasal incision in a trauma case involving extensive comminution of the nasoethmoidal complex. Small glabellar 'wrinkle' incisions (e.g. as in c) are very useful as a supplementary access during placement of nasal bone grafts in Le Fort 2 cases where the main access is by paranasal incisions of the type described (**603, 604**).

610 shows this combination as a planned access before Le Fort 2 osteotomy, and is one of the most used combinations. The nasal bridge 'flying bird' incision is the access of choice in those Le Fort 2 cases (usually cleft palate cases where maxillary elongation is contemplated) where the osteotomy is to be made anterior to the lachrymal apparatus and is shown at **608** (b). The subnasal 'flying bird' incision, **608**(d), gives useful access to the region of the anterior nasal spine and allows placement of a bone graft to advance this region together with columellar support; during closure skin can be transferred to the columella which may thus be lengthened by the V-Y technique. This is useful in Binder's syndrome. Similarly a mid-columella incision (e) or a vestibular intranasal incision (f) can be used to gain access to the nasal skeleton by subdermal blunt dissection, using curved blunt dissection scissors. Correction of alar deformities is usually performed through a higher 'flying bird' incision as shown at (g).

The V-Y incision (**611** and **612**) has been used by Converse and his co-workers (Converse *et al*, 1970), to assist in nasal lengthening, and may be combined with a variety of perinasal osteotomies, including the Le Fort 2 procedure. It is a poor incision for cosmetic healing (the case shown in **615** is 2 years postoperative), but certainly provides excellent access to the nasal architecture (**613**) and to the lachrymal region (**614**). Closure as a 'Y' increases nasal skin length by transfer from the undermined glabellar skin. It is not recommended where the underlying skeletal area is being advanced under tight nasal bridge skin, as closure may be difficult or impossible without unacceptable tension.

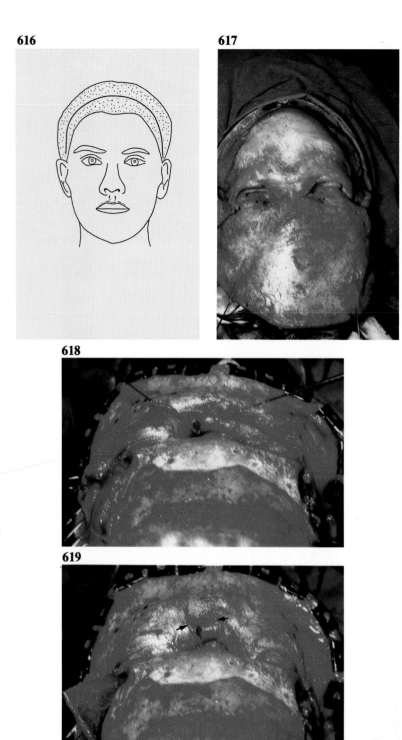

616

617

618

619

The bifrontal flap

This (**616, 617** and **618**) appears at first sight a rather drastic approach; it offers, however, the best access to the orbits, frontal area, and the zygomata, and has the enormous advantage of allowing direct comparison of the two sides so that symmetry can be monitored. It is the incision of choice in the Le Fort 3

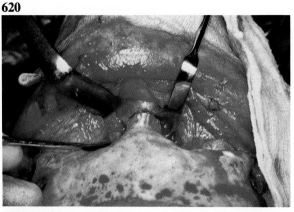

620

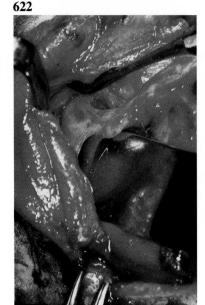

622

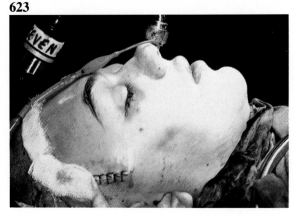

623

616 to 623   The bifrontal flap incision.

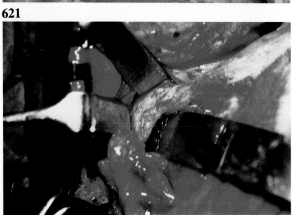

621

group of osteotomies, and provides the standard access for all combined craniofacial procedures.

The incision is made within the hairline and can be directly deepened to bone (**617**) or preferably initially to the pericranium (**618**). The scalp is thus dissected from the pericranium to the supraorbital region, and then, if not already incised, the pericranium is divided and the further dissection is carried over the supraorbital ridges subperiosteally. The supraorbital nerves emerge either through a supraorbital notch (from which they are dissected and thus carried down on the soft tissue flap without interruption) or through a closed foramen. In the latter case the foramen is converted into a notch by chiselling a small wedge of bone from the anterior aspect, and then the nerves can be delivered as before.

Laterally the dissection is carried to the anterior aspect of the temporal crest; the temporalis muscle is then dissected from bone deeply, and from the temporalis fascia superficially (**619** – left side) thus allowing the muscle to be rotated into a new position when the orbital walls are advanced. The periorbital tissues are raised carefully from the orbital roofs as far back as the junction of the posterior and middle thirds, thus securing the safety of the orbital apex. In craniostenotic deformity it must be remembered that the orbits will be very shallow anteroposteriorly, and due allowance made. The periosteum of the orbital roof is very thin and easily split, allowing escape of orbital fat into the incision. If this happens at the early stage of exposure, it is desirable to try to contain the split with a suture. As the dissection is carried down the nasal bones (**620**) the periosteum is divided in the midline to obtain sufficient tissue release (**619**, arrowed), and this completes the development of two triangular flaps of pericranium which can be used to cover any bone grafts or osteotomies in the immediate region of the supraorbital ridges.

Further dissection medially will expose the upper part of the lachrymal grooves, and can be made sufficient to visualise the whole of the medial wall. Laterally, dissecting beneath the temporalis muscle into the temporal fossa, the outside of the lateral orbital wall is exposed (**622**). The whole of the zygoma and zygomatic arch is exposed from the superficial aspect of the muscle, dissecting between the temporalis fascia and the temporalis muscle itself (**621**). Closure of the flap is in two layers, a deep layer of interrupted horizontal mattress sutures and a superficial layer of 3/0 black silk. Suction drains are placed beneath the flap and carried out laterally. The incision is dressed lightly (**623**) before a light pressure bandage is applied.

It is quite possible to expose the orbital floor from this approach (**622**) and thus complete circumorbital cuts entirely from the one incision, but it is often somewhat difficult to do with complete protection of the orbital contents. The author prefers the combination of bifrontal flap with subciliary incision, for full Le Fort 3 osteotomies. However, it is worthwhile exploring the full access from the former before exposing the latter.

SECTION 4

Treatment methods and techniques

Part 2

The techniques of facial bone osteotomy

The word 'osteotomy' will be used throughout the following descriptions as a general descriptive term to include all planned sectioning of the facial bones, including those procedures which involve the removal of a bony segment and which are more precisely termed 'ostectomies'. When a technical ostectomy is under sole discussion it will be described as such.

Corrective surgery of the mandible

Osteotomies of the mandible have been described at every part of the bone in order to achieve forward, backward, or rotational repositioning of the constituent parts relative to one another. A comprehensive review of the literature up to 1960 by Rowe shows many procedures which have fallen into disuse, mainly on account of postoperative instability. The review serves to illustrate both the variety of bony sections attempted and the long history of the field. Those operations which have survived, together with their more modern successors have been shown to be capable of producing stable results when chosen with due regard to the principles of assessment already outlined, especially in relation to the soft-tissue environment.

In this Section the operations found by the author to be most useful are discussed in detail, with briefer indications of some of the alternatives advocated by other surgeons. Many of these alternatives give excellent results and the choice is often one of personal preference. The beginner is advised to master a representative set of techniques properly, and the choice of

procedures singled out in this section is made to assist to that end. The commonly sought mandibular corrections are bilateral advancement or set-back for the correction of mandibular retrusion or protrusion respectively. The relevant techniques can be undertaken unilaterally or in combination to achieve individually tailored results where asymmetry is present; and they can also be combined with maxillary procedures in cases of bimaxillary anomalies.

The surgical alternatives in the mandible are (a) Ramus osteotomies, (b) Body and Angle osteotomies, (c) Anterior segmental and symphyseal procedures, (d) Genioplasty, (e) Condylar surgery, and (f) Camouflage techniques. The last two of this list will be discussed in relation to the treatment of asymmetries (see Section 5), although postcondylar cartilage grafts offer one method of mandibular advancement, and bilateral alloplastic augmentation is occasionally indicated. The ramus, angle, and subapical total alveolar osteotomies achieve movement of the whole dental arch as it stands, while body and anterior osteotomies usually involve interruption of the arch with rearrangement.

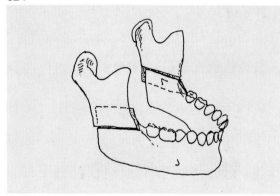

624

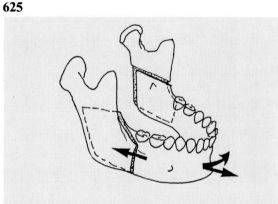

625

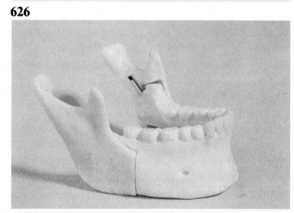

626

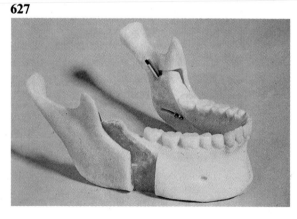

627

Ramus osteotomies

Sagittal splitting was introduced by Trauner and Obwegeser (1957) and by Obwegeser (1964), with later modifications by Dal Pont (1961) and Hunsuck (1968). The natural plane of cleavage between the buccal and lingual cortical plates of the ramus is used to develop a sagittal split separating the proximal (condylar) fragments from the distal (dentoalveolar) fragment.

In the original procedure (**624**) the split was confined to the ramus, but the most commonly practised variant (attributed to Dal Pont) brings the buccal cut downwards and forwards to a variable extent into the molar region (**625**), thereby increasing the area of bone-to-bone contact during the healing period. The cut is started on the medial aspect of the ramus above the lingula, carried down the anterior face and laterally to the lower border (**626**).

After the cortical plates have been split with an osteotome the anterior segment can be drawn forwards (**627**), pushed back (**625**), or rotated. The proximal fragments remain in their preoperative position in the anteroposterior plane (although slight medial or lateral rotation may occur about a vertical axis passing through the condyles). When the anterior segment is advanced a gap is developed in the buccal plate (**627**). When it is set-back a section of buccal plate is removed to allow good approximation of the buccal cortex of the proximal segment against the lingual cortex of the distal segment on each side (**628**).

628

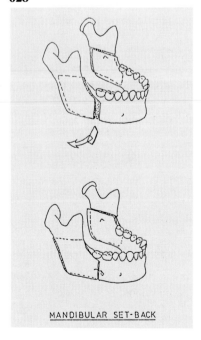

MANDIBULAR SET-BACK

624 to 628   Sagittal splitting.
Original split (**624**); extended split (**625** to **628**).

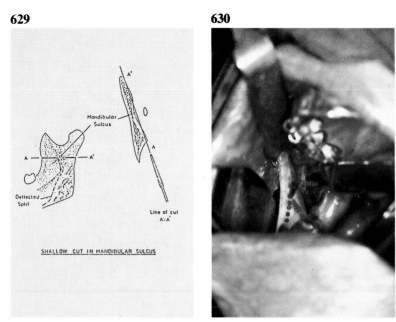

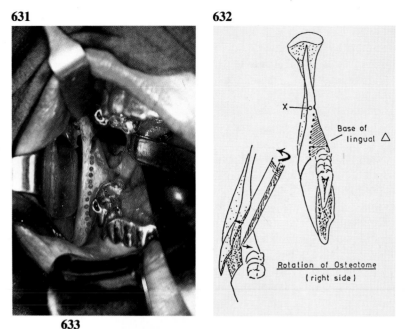

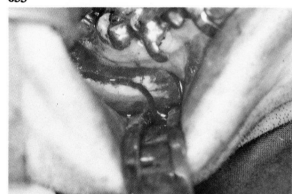

629 to 635 Sagittal splitting: surgical technique.

Technique

Incision and exposure are by intraoral approach to the ramus, medially and laterally, as described on pp. 148 and 149. The incision is carried forwards to the second premolar region, and the ramus is exposed fully with a Ward's third molar retractor laterally, a ramus retractor superiorly, and a long channel retractor medially, placed above the lingula. If desired the internal oblique ridge may be reduced at the level of the lingula to improve visual access to the mandibular sulcus and lingula (**549** and **550**). Good lighting and suction are essential.

Osteotomy (**629** to **635**). The first cut is a horizontal one on the medial aspect above the lingula and carried across the full width of the ramus through the cortex only. A Lindemann pattern spiral bur is ideal for this purpose, but must be allowed to 'find its own' cutting pressure while being moved gently backwards and forwards in the manner of a saw. Some prefer the Meisinger tapered fissure bur on a long shank, and others use a reciprocating air-driven saw. Care is taken to ensure that the cut is carried through the cortex in the region of the mandibular sulcus as the curvature may leave this area further from the long axis of the bur, resulting in incomplete cortical division behind and above the lingula (**629**). This will result in a split deflected down the medial aspect of the ramus along the mylohyoid groove or otherwise short of the posterior border (as intended in the 'short lingual split' modification, see pp. 174 and 175).

The lingual cut appears anteriorly through the internal oblique ridge (**630**). The second cut is carried down the anterior aspect of the ramus obliquely across the retromolar triangle to the commencement of the vertical buccal limb (if preferred the buccal cut can be made as the second cut and the

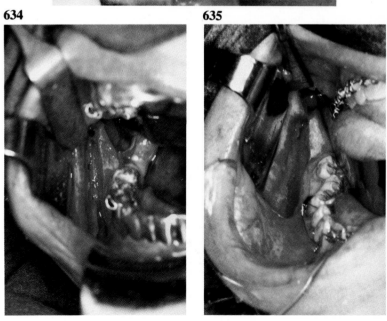

anterior section made to join the medial and buccal cuts last – the result is the same, but time may be saved by retaining the long bur for the buccal cut directly after the medial one). It is advantageous to mark this out with a spear-point drill first (**631**) connecting the holes with a Toller surgical fissure bur afterwards. In this way the tendency to 'wander' is avoided, and guidance of the handpiece by contact with the teeth or splints prevented. Only the cortex is penetrated, and care is taken to maintain a wide base to the lingual triangle of bone marked in the diagram (**632**) to minimise the danger of breaking off the lingual plate during splitting.

Similarly the strength of the buccal plate is maintained by preserving an adequate thickness of bone at the level of the medial cut (site marked X in diagram **632**). During splitting, the osteotome can thus be rotated while inserted in the anterior cut, rotation being anticlockwise on the right and clockwise on the left, always bearing on the stronger bony base.

The buccal cut is designed to achieve maximum bone-to-bone contact after the distal segment has been repositioned, which means that the extent of the split must be balanced against the feasibility of close apposition of the fragments. Too forward a cut may defeat the object if the angulation of ramus to body drives the anterior end of the proximal fragment out laterally after the distal fragment has been advanced (the problem is less in set-back operations). In general union is good with quite small degrees of overlap, and the buccal cut is better placed more posteriorly than too far forwards. In set-back procedures the first/second molar contact is usually about right, the section overlying the second molar itself being partially or wholly removed for the recession of the anterior fragment (**628**). In advancement procedures this is usually too far forwards, especially if there is much outward flare of the rami, and a cut made at the 2nd/3rd molar contact is about right. Alternatively the cut in either case can be moved to any position as far as the original Obwegeser/Trauner site (**624**).

The buccal cut is made with a channel retractor hooked under the lower border to protect and retract the soft-tissues (**633**). The cut is carried vertically to the lower border to the midpoint of the linguo-buccal width inferiorly, just penetrating the thickness of the cortex throughout. The dentoalveolar neurovascular bundle may be closely applied to the inner surface of the buccal cortical plate at a vertical level best assessed by reference to the radiographs. More nerves are damaged accidentally at the buccal cut than at the medial, or during splitting. The three component parts of the long cortical osteotomy (medial, anterior and buccal) have now been completed and are checked to confirm that the cortex is divided along the entire length, particularly where the parts of the cut connect together. A small cortical bridge of bone will prevent or misdirect splitting.

Either a slim but wide osteotome or thick one with acute bevels at the cutting edge may be used, according to preference, to split the mandibular ramus sagittally between the buccal and lingual cortical plates. A thick, acutely bevelled osteotome driven sharply between the cortices will usually effectively split the two apart by a 'wedge' action and is the recommended method. Others prefer to use a slim osteotome and progressively advance it through the plates. In both methods the osteotome should be directed laterally against the inner aspect of the outer cortex to minimise trauma to the neurovascular bundle, thus separating it towards the lingual cortex so that it is kept safely on the distal segment of bone.

Once the split has been started the osteotomes should be rotated as described previously (**632**) and the two cortices opened like the leaves of a book while the position of the nerve is determined (**634**). It will often be seen lying in the medulla between the plates, running from superomedially to inferolaterally. At other times (**635**) it will be closely adherent to the inner aspect of the buccal cortex, or even partially enclosed by a bony canal attached to the buccal cortex. On rare and unfortunate occasions it may be completely contained in a bony tunnel on the buccal cortex. Once identified the bundle must be dissected free from the buccal cortex and delivered over to the lingual side to move *en bloc* with the distal segment, backwards or forwards.

Where a bony overhang prevents access to the nerve (as in the anterior part of the split in **635**) a sharp chisel is used to open the roof of the bony canal and gain access to the nerve. At this stage the fragments are fully separated and the depths of the split examined. Any remaining bony spicules or soft-tissue connections between the cortices are detached especially at the posterior border, and an Obwegeser stripper is used through the split to finalise separation of periosteum from the posterior border. Separation of the medial pterygoid muscle from the medial aspect of the ramus is now attempted from the lingual side. Sometimes this is difficult and this difficulty is the author's main reason for preferring the short lingual split technique.

The short lingual split modification has been described by Dal Pont (1961) and by Hunsuck (1968), with recent improvements by Epker (1978) although the latter differs from the author in the treatment of the soft-tissues (*vide infra*). The observation that inadequate sectioning of the medial cortex at the mandibular sulcus leads to a deflected split which may adopt one of several directions but most commonly follows the mylohyoid groove (**636**), led to attempts to produce this modified split deliberately in an effort to avoid displacement of the musculature attached to the ramus.

If the sagittal split is carried out exactly as described above except that the medial cut is carried only as far as the area immediately above and behind the lingula and mandibular

636

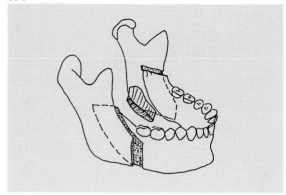

637

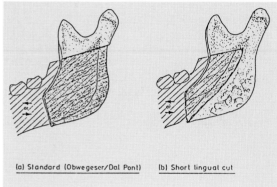

(a) Standard (Obwegeser/Dal Pont)   (b) Short lingual cut

638

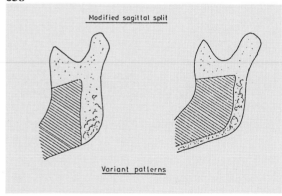

Modified sagittal split

Variant patterns

636 to 640   **The short lingual split.**

639

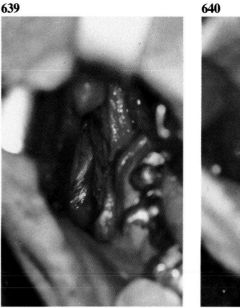

640

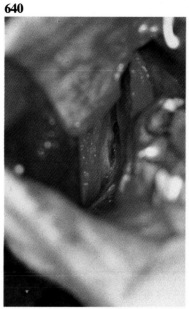

foramen, then the split almost always occurs in the modified form (**637**); nothing is lost if it occasionally travels back to the posterior border as for the full sagittal split. Other common variations in the direction of the split are shown in **638**. The medial pterygoid attachment remains untouched on the medial aspect of the mandible until the split is completed (**639**), when it is detached under direct vision *through the split*, (**640**).

This often requires considerable effort with a sharp dissector, and indicates the unreliability of attempting detachment 'blind' as in the standard procedure. It is important that the muscle be detached; if the mandible is to be set-back there must be space for the medial overlap, and if advanced there must be freedom for the periosteum to slide round the proximal segment or it will introduce an inextensible tether against the advancing distal segment. All periosteal tenting is eliminated. This procedure (carried out as described above) is in the author's opinion the procedure of choice for mandibular set-back, and for advancement provided the ramus is of good width (anteroposteriorly). In set-back cases it has the advantages of easy execution, less backward displacement of bone behind the ramus, easier detachment of the medial pterygoid, and probably greater stability.

The problem of the periosteal investment, which gives attachment to the pterygomasseteric group of soft-tissues, has already been identified (Section 2), and the question raised as to whether the periosteal envelope should be divided during intraoral sagittal splitting of the mandible. On the one hand there is some logic in opening the envelope along the posterior, angular and inferior borders to allow uninterrupted passage of repositioned bony fragments through the resulting gaps without tension. On the other hand, division of the periosteum in these circumstances involves scalpel dissection under relatively poor conditions of light and access through the mandibular split. Several moderately sized vessels lie immediately deep to this periosteum and if divided accidentally retract into the tissues away from the scalpel.

Control of bleeding may be difficult and the procedure undoubtedly increases postoperative oedema and haematoma formation in the parapharyngeal region. There is no evidence that later scarring is not as serious a source of postoperative contraction in the periosteal gaps as the original tension, although division of the periosteum seems effective in releasing tension at other sites. Therefore, when conditions of access are good but tension likely, division is recommended. The two cortices are stretched away from each other tensing the posterior and inferior periosteum, which is lightly stroked with the scalpel until divided along its entire length.

For most cases reliance is placed on the short split technique for set-back procedures (thus minimising periosteal tenting), and on wide soft-tissue detachment (allowing periosteal glide) in advancements.

In advancement cases no further bony work is required; the dentoalveolar fragment is brought forward into the planned occlusion developing a gap in the buccal plate (**626** and **627**) and fixed. When the mandible is to be set-back there is an overlap after the distal segment has been brought into its planned occlusion, and the overlapping bone is cut off after intermaxillary fixation has been temporarily applied. This is best done in the mouth at this stage, although some prefer to remove a planned segment marked out with a template prepared preoperatively. Minor rotations not predicted accurately often invalidate precise preoperative templates and it is preferable to tailor the cuts in the mouth. It is essential to maintain the proximal fragment in its correct position (condyle in the glenoid fossa and no forward rotation) while this is done.

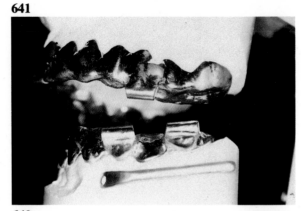

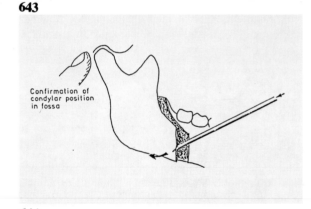

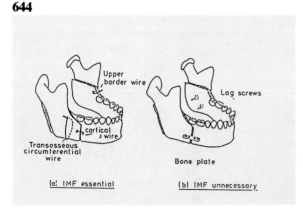

641 and 642 **Intermaxillary fixation:** Pin and tube system.

643 **Maintaining position of the posterior fragment.**

644 **Internal osteosynthesis.**

Fixation presents few special problems. Two aspects present separately, internal osteosynthesis and intermaxillary fixation. In general it is preferable to fix the teeth together in the planned occlusal correction, and the methods of arch bar fixation, cast cap splints or previously applied orthodontic fixed appliances are equally good, having advantages and disadvantages.

The author uses either arch wiring or orthodontic bands as a first choice, but also likes cast cap splints with a split tube and pin method of rapid IMF which can be applied, removed for pharyngeal toilet and pack clearance, and reapplied without loss of time. The pin system is shown (**641** and **642**), but has the disadvantage that the tubes may get in the way of closure after application of splints and before surgery.

Control of the posterior segments may also be achieved in several ways. Two requirements must be met. The condyle must remain in the glenoid fossa in its normal position (apart from minor rotations about the vertical axis introduced deliberately). There must be no forward rotation of the posterior (proximal) fragment allowing the segment to rise anteriorly around a transverse condylar axis, a real danger in advancement procedures. If forward translation occurs the planned degree of anterior movement will not, and when fixation is removed from the teeth the condyle will return to the fossa presenting an appearance of immediate relapse. The sequence of fixation is therefore to place the IMF first, securing the correct relationship of the anterior mandible to the maxilla, and second to position the posterior fragment correctly with the condyle palpably in the glenoid fossa, and forward rotation resisted by distal pressure on the front of the buccal cortical plate of the fragment (**643**). The fragments are then wired together. The possibilities for internal osteosynthesis are shown (**644**), and include upper border wiring, transosseous circumferential wiring, cortical wiring and bone plating. The use of lag screws through both cortical plates is much used in Europe.

The author advocates two methods, one for set-back procedures and one for advancements, and these are shown in **645** and **646**. The set-back (**645**) is secured by a figure-of-eight cortical wire, easy to apply as the wire is placed through corresponding holes in the buccal plates of both segments from the external surface of the bone. For advancements the method recently described by Epker (1978) and used by the author for over a decade is most reliable (**646**). Holes are drilled anteriorly on the proximal fragment through the buccal plate, and posteriorly on the distal fragment through the lingual plate. A direct upper border wire is applied through these two holes and tightened after IMF is in place. This pulls the condyle back into its proper position directly, and works well provided IMF is used to supplement it.

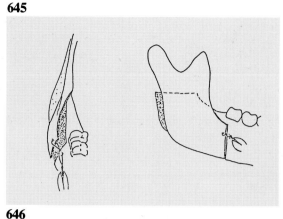

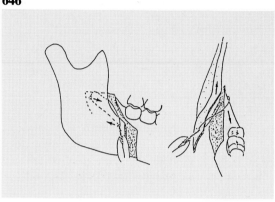

645 and 646 **Internal osteosynthesis:** method for set-back procedures (**645**) and for advancements (**646**).

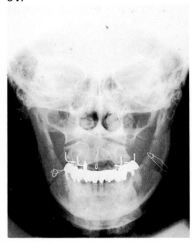

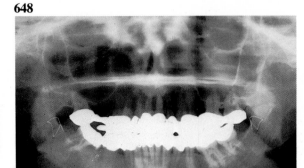

647 Upper border wire on the right; **transosseous circumferential wire** on the left.

648 Upper border wiring and splints.

649 Bilateral plating.

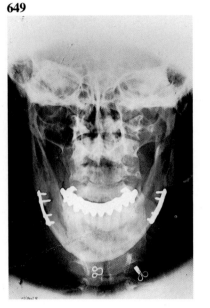

Intraoral bone plating is technically difficult, the screws being applied through stab incisions in the skin, as are lag screws. IMF may not be necessary after the application of plates or lag screws, but must be applied during their placement. Unfortunately many of these devices require removal a few months later, and for this reason are not recommended.

Postoperative radiographs illustrate the wiring and plating methods. **647** shows a case of bilateral mandibular advancement secured on the right by an upper border wire and on the left by a transosseous circumferential wire. The latter brings the two cortical plates into good apposition but allows rotation around the hole in the buccal plate; it is effective with IMF, but the long wire often requires removal a few months postoperatively. **648** shows a typical bilateral advancement secured by upper border wiring and splints, while bilateral plating is shown in **649**. The IMF was released in the plated case soon after operation and the jaws allowed to function freely.

At operation the figure-of-eight cortical wire can be seen to hold the buccal cortex of the proximal fragment in good apposition with the distal fragment (**650**). This case illustrates the use of orthodontic banding applied during the preoperative phase of orthodontic preparation.

650

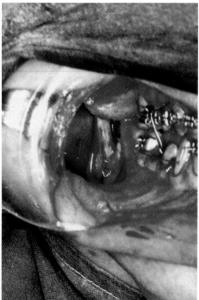

650 Figure-of-eight cortical wire.

Postoperative swelling is sometimes severe after sagittal splitting (**651**),and may be due to oedema or haematoma formation. The latter can be significantly reduced by the use of vacuum drains inserted below the lower border of the ramus well away from the intraoral incision, and brought out below the angle of the mandible through a stab incision (**652**). The use of steroids perioperatively certainly reduces oedema. The increased speed which comes with experience markedly diminishes the amount of postoperative swelling which is clearly exacerbated by prolonged retraction and operative manipulation.

Indications for sagittal splitting of the mandible

1. *Mandibular retrusion.* The modified sagittal split (short lingual cut) is the operation of choice when the ramus is wide and the full split when it is narrow, and in both cases can be combined with genioplasty carried out simultaneously allowing wide detachment of soft-tissue. Alternative operations are the inverted L-osteotomy with bone grafting and the C-osteotomy, which are both best carried out extraorally, and are indicated when intraoral access is poor (see, for example, **688** to **692**).

2. *Mandibular protrusion (prognathism),* of the horizontal growth pattern, but not in the presence of anterior open bite (unless carried out as part of a bimaxillary correction aimed at correction of vertical dysplasias). The main alternative is vertical subsigmoid (or for some operators oblique subcondylar osteotomies) with the disadvantage of an avoidable extraoral scar. For set-back procedures the short split modification is recommended. Displacement of large degree is always more likely to be unstable than small degree, and if movement in excess of 15–20 mm is contemplated, bimaxillary alternatives should be considered. Other factors must be taken into account. A large mandible with concomitant soft-tissue enlargement, a low tongue posture, and normal gonial and SM:MP angles may well take a 20 mm set-back, while 15 mm might be maximum for a narrow ramus, high angle, high tongue posture case.

3. *Mandibular asymmetry* usually requires operation bilaterally and often in the maxilla also, but unilateral or bilateral sagittal splitting is useful to obtain rotations and other asymmetric adjustments of mandibular shape.

4. *Compensatory repositioning of the occlusal plane* is sometimes necessary to allow other osteotomies to take place especially vertical adjustments in the mid-face. Short split sagittal splitting is suitable provided no increase in ramus length is involved.

651

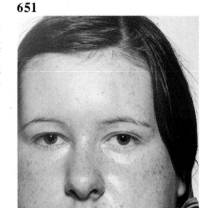

651 Postoperative swelling after sagittal splitting.

652 Insertion of vacuum drain to reduce haematoma formation.

652

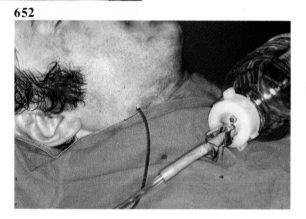

Correction of mandibular protrusion by bilateral sagittal splitting of the rami and set-back is illustrated in **653** to **657** which show the typical profile changes of mandibular set-back procedures, whether carried out in the ramus or body. A balanced improvement in facial appearance occurs combined with correction of the malocclusion (not illustrated here).

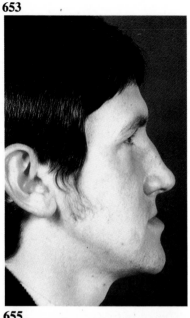

653

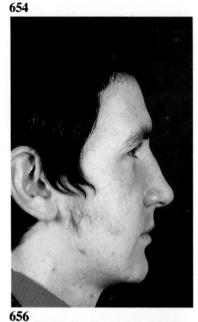

654

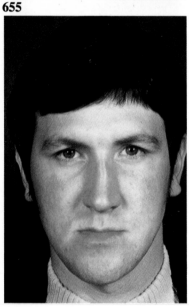

655

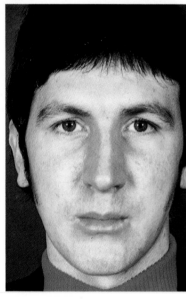

656

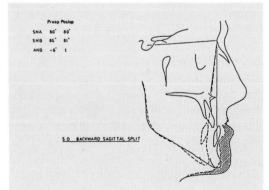

657

Profile changes associated with mandibular set-back (657):

1. The stomion moves down and lingually.

2. Hence the upper lip *lengthens and straightens*, and the nasolabial angle increases.

3. More vermilion border shows on the upper lip and less on the lower lip.

4. The projection of the upper lip (F point) falls back by about 1mm–2mm (rarely more, regardless of the amount of set-back).

5. The soft-tissue pogonion and soft-tissue supramentale fall back in a 1:1 proportion with the hard-tissue counterparts (Po and B point), but the lower lip is held forwards by contact with the upper incisors, thus only moving about two thirds to three quarters of the movement of the lower incisor tips.

6 Hence the concavity of the labiomental curve is increased.

Correction of mandibular retrusion by bilateral sagittal splitting of the rami and advancement of the dentoalveolar segment (**658** to **664**) produces very satisfying results and represents the operation of choice. Stability is more difficult to ensure than with set-back procedures and over-correction or prolonged fixation is advisable. The occlusal correction is shown here (**662** and **663**) together with the typical profile changes of advancement (**658** and **659**). To some extent the latter can be simulated preoperatively by forward posturing of the mandible, but this can be misleading by producing a posterior open bite as a result of incisal guidance.

Profile changes associated with mandibular advancement:

1. No effect on the upper lip. This is only true when a straight anteroposterior movement is carried out. Superadded vertical or rotational movements may modify this statement. Discussed on p. 282.

2. The stomion is advanced and may be lowered.

653 to 657   Correction of mandibular protrusion by bilateral sagittal splitting and set-back (**653** and **655,** before operation; profile changes, **657**).

658

659

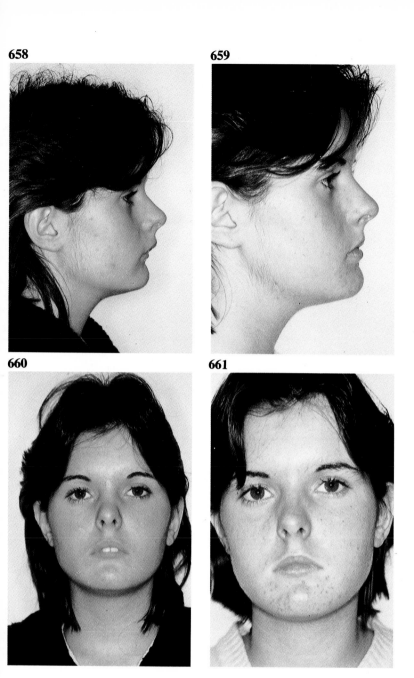

660

661

662

663

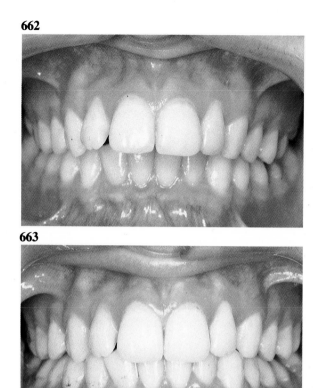

658 to 664   Correction of mandibular retrusion by
bilateral sagittal splitting and advancement (**658, 660,
662** before operation; profile changes, **664**).

664

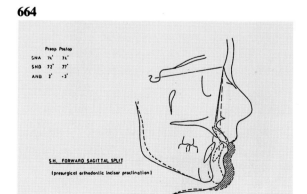

	Preop	Postop
SNA	76°	76°
SNB	72°	77°
ANB	2°	-3°

S.H. FORWARD SAGITTAL SPLIT

(presurgical orthodontic incisor proclination)

3. The pogonion and B point are matched 1:1 with the soft-tissues (soft-tissue pogonion and supramentale). This may be modified if a genioplasty is carried out at the same time, a common requirement (**668** to **670**).

4. The lower lip (H point) is advanced less than the chin and supramentale, usually about two thirds of the movement of the lower incisor tip. Hence the concavity of the labio-mental curve is reduced, especially if there was the typical rolled forward lower lip when caught below the protruding upper incisors, as in the case shown in **328** to **331**. The less the preoperative roll, the nearer to a 1:1 change occurs; occasionally a flat lip will show an improved curvature by increasing the concavity.

5. The vermilion of the upper lip exposure is decreased while more vermilion comes into view in the lower lip (which is seen in the full face view also).

6. In cases with a low SN:MP angle the lower facial height is increased but not in high angle cases. This patient in fact is neither high nor low and facial height is only marginally affected by advancement (see also pp. 100 to 103).

This patient underwent presurgical orthodontics to expand the maxillary arch and correct the proclination of the upper incisors. The latter is seen in the postoperative tracing together with the effect on the upper lip of this orthodontic movement. It is seen to be slight but definite and confined to the lower part of the lip (**664**).

A common combination of procedures in the correction of Class 2 division 1 cases is that of forward sagittal split and premaxillary set-back, the latter usually by the Wassmund technique. Such a case is illustrated here (**665** to **667**). Presurgical orthodontic treatment had failed as the lower lip constantly worked under the upper incisors. During the patient's 17th year, therefore, a preliminary anterior segmental procedure was carried out, setting the lower labial segment down by 3mm and back by 8mm with extraction of the first lower premolars. This was combined with a premaxillary set-back (by the Epker downfracture method) elevating the premaxilla by 3mm and setting it back by 8mm, again with extraction of first premolars. Three months later the mandible was advanced by forward sagittal split and the total correction is shown in profile and tracing. This kind of combined anterior segmental and ramus surgery is often necessary and can produce very pleasing and balanced results.

When mandibular advancement is combined with augmentation genioplasty, as in the case shown in **668** to **670,** the profile effects are those of the combined procedures by simple summation of effects. The increase at the soft-tissue pogonion is usually that of the mandibular advancement (bilateral forward sagittal split in this case) plus about 4mm–6mm due to the forward sliding genioplasty (as here). Other types of

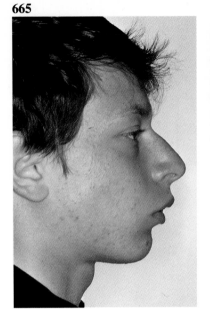

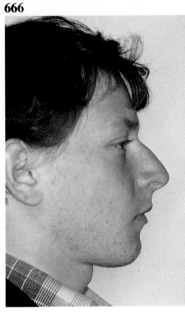

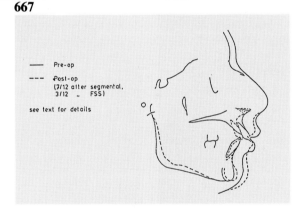

665 to 667   Class 2 division 1 case (**665**) corrected by forward sagittal split **with preliminary segmental surgery.**

genioplasty will vary the effect (see p. 216 et seq. for a discussion of chin management). The soft-tissue supramentale tends to be affected also by the genioplasty, moving forwards by about 1mm in excess of the movement caused by the mandibular advancement. Some retroclination of the upper incisors has occurred postoperatively, without orthodontic activation.

Ramus osteotomies

The vertical subsigmoid osteotomy is one of the simplest mandibular osteotomies to perform and enjoys wide popularity. The approach may be extraoral or intraoral, although slightly different principles apply to the two approaches. In both cases the bony cuts are the same (**671**), the object being to

668

669

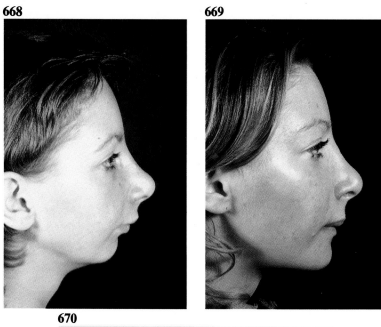

670

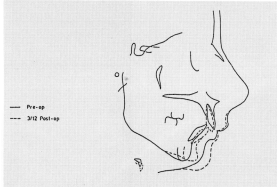

— Pre-op
--- 3/12 Post-op

668 to 670 **Mandibular advancement combined with augmentation genioplasty** (**668,** before operation).

671

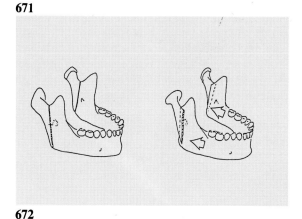

672

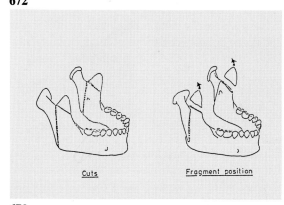

Cuts   Fragment position

673

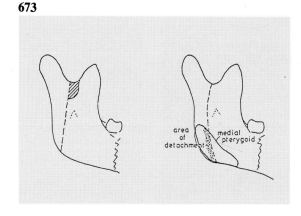

area of detachment   medial pterygoid

671 **Vertical subsigmoid osteotomy.**

672 **Coronoidotomy.**

673 **Moule modification** (left) and **Walker modification** (right).

move the distal segment backwards with the proximal segments overlapping laterally. The procedure is better for set-back cases although an interpositional bone graft can be used to increase ramal width and advance the distal segment. The inverted-L osteotomy is preferred for advancement cases, see p. 187.

It is hoped to maintain the proximal fragments in the preoperative position although most operators concede that some forward rotation occurs. When the distal segment is set-back there is frequently some resistance, partly due to impaction of the coronoid process on the proximal fragment, and partly due to muscle pull from the temporalis muscle attached to the coronoid process. Coronoidotomy (**672**) is recommended in these circumstances, and indeed there is an argument for employing it in all cases. It should certainly be used when there is a major set-back (1 cm plus). Coronoidotomy effectively removes the influence of the temporalis on the distal segment; some think this a good thing, while others argue that the natural balance of muscle forces is upset and may induce relapse or temporomandibular joint dysfunction.

The author feels that coronoidotomy is advisable in *all* vertical subsigmoid procedures where the slightest resistance to repositioning the distal segment is experienced.

A further modification introduced by Moule of Manchester is seen in **673**. The shaded area of bone in the region of the sigmoid notch is removed when this area impacts on the proximal fragment during repositioning. This is not uncommon, and careful observation of the area of resistance will show when the modification is appropriate. It is not recommended as a routine.

Finally, the most recent modification, attributed to Walker by Bell (1980) is especially applicable to the intraoral approach. This involves a slight curvature to the vertical line of osteotomy designed to clear the region of the mandibular foramen on the medial aspect but to allow a reasonable (about 1 cm) amount of bone at the lower border (**673**). In theory this allows a wider pedicle of medial pterygoid muscle to be left attached to the proximal fragment – *vide infra*. However, there are many cases when the shape of the mandible renders this a token exercise only. Nevertheless it is a worthwhile shape of cut and is recommended where appropriate.

Technique

Incision and exposure may be either extraoral or intraoral.

(a) *Extraoral.* This is the traditional approach and offers good access with an opportunity to divide the pterygomasseteric tissues with good access and also the chance of contouring the angle of the mandible under direct vision. The submandibular approach (see pp. 160 to 163) is used, keeping to the area below the ramus. The whole of the lateral aspect of the ramus is exposed subperiosteally, although the posterior margin is not freed, in order to maintain as large a soft-tissue pedicle as possible to aid blood supply to the proximal fragment (Bell and Kennedy, 1976).

For the same reason minimal detachment of the medial pterygoid insertion at the lower part of the ramus on the medial aspect is undertaken from below, to allow a slim protector to be passed towards the sigmoid notch. A retractor with the handle bent at an angle to the instrument and having a tip which can be hooked into the sigmoid notch above is essential; The Rayne retractor or the Henderson Long Channel retractor are suitable, the latter having a long handle at a less acute angle but the length suffices to prevent obstruction of the operator's view. Fibreoptic illumination along these retractors (as in the Withington patterns) is also very helpful. A small elevation on the lateral aspect of the ramus commonly indicates the position of the lingula on the medial side – the so-called antilingular prominence.

(b) *Intraoral.* The ramus is exposed as for sagittal splitting. For intraoral vertical ramus procedures special retractors are available to hook round the posterior border, sigmoid notch, or antegonial notch, and it is important that the design holds the soft-tissues away from the ramus during manipulation and osteotomy.

674

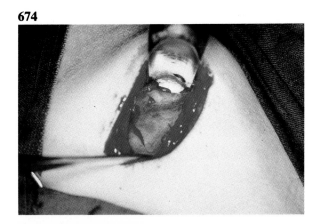

675

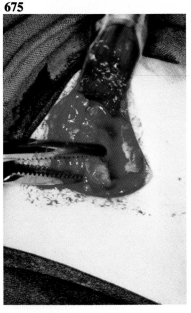

674 to 677 Vertical subsigmoid osteotomy: surgical technique.

676

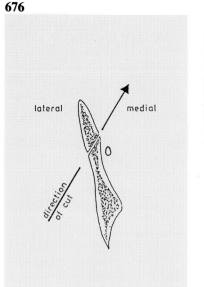

677

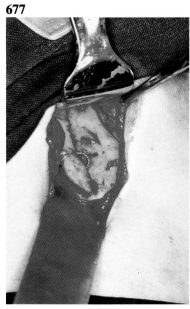

678

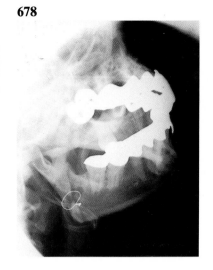

679

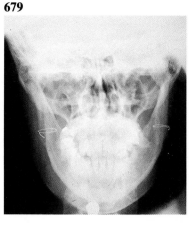

678 and 679   Postoperative radiographs.

Osteotomy. In **674** the exposure of the ramus is seen and the position of the antilingular prominence. The vertical cut is made from the depth of the sigmoid notch above to the angle below, tailoring the angulation to the case, but always keeping posterior to the position of the lingula. The cut may be curved or straight and should be angled transversely towards the posterior pharynx to achieve a bevel in the direction of the proposed movement of the anterior fragment (**675** and **676**). Some operators prefer to decorticate the distal fragment below the proposed overlap, in order to expedite union, but it is not essential. The medial pterygoid is separated from the proximal fragment in the area of overlap only, maintaining a pedicle of muscle behind that area (**673**).

Bell and his co-workers (1976) maintain that this muscle pedicle is sufficient to maintain contact of the fragments, but most prefer to wire the fragments together. The positioning of the wire holes will vary from case to case. If a coronoidotomy is *planned* the cut is made with a bur or saw before the vertical cut is completed, as this makes separation of the coronoid fragment easier; some use an osteotome for this cut. The bur or reciprocating saw is used for the vertical cut itself. When the approach is intraoral a special rightangled curved saw blade is almost essential (Stryker pattern). In other respects the cuts are the same. **678** and **679** show postoperative radiographs which indicate the osteotomy well. IMF is applied prior to any internal fixation of the proximal to the distal segments.

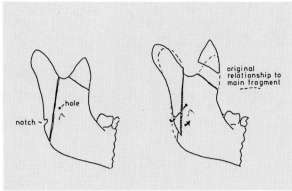

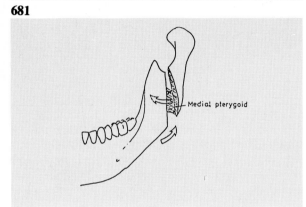

680 Interosseous fixation for vertical subsigmoid osteotomy.

681 The medial pterygoid maintaining bony contact in the intraoral approach.

Fixation follows the usual pattern of intermaxillary fixation, by any preferred method, supplemented by interosseous wires. The condyle tends to remain in position for backward displacements of the mandible in the correction of protrusion, but wiring is *essential* in all other cases; if the ramus is increased in length by more than a few millimetres it is essential, and the distal hole is drilled 3mm anterior to the osteotomy after protection of the neurovascular bundle. A notch is made at a lower level in the condylar fragment (**680**) and the wire passed as shown. This method secures the condylar fragment in an upward and backward position ensuring that there is no distraction from the glenoid fossa. The wire is passed round the posterior border through the soft-tissues without further detachment of the muscle pedicle (**680**). In intraoral cases the attached remnant of the medial pterygoid is relied upon to maintain bony contact (**681**); a wire can be placed from the intraoral approach only with difficulty. The soft-tissues are closed in layers without tight approximation of the pterygo-

masseteric tissues (extraorally); in the intraoral approach the periosteum should be split where necessary to relax periosteal tension.

Indications for vertical subsigmoid osteotomy (VSO)

These are very similar to the sagittal split in the treatment of mandibular protrusion, and there is little apart from personal preference to determine which is undertaken. The sagittal split is preferable in the treatment of mandibular retrusion unless it is desired to increase the mandibular width and/or length with a bone graft, when the inverted-L is probably the better choice. The author considers the main indications for VSO are:

1. *Mandibular protrusion (prognathism)* with a prenormal incisor relationship and a wide ramus (at least three times the extent of the proposed set-back), with no element of anterior open bite. Best cases are those with mandibular enlargement and concomitant soft-tissue excess.

2. *Mandibular protrusion or retrusion* with restricted intraoral access making sagittal splitting technically difficult or impossible.

3. Cases where there is a need for *contouring* the *shape* of the angle or even adding bone laterally.

Comparison of VSO with sagittal split:

VSO	Sagittal Split
More suitable for set-back than advancement.	Suitable for set-back or advancement.
Stability as for sagittal split.	Stability as for VSO.
Less danger of damage to inferior dental nerve and more danger of damage to facial nerve (extraoral).	Slightly greater danger of damage to ID nerve (but probably not with experience of the technique). Minor danger to facial nerve.
Extraoral scar (EO only).	No external scar.
Allows direct division of pterygomasseteric sling.	Division confined to periosteum.
Simple technique.	Technique requires more learning.
Less bone-to-bone contact.	More bone-to-bone contact.
Allows shaping of angle by extraoral approach.	No contouring of angle possible.

Correction of mandibular protrusion by vertical subsigmoid osteotomy shows changes in facial form almost identical to those obtained with other ramus procedures, apart from the external scar in cases approached extraorally. The profile

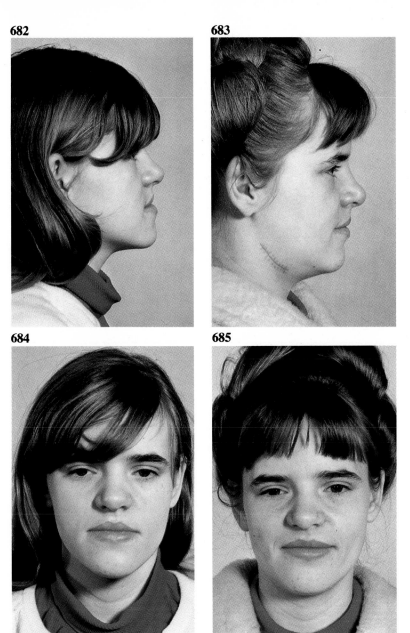

682   **683**

684   **685**

682 to 685   **Mandibular protrusion** (**682** and **684**) **corrected** by vertical subsigmoid osteotomy.

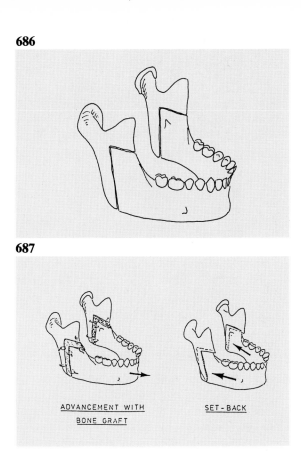

686

687

ADVANCEMENT WITH BONE GRAFT   SET-BACK

686 and 687   **Inverted L-osteotomy.**

changes are therefore the same as those described for backward sagittal splitting. The case illustrated (**682** to **685**) shows early scarring at the 'red stage', and this settles into the creases of the neck quite inconspicuously in the majority of cases.

The inverted-L osteotomy (**686**) was introduced by Trauner and Obwegeser in 1957 and is particularly suited to mandibular advancement where there is deficient ramal width (**687**). The operation is essentially a variant of the vertical subsigmoid, and maintains muscular attachments to the proximal fragments although the periosteum may require splitting for advancements and the medial pterygoid must be partially detached for set-backs. Where the jaw is brought forward L-shaped cortico-cancellous grafts are cut from the ileum with a preformed template, and inserted upside down into the defects in the mandibular rami.

During set-back procedures the proximal fragments overlap the distal fragment laterally, as in the VSO (**687**). The grafts are wired by direct interosseous wires after placement of IMF. Displacement of the distal segment forwards is usually easy, but backward movement may require some tailoring of the bone contact at the level of the horizontal cut. Careful model planning helps to avoid trouble here, and is also useful in the production of accurate templates. A bone graft may substantially recontour the deficient angle in micrognathic cases (see **689**). Access is the same as that for the VSO, being either intraoral or extraoral, preferably the latter.

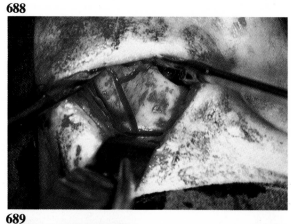

688

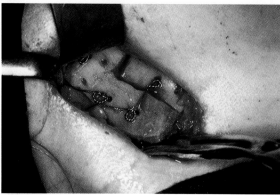

689

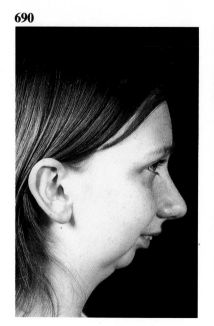

690

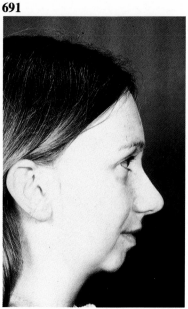

691

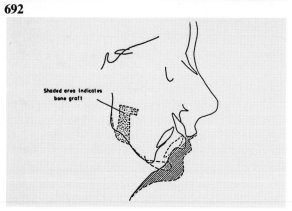

692

Shaded area indicates bone graft

688 to 692   Correction of mandibular hypoplasia by inverted-L osteotomy (and augmentation genioplasty) (**690,** before operation).

Indications for inverted-L osteotomy

1. *Mandibular hypoplasia* where the mandibular rami are deficient both vertically and horizontally (the soft-tissue investment being adequate, or capable of stimulated growth). The case illustrated (**688** to **692**) shows a girl suffering from Still's disease in whom mandibular opening and neck movements were very limited mainly due to involvement of the cervical spine, but joint movement in the TMJ was potentially good. The operative pictures (**688** and **689**) show the placement of the bone graft and the effect on profile is clear. An augmentation genioplasty was performed at the same time. (Joint operation with K.F. Moos, Esq). The profile changes (**692**) are very similar to those for forward sagittal split plus genioplasty, and indeed all ramus movements have a similar profile effect, forward or backward. However, the angle contour is better than would be obtained by any other method.

2. *Mandibular protrusion* as an alternative to VSO, especially when intraoral access is difficult (using the extraoral approach).

693

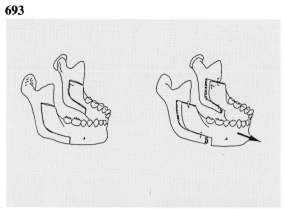

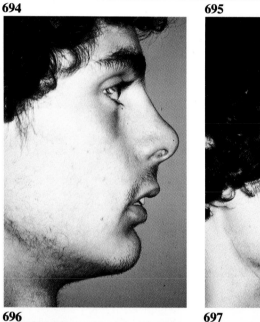

694

695

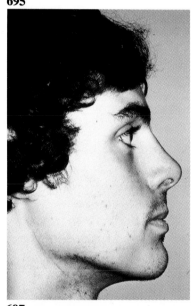

696

697

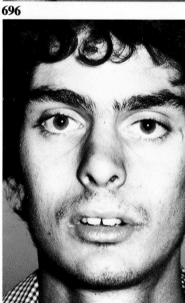

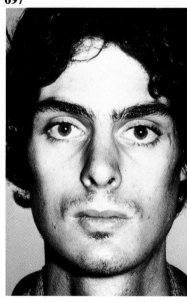

Other ramus osteotomies include the C-osteotomy (**693**) popularised by Caldwell, Hayward and Lister (1968) which is performed extraorally; and the oblique subcondylar osteotomy (**699**) commonly used in the United States and advocated in the UK by Winstanley (1968).

The C-osteotomy requires careful planning on mandibular models if embarrassing three-dimensional problems of contact are to be avoided at operation, and the radiographs must be studied to determine the course of the inferior alveolar bundle as the osteotomy cut must be arched behind it. Some surgeons advocate the use of a sterilised template to indicate the course of the nerve. The operation allows good bone-to-bone contact if properly planned and bone grafting is rarely necessary. It is indicated in mandibular advancement cases only, as in **694** to **698** (case of Mr Gordon Fordyce, FDSRCS).

The *oblique subcondylar* is easily performed intraorally but allows little bone-to-bone contact. Relapse is denied by its advocates; the author uses it mainly when requiring a simple 'relieving' incision in the correction of asymmetries, where the principal correction is required on the contralateral side.

698

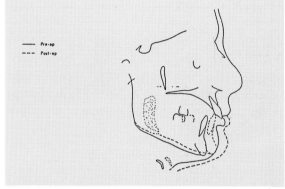

699

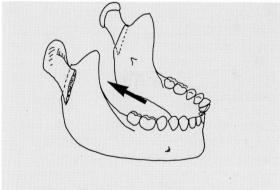

693   C-osteotomy.

694 to 698   Mandibular advancement using the C-osteotomy (**694** and **696** before operation).

699   Oblique subcondylar osteotomy.

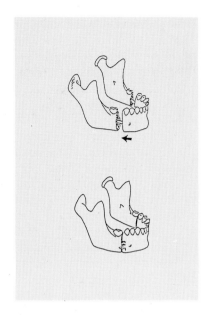

Horizontal sections of the ramus, either extraorally (Blair, 1907) or by blind division with a gigli saw (Kostechka, 1931) undoubtedly lead to an unstable postoperative result, and are rejected today. The same applies to horizontal ramisection by intraoral subperiosteal exposure (Ernst, 1927; Ginestet, 1939), or by combined intraoral and extraoral access (Skaloud, 1951).

Body and angle ostectomies

Operations on the mandible centred on the angle and the body are most useful for mandibular set-back procedures. Advancement operations, with rare exceptions in asymmetrically distorted mandibles, are much better performed on the ramus. Of these, as we have seen, the forward sliding sagittal split is perhaps the most universally applicable and the most logical, provided that the mouth can be opened and the neck extended to allow proper intraoral surgical access. Otherwise the inverted L-osteotomy with bone grafting or the C-osteotomy provide the best options. Discussion of the body and angle ostectomies will therefore be mainly concerned with the body ostectomy and its counterpart at the angle.

Body ostectomy of the mandible (**700**) was first described by Blair (1907) as an extraoral operation. The technique passed through various stages of development directed towards preventing the extraoral wound becoming compound into the mouth (inevitable if teeth are removed from the ostectomy site at the time of operation), and later towards the preservation of

the neurovascular bundle. Dingman (1944) described a method of two-stage combined intraoral and extraoral access with preservation of the neurovascular bundle. Some operators believe that preservation of the bundle is unnecessary and claim that regeneration of the involved nerves always occurs, but this is not the author's experience. The literature is reviewed by Rowe (1960). The method to be described here is simple, performed in one stage, preserves the nerve and vessels, results in rapid bony union, and avoids external scarring.

The object of body ostectomy is to remove a preplanned segment of the mandibular body allowing the anterior segment of the jaw to be set-back, and usually the posterior (proximal) segments to be rotated internally to a minor degree. This is necessary for two reasons. First there is often a lateral molar crossbite which involves the dentition behind the site of operation. Second, the curvature of the mandible increases as the anterior part is reached and the symphysis formed. Therefore if a segment is removed and the anterior segment set back the posterior part of the anterior segment will fall within the larger span of the posterior segments. Again, in cases with a steep mandibular plane relative to the occlusal plane (along which the anterior segment must be displaced) the posterior edge of the lower border of the anterior segment will tend to lie at a higher level than the lower border of the anterior surfaces of the posterior segments.

Both these effects reduce the area of bone-to-bone contact and tend to result in delayed union. The first is substantially avoided by inward rotation of the posterior segments in most cases. Where this is not possible without unwanted opening of the vertical dimension, or where the occlusal plane and the mandibular plane diverge steeply, the choice of body ostectomy should be reconsidered. In cases of open bite the anterior segment will not be displaced along the occlusal plane and the vertical problem may not occur.

The degree to which medial rotation of the proximal segments is possible will depend on the amount of space present between the coronoid processes and the underlying maxilla and posterior molar teeth. This should therefore be assessed carefully before embarking on body ostectomy. The condyles appear to bear considerable medial rotation without longterm ill-effects, although there is sometimes mild TMJ discomfort in the immediate postoperative period where much rotation has occurred. It is probable that the condyle remodels to establish its preoperative relationship to the glenoid fossa.

For the reasons discussed above it is helpful to have an accurate model of the total mandibular shape including the relationship of the condyles to the anterior mandible and to each other when planning body ostectomy, and the same applies to ostectomy of the symphysis (see **767, 768** and **769**).

Technique. The mandibular body is exposed intraorally as described on pp. 148 and 149. The planned ostectomy will have been previously performed on the prepared mandibular model

701 Body ostectomy: mandibular model and template with screw attachment.

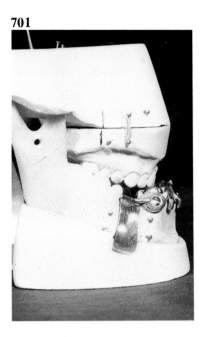

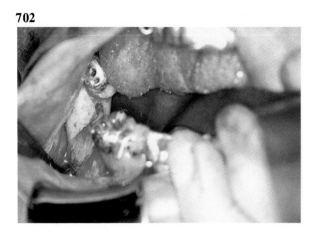

702 to 704   **Body ostectomy:** surgical technique.

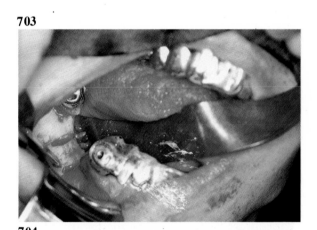

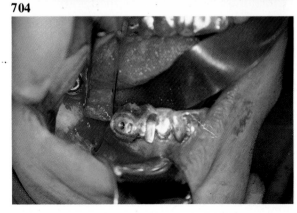

and a template prepared to indicate the exact extent of the resection intended. If cast cap splint fixation is to be used, the template can be prepared with a screw attachment for fixation to the anterior splint section (**701**). The same locking plate will later be used for placement of a connecting bar. The template indicates only the extent of resection required in the buccal plate.

For simplicity the model operation should be planned to provide cuts from buccal to lingual at right angles to the buccal plate; when this is done the template is indicative of the amount of bone to be removed throughout the entire depth of the body. Occasionally the shape of the mandible will indicate that a section of more wedge-shaped pattern must be removed. The operator must be aware of this while making the bony cuts or difficulty will be experienced in matching the cut segments for fixation. The template is fabricated in a malleable metal for close adaptation to the buccal cortical surface of the bone when it has been exposed and the template screwed into place.

Stages of the intraoral operation. If a tooth has to be sacrificed this should either be extracted several weeks prior to operation or during the operation itself; extraction the night before will result in troublesome reactive hyperaemia. After incision and exposure of the body the template is secured in place, adapted to the mandible, and the area to be removed marked out with the flat surface of a chisel placed flush against the edges of the template (**702**). The template is then removed and discarded.

Keeping inside the guidelines thus established a Lindemann bur is used to carry two cuts through the full buccolingual depth of the bone from the upper border to the level judged to be just above the position of the inferior alveolar bundle. (**703**). This segment is removed with a chisel (**704**).

705

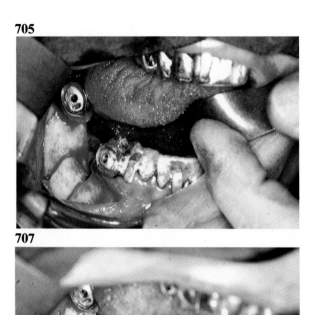

706

707

708

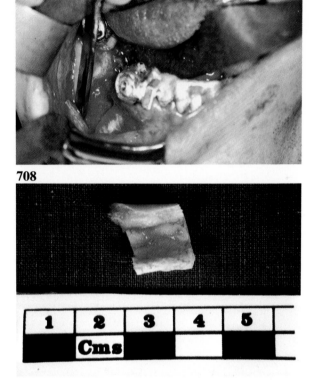

A channel retractor (**705**) is hooked beneath the lower border and the two cuts delimiting the segment are carried through the cortex only to the lower border and as far underneath it as possible towards the lingual aspect of the body.

The cuts are checked to see that no cortical bridges remain and a chisel is inserted from above, separating the buccal cortex to the lower border (**706**).

The nerve itself is located (**707**), with good light and suction, scooping cancellous bone from the medullary cavity. Sometimes the nerve will be found to be contained in a definite tube of bone (which gives a clearer white line on both sides of the radiographic shadow marking the site of the bundle). This can be gently split along its longitudinal axis with a 5mm Ward's nasal chisel and the nerve 'peeled' with a Warwick James elevator (which is an ideal shape for this without being too sharp). The nerve invariably lies nearer to the lingual plate than the buccal, but there are always exceptions to every rule, and great caution is needed until the location is clear.

Once the bundle is clearly exposed the remaining bone (**708**) can be removed from the lower border by separation with a sharp chisel blow, provided the limiting cuts have been made through its full thickness. Warwick James elevators are again useful applied on either side of the segment to be removed to facilitate its delivery.

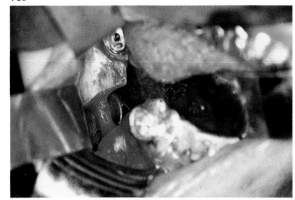

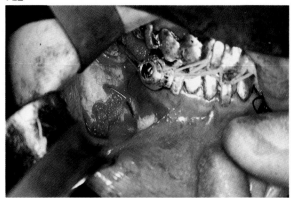

712   Fixation.

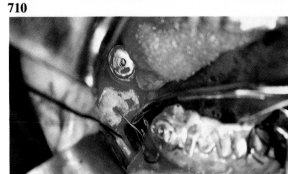

705 to 710   Body ostectomy: surgical technique.

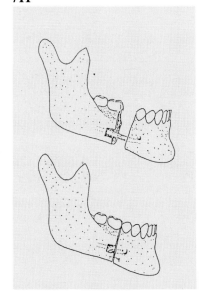

711   Inferior neurovascular bundle: window.

Finally only a small lingual bridge of bone remains on the infero-medial surface (**709**). In bilateral cases this is a good time to drill two holes in the buccal cortices opposite the final position of the segments and as low down on the buccal aspect as possible. A cortical wire is placed and tightened (**710**). Should this lingual bridge break during section of the contralateral side the wire will reduce the danger of damage to the bundle by distraction of the bony ends. The other side is next sectioned to the same stage. The anterior segment is then manipulated to break the two lingual bridges which can be trimmed flush with the rest of the sections, using bone shears or a bur.

The author rarely constructs a bony window to accommodate the excess length of neurovascular bundle in the buccal plate (**711**). In most cases cancellous bone can be scooped from around the bundle in both anterior and posterior segments, taking care to pass right up to the nerve itself including any thicker bony tube. The space thus created is adequate to accommodate the excess bundle. Sometimes the cancellous bone is sparse and the medullary cavity filled with dense bone. In these cases a window is cut in the buccal cortex, but great care is necessary to ensure that the nerve actually occupies this space when the segments are wired together.

The anterior segment and the posterior segments are placed in the planned position of intermaxillary fixation, the cortical wires are tightened and secured, and the preplanned connecting bars are screwed into place (**712**). Cancellous bone chips from the ileum, taken by the method described by Flint (1964) are packed around the ostectomy site. These provide a rich reservoir of osteogenic material which results in firm bony union within 4 weeks. Without bone grafting in this way union may take up to 3 months. The incision is closed without drainage.

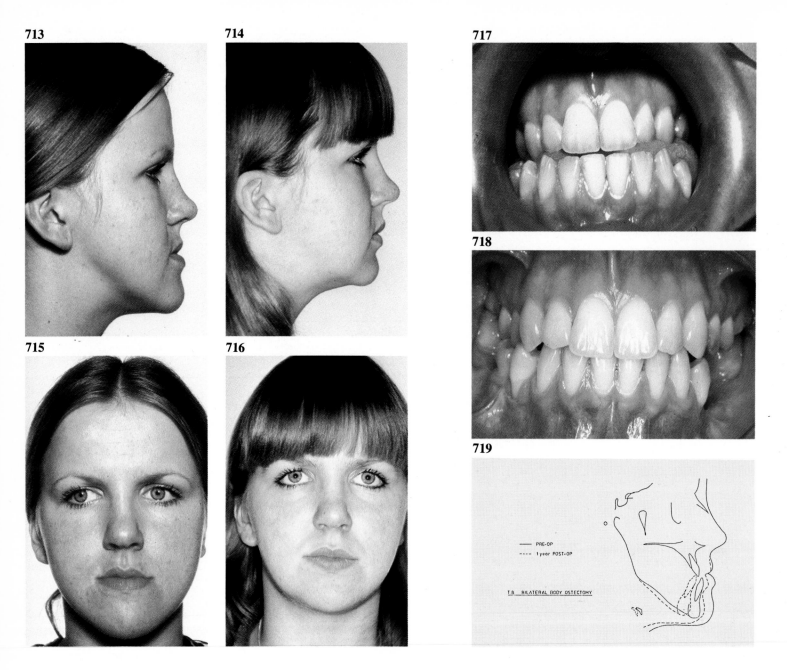

713   **714**

717

715   **716**

718

719

PRE-OP
1 year POST-OP

T.B BILATERAL BODY OSTECTOMY

Indications for body ostectomy include both bilateral and unilateral mandibular set-back for the correction of bilateral or unilateral mandibular protrusion. It is best suited to cases where the abnormality is primarily located in the mandibular body itself, where the length of the body is disproportionate to the length and width of the ramus. This is especially the case where the gonial angle lies within normal limits and the mandibular body is intrinsically long, or where there is anterior open bite (with posterior molar contact) in patients with a low tongue position and absolutely no suspicion of endogenous tongue thrusting. The latter type of case is likely to end up with disastrous 'bucket handle' displacement if treated by bilateral body ostectomy. It is particularly useful where:

713 to 719   **Correction of mandibular protrusion** by body ostectomy (**713, 715, 717,** before operation).

(a) The dental arches are not capable of being fitted together in a corrected relationship without breaking the integrity of the arch in the lower jaw.

(b) Where saddle areas already exist in the molar/premolar areas, or

(c) Very heavily filled, carious or abscessed teeth occupy the molar/premolar areas.

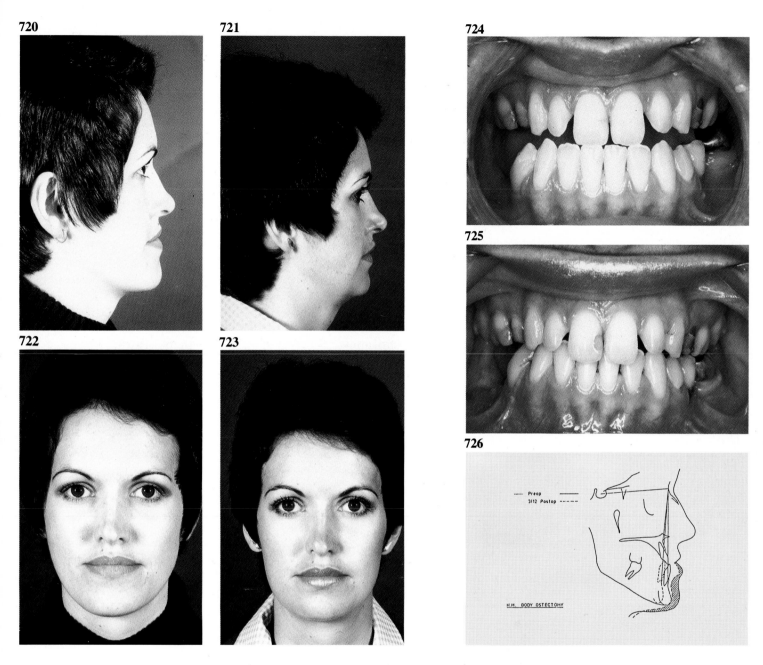

720   **721**   **724**

722   **723**   **725**

726

(d) Where it is desirable to exercise the maximal postoperative effect of the tongue in repositioning retroclined lower anterior incisor teeth to normalise the axial inclinations postoperatively, room having been allowed for this in planning the overbite.

(e) Where it is necessary to remove a wedge-shaped piece of bone in order to retract the chin to a different degree to the retraction of the lower incisor tips, assuming that the occlusion of the anterior dentition allows this.

The procedure is contra-indicated in edentulous cases, and in cases where the thickness of the neck causes the jaw line to

720 to 726   **Poor chin correction** in a case of mandibular set-back by body ostectomy (**720, 722, 724,** before operation).

project from the neck anteriorly to only a minor extent despite a prenormal dental and skeletal relationship (see **720** to **726**).

Results are shown in a typical and well selected case (**713** to **719**). Body ostectomy is a stable procedure, but there is a tendency to the production of a 'double chin' effect, rather more than in the ramus procedures. Hence it is more appropriate to the type of case shown here with a good line to the neck and jaw prior to operation albeit with real mandibular protrusion. Over the first postoperative year the neck tissues adapt and usually the 'double chin' disappears.

195

Compare the results of the case illustrated in **713** to **719** with those shown in **720** to **726.** This is a case with inadequate chin projection from the neck and would probably have been more pleasing had a maxillary advancement been undertaken. The patient however opted for mandibular set-back, and, while there is a great improvement, the poor chin projection (in contrast to the facial profile from menton to glabella) detracts from the result. Otherwise the profile changes are identical with those obtained by set-back procedures in the ramus.

Angle ostectomy of the mandible (**727**) differs very little in principle from the body procedure, except that it is performed behind the tooth-bearing part of the jaw. Like the body ostectomy it involves the removal of a preplanned segment of bone, from the angle region in this instance. The neurovascular bundle must be preserved, and the operation is a stable one as no attempt is made to lengthen the ramus against its soft-tissue investment.

The procedure is possible by the intraoral route, as described by Obwegeser (1971), but in this technique an area of buccal plate larger than the proposed ostectomy is first split away from the mandible, the planned section is removed from the lingual plate (with preservation of the now visible bundle), the lingual plate is wired and the fragments positioned. The buccal plate is then trimmed and replaced as a free bone graft. The technique is not easy to perform, and the postoperative stability of free bone grafts in this region cannot be guaranteed. It is also more difficult to tailor the shape of the angle.

Indications

The main indication is in the treatment of severe anterior open bite cases where posterior contact is confined to the last standing tooth on one or both sides, but most of these cases also require extensive maxillary surgery (see Section 5). Here the function of the mandibular procedure is to correct the large gonial angle, elevating the mandibular plane anteriorly to allow restoration of occlusion and correction of the occlusal plane as an adjunct to correction of vertical maxillary abnormalities. The illustrative case (**731** to **736**) shows several points of importance in this respect.

727

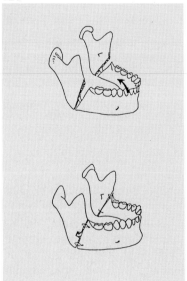

727 Angle ostectomy of the mandible.

728

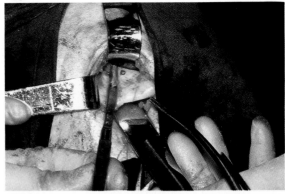

729

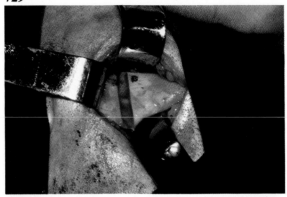

730

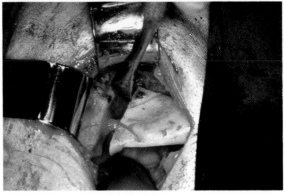

728 to 730 **Angle ostectomy:** surgical technique.

The technique is therefore by extraoral access by choice. The angle is exposed by the submandibular approach, and the ostectomy is marked out with a template constructed on the preoperative mandibular models. The angle ostectomy is one operation where construction of full mandibular models is advisable. Working similarly to the technique for body ostectomy already described, but with access from below rather than above, the buccal plate is removed between the cuts **(728)**, and the nerve identified between the buccal and cortical plates **(729)**. The thickness of the mandible is much less here than in the body, and care must be taken in the region of the bundle, which can usually be located easily with the aid of the preoperative radiographs which indicate the level at which it should be sought. The rest of the ostectomy is then removed from the lingual plate **(730)**.

A window is usually necessary to accommodate the nerve in this procedure as there is insufficient depth of cancellous bone for it to be placed between the plates. Bone grafting is advisable (by Flint's method, 1964) to expedite union, but it is less essential than in body ostectomy.

731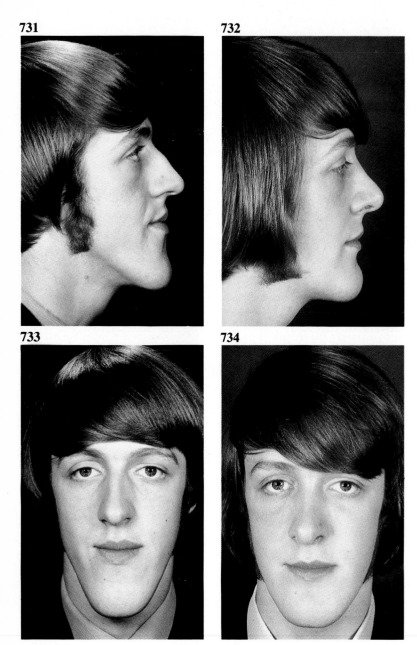

732

733

734

735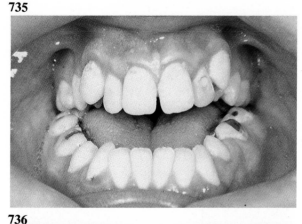

736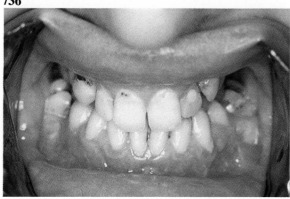

731 to 736   Anterior open bite: a case treated by angle ostectomy of the mandible alone (**731, 733, 735,** before operation).

The problem of anterior open bite and treatment by angle ostectomy of the mandible *alone,* a technique which the author would not undertake today, is shown in **731** to **736.** The case shows many of the compromises which characterised correction by this method some years ago. It is included, however, to illustrate the effect of angle ostectomy on the mandibular plane angle and the occlusion which has remained stable over 10 years. A reduction genioplasty was performed to correct anterior lower-facial height and the labiomental curve, and a rhinoplasty was undertaken (the latter by G.L. Lister, Esq, FRCS). Compare this case with the similar one shown in **1071** to **1077,** which also had the necessary primary correction of maxillary height. Incidentally, this case was carried out intra-orally, and there is therefore no extraoral scar.

Other body procedures have been advocated. Step sections of the body for both advancement and set-back have little advantage over bonegrafted body ostectomy for set-back or sagittal splitting for advancement, and they complicate the surgery unnecessarily. The author finds the operations described here in combination with anterior mandibular procedures to be described next are quite adequate to correct the vast majority of cases; it is better to master a few techniques than to experiment with numerous options, unless there is a demonstrable indication.

Anterior mandibular osteotomies

Lower labial segmental osteotomies

Osteotomies performed on the anterior mandible have in common the separation of a labial segment of alveolar bone bearing the anterior teeth, usually from canine to canine or from first premolar to first premolar. This segment derives its blood supply from the soft-tissues attached to the lingual aspect and it is of paramount importance that this attachment is maintained during the surgical procedure. There is much experimental support for this clinical practice (Bell and Levy, 1970; Bradley *et al*, 1974; Banks, 1977) although it has been shown that the teeth contained in the lower labial segment undergo impaired cellular differentiation including loss of normal innervation. The pulps remain alive, and there is evidence that some reinnervation occurs by apical ingrowth of nerves (Poswillo, 1972; Robinson, 1980, 1981).

The lower labial segment may then be repositioned superiorly to correct anterior open bite confined to the anterior dentition, inferiorly (after subapical ostectomy), posteriorly (after alveolar ostectomy), or it may be rotated in combination with any of these movements to produce desired axial incisor inclinations. These procedures are often combined with anterior maxillary osteotomies, particularly in the correction of bimaxillary alveolar protrusion.

Anterior mandibular subapical osteotomy or ostectomy (**737** and **738**) may be combined with vertical alveolar ostectomy, usually following extraction of the first premolars on each side, to produce varied repositioning of the lower labial segment. In the UK the term 'lower labial segmental surgery' is used to describe these movements with adjunctive descriptions such as 'lower labial set-back', 'set-down' or 'set-up' to indicate the direction of movement. Further modifications are those of Köle (**747** to **751**) which maintains the right/left integrity of the mandible; and the symphyseal ostectomy or the anterior mandibuloplasty (**767** to **769** and **775** to **777**) which break left/right mandibular continuity and require intermaxillary fixation during at least a part of the healing period.

737

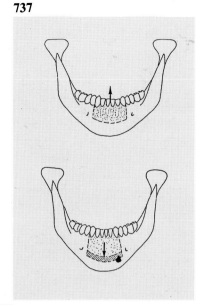

738

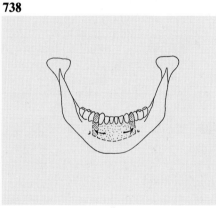

737 Anterior mandibular subapical osteotomy (top) and ostectomy (bottom).

738 Anterior mandibular subapical osteotomy combined with vertical alveolar ostectomy (lower labial set-back).

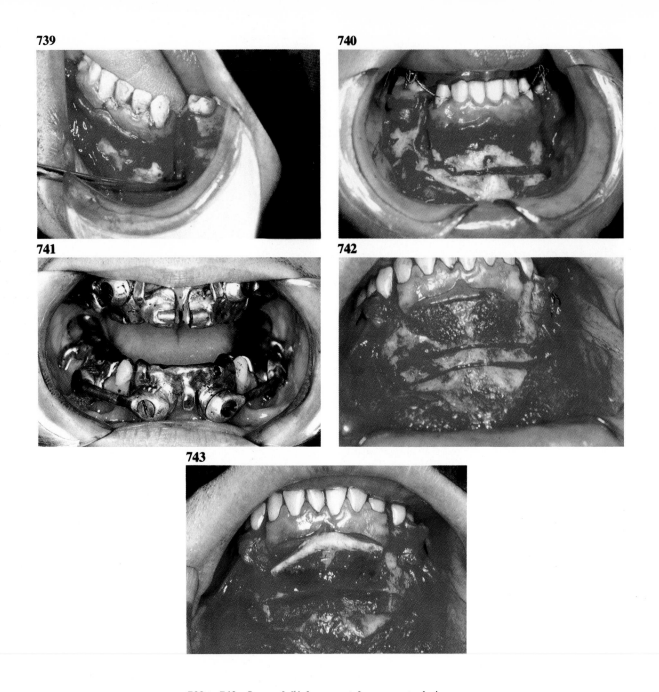

739 to 743   Lower labial segmental surgery: technique.

Technique. The symphysis is exposed as shown in **536** to **544**, using the mucogingival approach except where substantial upward displacement of the labial segment is proposed. In the latter case the labial incision is used. The osteotomy lines are marked out with a bur or saw blade. The subapical horizontal cut may be made with the Stryker saw blade through the depth of the mandible, or if preferred the labial cortex may be cut in this way and the bur used to take the cut through to the lingual side. Care is taken to remain below the apices of the teeth, the position of which can usually be assessed by reference to the contour of the labial cortical plate and to the radiographs. When a vertical alveolar segment is to be removed the exact amount of bone is determined on preoperative models and a template provided as a guide in the theatre. The tooth is extracted at operation and the planned segment excised with bur and chisels, avoiding detachment of lingual soft-tissues (**739**). When the subapical and vertical cuts have been connected the labial segment is placed in the planned position and held there by splints or an occlusal acrylic wafer (**740**).

In anterior segmental surgery the axial inclination of the incisor teeth is often very important and the use of segmentalised cast cap splints with precise locking plates is the best means of ensuring that preplanned axial inclinations are achieved at operation. Several authors have described methods of model planning and splint construction designed to this end (see, for example, Lockwood, 1974; Fitzpatrick, 1974; Barton, 1973). The latter author points out that it is important to cement both the posterior splint sections to the teeth while they are connected together in their correct relationship. Otherwise the placement of connecting bars to the anterior segmental splint may prove impossible or inaccurate due to variation in the thickness of the cement layer of separately positioned posterior splints. Similarly, too thick a cement layer will affect the planned position of the anterior segment. A temporary labial connecting bar is therefore constructed for use during cementation of the sections (**741**), and a thin mix of cement is used.

The same applies in the cementation of splints for anterior maxillary segmental surgery. Removal of bone for subapical ostectomy is most easily done by marking out the segment planned for removal and cutting this out of the labial plate first (**742**). The cancellous bone can then be removed from the area and the lingual plate sectioned under direct vision (**743**). This technique is also used for the removal of wedge-shaped sections in reduction genioplasties or anterior mandibuloplasties.

Vertical alveolar osteotomies between adjacent teeth are difficult to place without endangering the roots of the teeth. The relationships of the roots to each other and to the proposed line of osteotomy must be very carefully studied with the aid of undistorted intraoral radiographs preoperatively, and the presumed position of the roots is marked on the study models (**744**). At operation, if the roots are not obvious

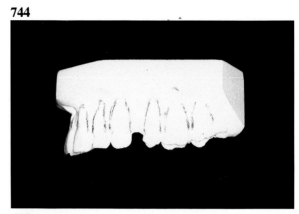

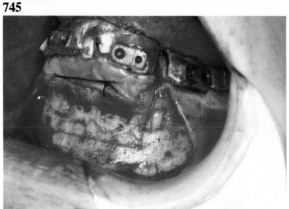

744 and 745   Vertical alveolar osteotomy. Model with position of roots marked (**744**); cortical window over the roots (**745**).

through the labial cortical plate, a small cortical window is removed over the middle third of the root(s) (**745**), and in this way the position can usually be identified by direct vision and the exact line of osteotomy determined with precision.

When the teeth are close together it is usually necessary to elevate the lingual periosteum along the line of cut and *posteriorly*, taking care not to elevate it from the lingual aspect of the anterior segment. A vertical bur cut is made through or nearly through the cortex only, and the osteotomy is completed with very fine osteotomes. In this way damage to the roots can be avoided. Minor damage to the cementum does not seem to matter, but if a deep cut into the root is made there is a real danger of losing a tooth.

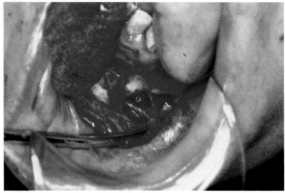

746 The incisive branch.

Proximity of the mental foramen and emerging mental nerve to the proposed line of osteotomy indicates the need to reposition the foramen posteriorly. The technique is described with the operation of anterior mandibuloplasty (pp. 209 to 211), but the distance the nerve is moved is much less – just sufficient to allow the cut to be made without damage to the main part of the mental nerve. The incisive branch (see **746**) is identified and must be divided before the main trunk can be displaced posteriorly. Neither this nor the rather ragged hole in the cortical bone which remains is of the slightest importance.

The Köle procedure

This (Köle, 1959) (**747**), is used to correct minor degrees of anterior open bite characterised by downward inclination of the mandibular occlusal plane from the premolar region, with associated increase in anterior lower-facial height. It is ideal where a Class 3 incisor relationship also exists because the removal of a premolar and appropriate bony segment allows not only superior repositioning of the labial segment but also set-back to correct the incisor relationship (**748**). The upward movement of the labial segment does not correct the increased anterior lower-facial height, it simply transfers the site of abnormality from the open bite (reverse overbite) to the subapical mandibular bone.

The Köle procedure therefore transposes the inferior border of the symphysis into the defect created by upward movement of the labial segment. This not only corrects the excess anterior mandibular height (ALDH), but theoretically provides an opportunity for chin augmentation by bringing the lower border free bone graft forwards. The stages of the operation are seen in **749** to **751.** In the author's experience the degree of improvement in labiomental curvature which can be obtained in this way is limited unless additional bone is onlaid, and the anterior mandibuloplasty is preferred (Foster and Henderson, 1981).

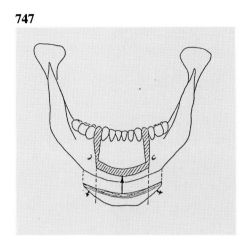

747

748

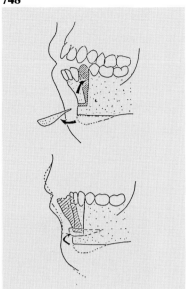

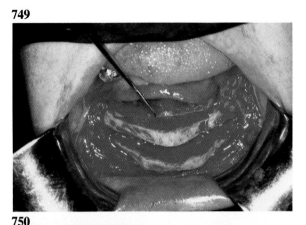

749

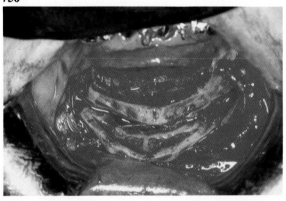

750

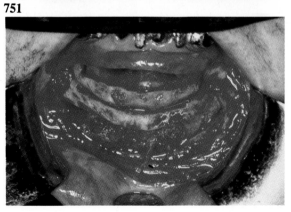

751

747 to 751 The Köle procedure.

Indications for anterior mandibular subapical osteotomies and ostectomies

These, with the Köle procedure, include the following:

1. *Inferior alveolar protrusion,* correctable within one premolar width, in the presence of a good chin to cranial base profile relationship. These cases require a straight anterior alveolar set-back.

2. *An exaggerated curve of Spee* with relative overeruption of the mandibular incisor teeth. This commonly occurs in association with mandibular retrusion and a Class 2 (Division 1 or 2) incisor relationship. Mandibular advancement is required, usually by bilateral sagittal split. Incisal guidance will prevent correction of the occlusion, resulting in bilateral lateral openbite. In a young child, below 18 years of age, this may close without additional surgery provided there is no crowding in the premolar region. In a person over 20 years of age the anterior labial segment should be depressed by subapical ostectomy at the same time as the mandibular advancement.

3. Some cases of anterior open bite are well treated by the Köle procedure. This will be discussed further in connection with vertical facial dysplasias.

4. As part of the correction of bimaxillary alveolar protrusion.

5. As a part of more extensive corrections to the facial bones where the incisor angulation is incorrect for proper labial contour in the postoperative prediction for the main procedure, and where orthodontic correction is inappropriate for any reason.

752

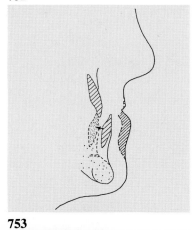

752 Lower labial segmental set-back: profile changes.

753

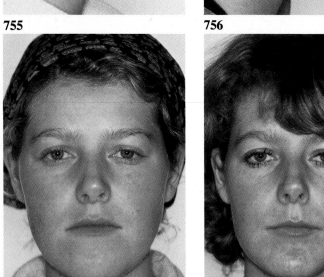

754

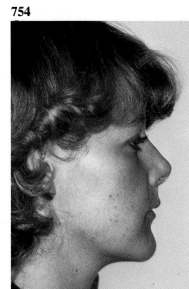

755

756

757

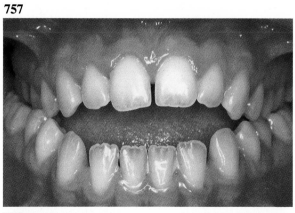

758

759

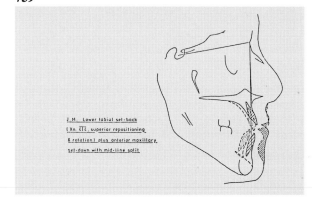

J. M. Lower labial set-back
(Xn ⟨⟩ , superior repositioning
& rotation) plus anterior maxillary
set-down with mid-line split

753 to 759 A case treated by lower labial segmental set-back combined with pre-maxillary set-back and correction of anterior open bite (**753, 755, 757**, before operation).

760 Köle procedure: profile changes.

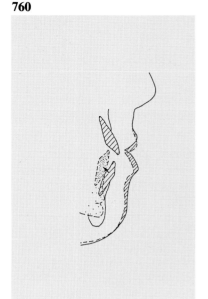

760

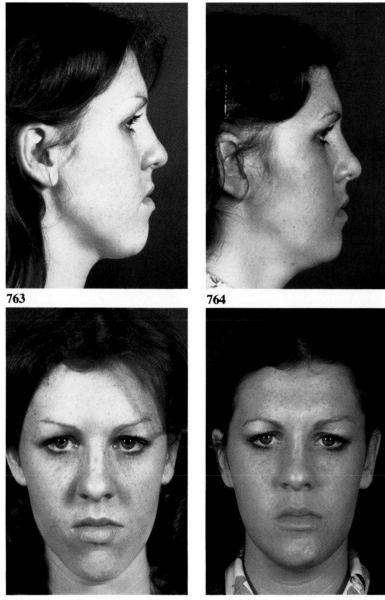

761

762

763

764

Profile changes after lower labial segmental surgery depend largely on the type of segmental movement undertaken (set-back, set-up, set-down, or rotational) and the main effect is seen on the labiomental curve. The main results of the operation are at the occlusal level.

The profile changes following simple set-back are as follows (**752**):

1. The chin remains unaltered, as does the pogonion beneath the soft-tissue contour.

2. Otherwise the changes resemble those of mandibular set-back; the upper lip is slightly lengthened and flattened, the lower lip moves back rather less than the underlying lower incisor tip (from 60% to 75%, depending on the relationship to the upper lip and upper incisor), and the labiomental curve is increased.

The case shown (**753** to **759**) illustrates a common use of the lower labial segmental procedure, in combination with pre-maxillary set-back and correction of anterior open bite with occlusal movement of both upper and lower anterior segments.

761 to 766 **Correction of anterior open bite** by the Köle procedure (**761, 763, 765,** before operation). (See next page for **765** and **766**.)

765

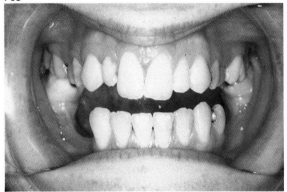

766

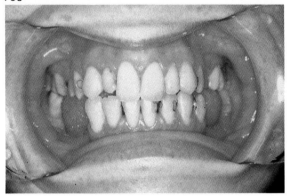

Profile changes after the Köle procedure (**760**) consist of the following:

1. Decreased anterior lower-facial height, but less than might be expected.

2. No effect on chin prominence, a consistent occurrence in the author's hands with this operation. It is not always sought (as in the case shown in **761** to **766**).

3. The lip again reflects the changes seen in mandibular set-back. As the pogonion remains where it was the labiomental curvature is improved.

An illustrative case is shown where the saddle spaces already present in the premolar regions invite anterior segmental movement. The anterior segment is pushing the lip forwards, there is an anterior open bite but good upper lip to upper incisor balance (**761** to **766**). For practical purposes this operation has been abandoned in favour of the much more versatile and effective anterior mandibuloplasty.

767

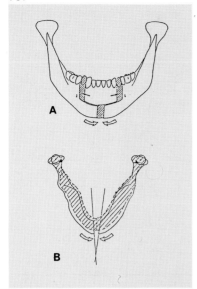

768

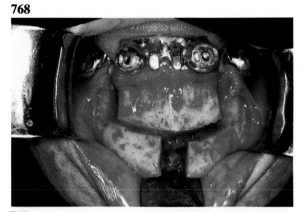

769

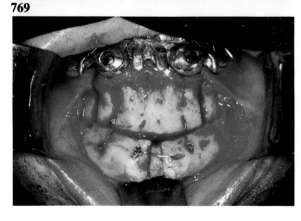

767 to 769   Symphyseal ostectomy.

Symphyseal ostectomy (Sowray and Haskell, 1968) is a lower labial set-back, usually involving extraction of the two first premolars, combined with the removal of a central segment of bone at the midline, carried down from the subapical horizontal osteotomy line to the lower border (**767A**). This is a logical extension where there is mild mandibular protrusion associated with bilateral molar crossbite. The medial rotation of the proximal segments (**767B**) does not seem to produce longterm problems with the temporomandibular joints, presumably as a result of remodelling; short-term TMJ discomfort is not uncommon postoperatively.

The operative technique is illustrated (**768** and **769**). The only technical point of importance relates to the angulation of the cuts at the symphysis (**767B**) as there is a strong tendency to underestimate the obliquity of the cuts required if the cut surfaces are to approximate exactly after medial rotation; if a gap should result in the labial cortex when the segments are correctly located, then a piece of the bone removed is tailored to occlude the gap (which has happened in **769**).

770 Symphyseal ostectomy: typical profile changes.

771 to 774 Full face and profile changes. (**771** and **773**, preoperative.)

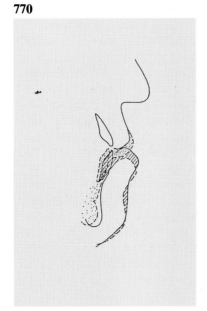

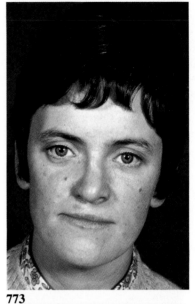

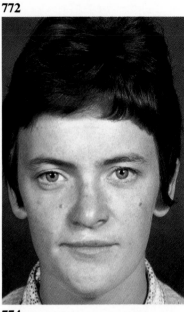

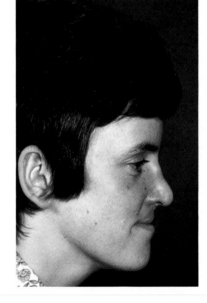

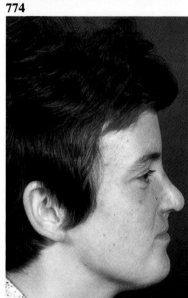

The results of symphyseal ostectomy when seen in profile (**770**), are important in relation to some cases of secondary cleft lip and palate. The procedure repositions the pogonion only to a slight extent, and hence the indication in mild protrusion of the mandible rather than severe prognathism. In contributing soft-tissue relaxation to the upper lip, by reducing perioral tension as a result of the medial rotation of the lateral segments, the operation is invaluable in correcting the tense, stretched appearance of many otherwise nicely restored upper lips following hare lip surgery.

As a final procedure after lip revision, fistula repair, etc, the effect on the full face and lateral view in these cases is out of all proportion to the bony movements achieved. The case shown (previously corrected to this point by I.T. Jackson, Esq, FRCS) was referred for correction of the residual mild Class 3 occlusion, a maxillary osteotomy having been felt unnecessary. The surgical technique makes additional minor modification to the chin very simple if required.

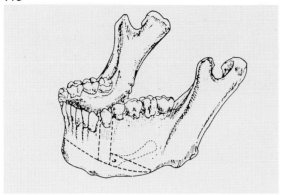

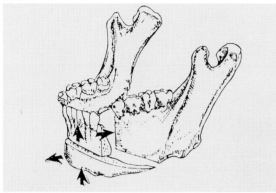

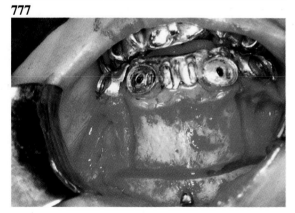

775 to 777   **Anterior mandibuloplasty.**

Anterior mandibuloplasty (775 to 777) (Foster and Henderson, 1981) is another extension of anterior mandibular surgery which is exceedingly flexible to cope with a number of common abnormalities of the anterior lower-face. The Köle procedure and the total subapical mandibular osteotomy (McIntosh and Carlotti, 1975; Fitzpatrick, 1977) allow limited correction of chin position but lack the flexibility required to produce good chin aesthetics in many cases. Bell and Condit (1970) indicated the three-dimensional flexibility required in many anterior mandibular problems. Anterior mandibuloplasty effectively combines lower labial segmental surgery with simultaneous genioplasty, all the cuts being continuous. Thus the anterior teeth and the chin point can be independently moved as the case demands, vertically or anteroposteriorly. Like the Sowray Haskell procedure the operation also allows medial (or lateral) rotation of the proximal mandibular fragments.

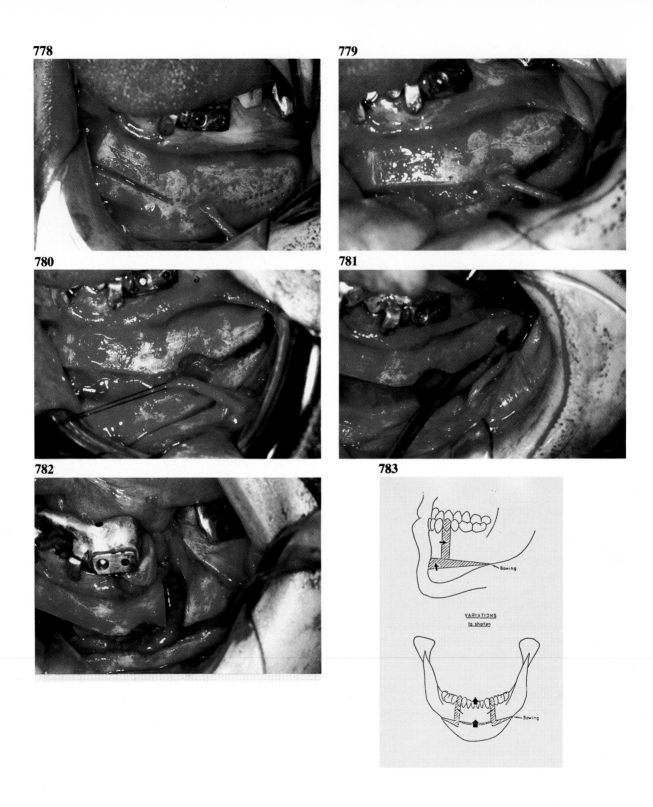

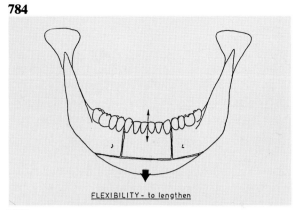

FLEXIBILITY - to lengthen

785

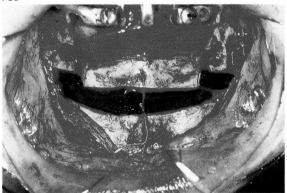

786

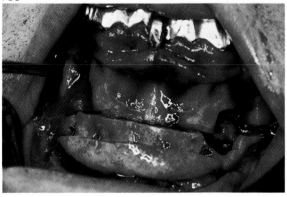

778 to 786   Anterior mandibuloplasty: surgical technique.

Technique. The mandible is degloved anteriorly by a labial or mucogingival incision, the mental nerves are identified and freed from their epineural sheaths. The mental nerve usually requires retropositioning, because the genioplasty cut is to be directed quite far posteriorly in order to achieve good lower border contour. This is particularly indicated when vertical reduction genioplasty is a part of the mandibuloplasty.

The inferior dental canal is approximately outlined with a series of cortical bur holes (made with a fine spearpoint drill) which also enclose the mental foramen and outline the proposed new site for the foramen (**778**). In the case illustrated a wedge is also to be removed subapically in the symphyseal region and the pictures show this at the same time. The holes are joined with a fine chisel, and the cortical bone thus outlined is removed with a small elevator (Warwick James pattern is good for this) (**779**). The circular bone surrounding the foramen is delivered last as a ring around the nerve along which it is eased buccally, divided with shears and separated in two parts.

The neurovascular bundle is identified from the front, the incisive branch (marked with a suture, **780**) is divided, and the whole bundle delivered from the mandible and repositioned posteriorly (**781**), being retained with a small chip of bone wedged into the cortical channel in front of the definitive position. The appropriate bony cuts and/or ostectomies are completed according to the requirements of the case (**782**), and the fragments positioned and wired together by direct wiring to supplement occlusal splintage, wiring or arch wiring. Intermaxillary fixation is essential.

In cases with a bowed lower border, viewed from the side, the genioplasty cut is carried to the point at which bowing starts (**783**). Excision of an appropriate subapical wedge thus corrects the mandibular plane and improves the SN:MP angle where this is too great. This can be combined, as shown in **783**, with lower labial segmental set-back. Conversely (**784** and **785**), deficient anterior mandibular height can be increased by cutting a single genioplasty line, rotating the lower border downwards and inserting bone or proplast. The illustrations show the common combination of this procedure with lower labial set-down. Advancement, or right/left rotational genioplasty can also be incorporated (**786**). There is adequate access for suprahyoid myotomy if the operation involves much increase in the distance from symphysis to hyoid bone.

Indications for anterior mandibuloplasty vary widely because of the inherent flexibility of the procedure, but share in common three-dimensional abnormality in the region of the anterior mandible. There are those cases with increased anterior lower-facial height and increased anterior lower dental height, a reduced overbite (or anterior open bite), a reversed curve of Spee, and a very flattened labiomental curve with or without lip competence. This group is inevitably the reflection of vertical growth abnormalities, the effects of which are seen mainly in the lower-face, and usually requires maxillary surgery also.

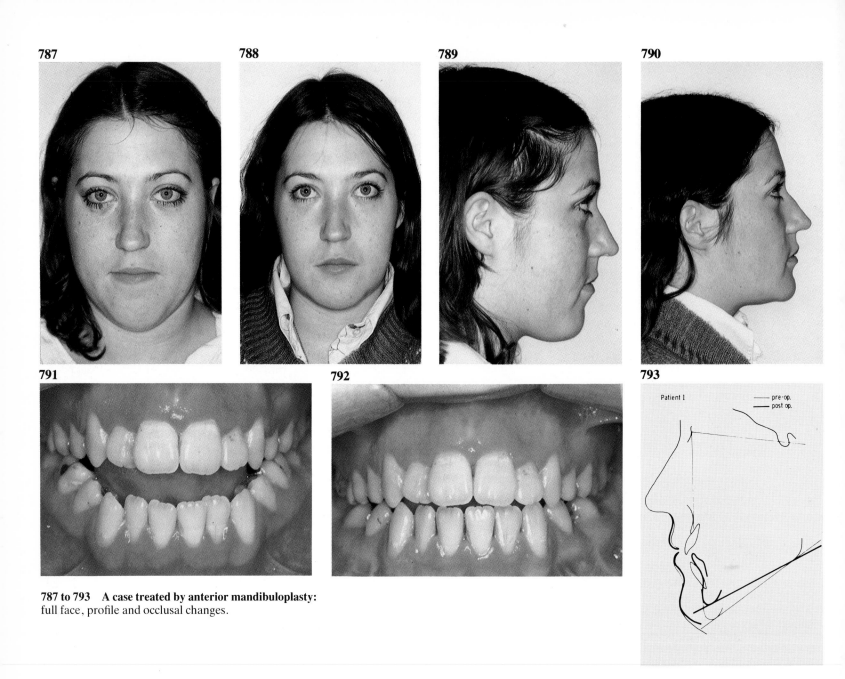

787 **788** **789** **790**

791 **792** **793**

Patient I
— pre-op.
— post op.

787 to 793   A case treated by anterior mandibuloplasty:
full face, profile and occlusal changes.

Two examples are shown (**787** to **793**, and **794** to **800**) which illustrate the range of applications to this group quite well. In the first there was an anterior mandibuloplasty alone, while in the second anterior maxillary osteotomy was also indicated; the tracings illustrate the changes.

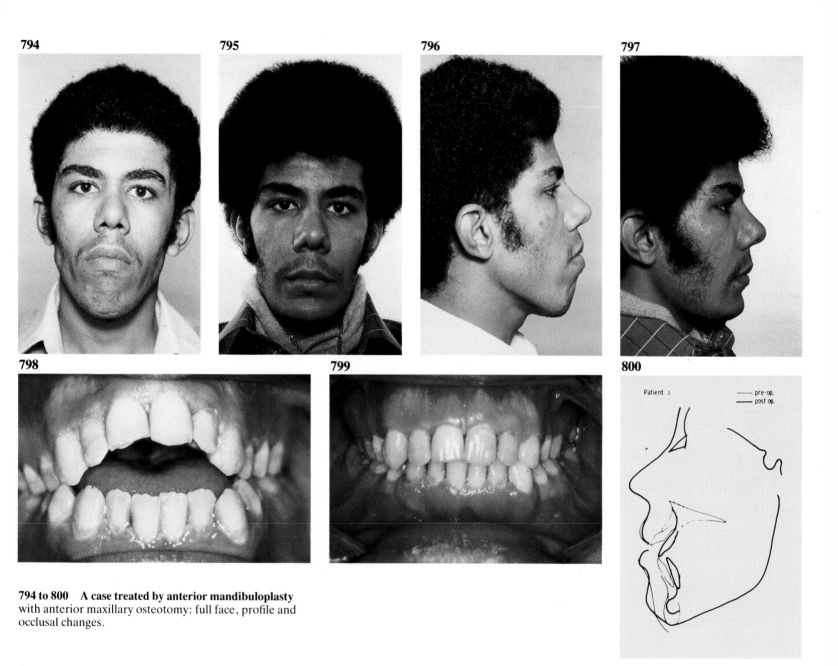

794 to 800   A case treated by anterior mandibuloplasty with anterior maxillary osteotomy: full face, profile and occlusal changes.

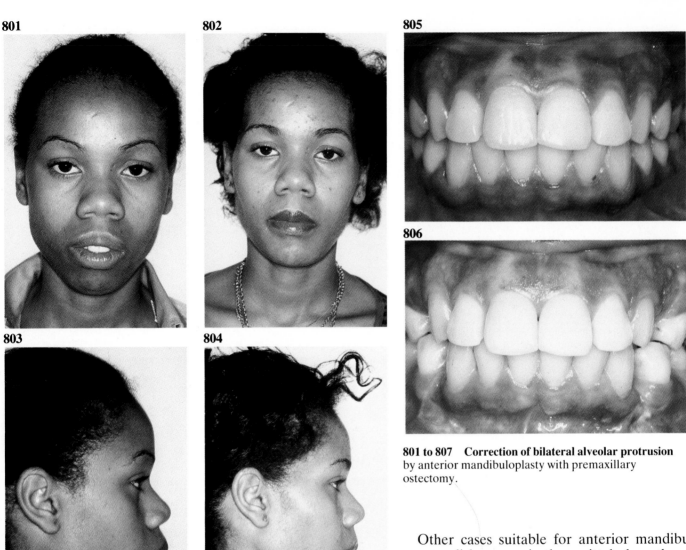

801 to 807 **Correction of bilateral alveolar protrusion** by anterior mandibuloplasty with premaxillary ostectomy.

Other cases suitable for anterior mandibuloplasty show a greater disharmony in the sagittal plane than the vertical, and often include cases of racial bilateral alveolar protrusion. Nice results can be obtained in these cases by combining premaxillary ostectomy with anterior mandibuloplasty as illustrated in the case shown in **801** to **807.** The two first premolars have been extracted from the maxillary arch and two premolars from the mandibular arch, thus allowing a premaxillary ostectomy and set-back together with a sliding genioplasty built into the planning of the anterior mandibuloplasty. In this way the lower anterior segment has been set-back to provide good occlusal and labial relationships, and the lower border has been brought forwards actually increasing chin prominence in a controlled fashion. The resulting facial change is sometimes sought by those of negro origin living in a Caucasian environment; but it is by no means confined to this group. Indian and oriental facies are both amenable to similar changes by using anterior mandibuloplasty intelligently. It is important to plan carefully with the patient, and most useful to have previous cases of similar ethnic origin so that no misunderstanding can arise as to the objective being sought.

808

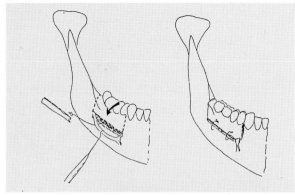

809

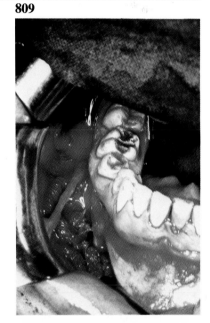

811

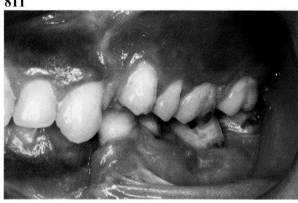

808 to 811   Posterior mandibular segmental osteotomy. 809, delivery of inferior alveolar bundle; **810 and 811,** difficulty in achieving a pleasing occlusal line and arch form (with posterior maxillary osteotomy).

810

Posterior segmental mandibular osteotomy

Other mandibular segmental osteotomies are rarely performed, but are sometimes useful to correct particular problems. **Posterior mandibular segmental osteotomy (808)** is technically quite demanding. Described by Peterson (1978) it is most often used in the correction of lingually inclined posterior mandibular segments; less often buccally tilted or over-erupted segments may be repositioned with this method, and endentulous gaps may be closed.

The technique is similar to anterior mandibular osteotomy, but with the problem of the dentoalveolar neurovascular bundle adding to the technical difficulties. Care must be taken with the vertical posterior limb of the osteotomy to ensure that the cut is not bevelled from the anterobuccal to the posterolingual, which tends to occur and will prevent buccal movement of the segment without the removal of additional bone from the lingual side.

The author prefers to deliver the inferior alveolar bundle completely (as described for anterior mandibuloplasty) prior to making the lingual cut with bur or chisel (**809**). Final detachment of the segment is made with an osteotome inserted into the buccal cut and used as an elevator to complete fracture of the lingual plate, taking care to retain the soft-tissue attachment to the lingual aspect of the segment, thus maintaining viability. The example shown (**810** and **811**) had a simultaneous posterior maxillary osteotomy and illustrates the difficulty in achieving a pleasing occlusal line and arch form.

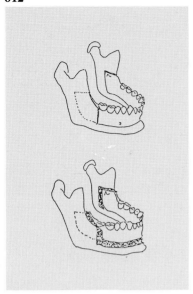

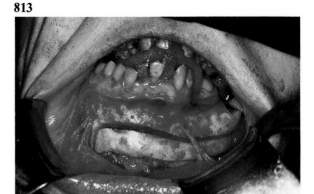

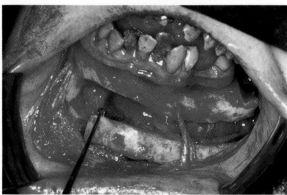

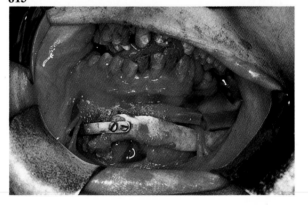

Total subapical mandibular osteotomy (812)

This is indicated when it is desired to retain the chin to cranial base relationship and to move the whole lower dentition forwards on the mandibular basal bone. Thus it will correct the Class 2 dental relationship where the pogonion is in good position; and it can be modified, by the insertion of subapical bone or proplast, to increase lower-facial height both anteriorly and posteriorly.

Introduced by McIntosh and Carlotti (1975) the procedure is self-explanatory from the diagram, which shows the modification advocated by Booth *et al* (1976) involving extension of the osteotomy to include a short lingual cut sagittal split of the ramus on each side. If this is done (instead of a simple vertical osteotomy through the alveolus distal to the last tooth) the subapical osteotomy should be carried through to the lingual aspect of the body of the mandible prior to osteotome splitting of the ramus.

This is greatly facilitated by delivery of the inferior alveolar bundle as described for anterior mandibuloplasty and posterior segmental osteotomy, and is advocated by Fitzpatrick (1977). The illustrated sequence (**813** to **815**) shows the method adapted to the asymmetric case requiring left-sided increase in vertical mandibular height together with rotational centralisation of the chin. Fixation here is by bone plating, and bone has been inserted. On the right the vertical cut has been brought forwards to the premolar region.

Genioplasty – the management of the chin

The assessment of chin prominence and contour in relation to the total facial profile has already been discussed (p. 61). In profile the chin may be recessive or protrusive, and it may display displeasing contour, especially in relation to the height or level of the most prominent part (soft-tissue pogonion). From the front the chin may be asymmetric with deviation to right or left; sloping of the lower border up or down is more likely to reflect mandibular asymmetry on a wider base.

816

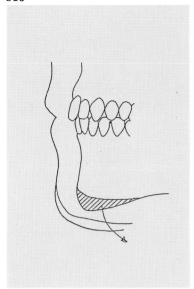

816 to 819 **Vertical reduction genioplasty:** by lower border reduction (**816**); by removal of subapical wedge of bone (**817** and **818**); in combination with horizontal correction (**819**).

817

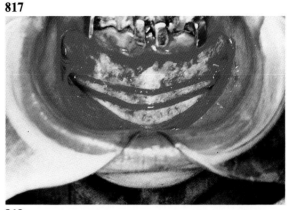

818

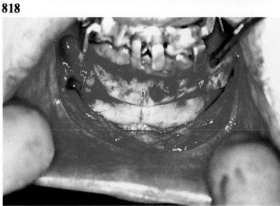

819

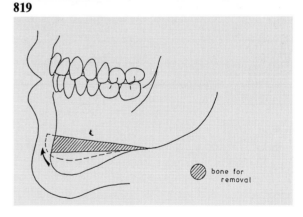

bone for removal

Methods of correction include simple reduction or recontouring by bone sculpture, augmentation by bone onlays or the addition of alloplastic materials, and various forms of sliding osteotomy of the lower border.

The recessive chin often reflects deficiency of total mandibular growth rather than failure of growth in the mental region itself. Indeed, the receding chin is often quite normal in size and shape, apart from its backward position and sometimes posterior rotation. If the whole anterior complex is rotated forwards with the advanced mandible, a normal contour results. Therefore the importance of assessing the chin in relation to the whole pattern of mandibular growth and form cannot be over-emphasised, before 'simple cosmetic' chin augmentation is undertaken. The author has seen several cases where previous chin augmentation has had to be reversed before total mandibular reconstruction was undertaken.

Many patients with receding chins have, on close inspection, perfectly normal shape at the lower border of the mandibular symphysis. The best results are obtained if this normally contoured (but posteriorly placed) lower border area can be brought forwards to constitute the new chin prominence, rather than by the addition of autogenous or alloplastic materials to simulate the normal.

Reduction genioplasty may be necessary in the vertical or the anteroposterior planes, and the term 'vertical reduction genioplasty' will be used for the first, 'horizontal reduction genioplasty' for the second. Reduction of the vertical height of the chin is indicated when the anterior lower dental height (ALDH) is high in relation to the other linear and angular measurements indicative of anterior facial height (p. 58). The simplest method is to deglove the anterior mandible and reduce the lower border with a bur (**816**). Unfortunately this removes all or most of the cortical plate of the lower border and often results in poor contour and irregularity on palpation, worse if there is irregular resorption. The correct method for all but the most minor recontouring is to remove a subapical wedge of bone and reposition the lower border superiorly, using simple wire fixation between the cut surfaces of the labial cortical plate. The soft-tissues are not detached from the inferior surface in order to maintain viability and improve the postoperative contour (**817** and **818**). This technique, while time-consuming also has the advantage that horizontal correction can be undertaken at the same time (**819**), and this is frequently of benefit.

820

821

824

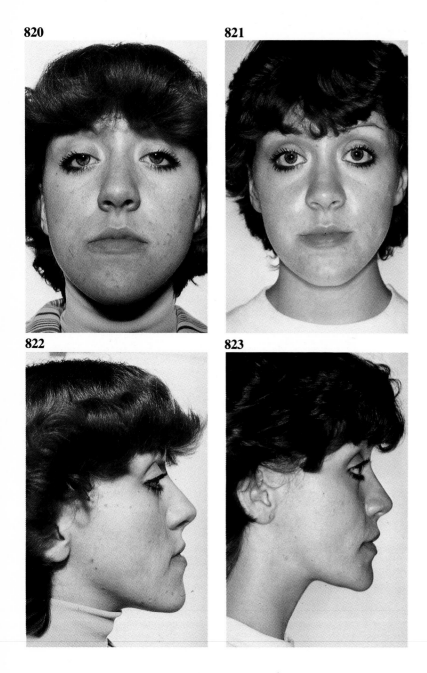

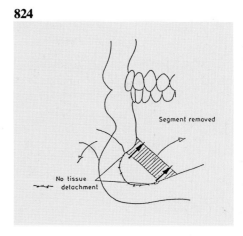

822

823

825

826

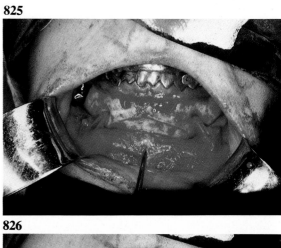

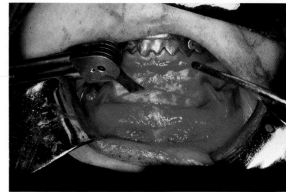

820 to 823 **Combined vertical and horizontal reduction genioplasty** plus Le Fort 1 maxillary advancement: full face and profile changes (**821** and **823**, three years after operation).

The case shown in **820** to **823** illustrates the result of combined vertical and horizontal reduction genioplasty by the method described (**816** to **819**) plus Le Fort 1 maxillary advancement, a common combination. Note the improved vertical balance and the better chin contour from both the anterior and side views. The postoperative views were taken 3 years after operation, and confirm both the stability and the adaptation of the soft-tissues to the reduced skeletal base. A further example of this type of problem is illustrated (**303** to **307**).

824 to 828 **Horizontal reduction genioplasty:** surgical technique.

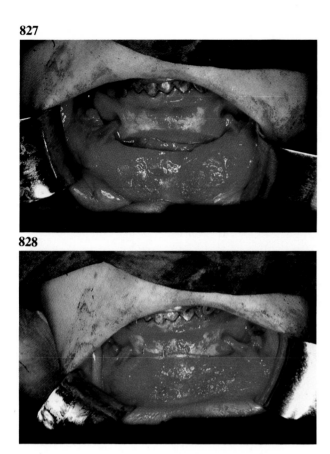

827

828

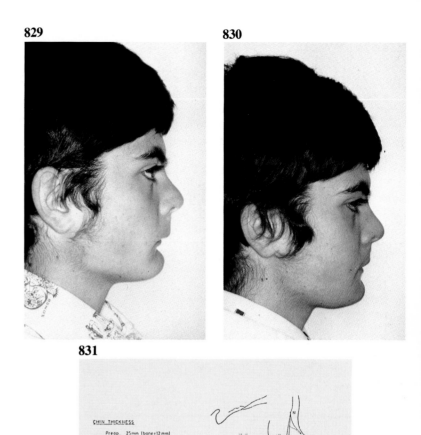

829   830

831

CHIN THICKNESS

Preop. 25mm (bone=12mm)
Postop. 21mm (· 5mm)

ie bony reduction of 7mm produced
only 3mm reduction in total chin thickness
or approx. ⅖ th.
The soft tissue thickness is always increased.

S.M. Case treated by FSS & HORIZONTAL

REDUCTION GENIOPLASTY

829 to 831   Horizontal reduction genioplasty with mandibular advancement: profile changes.

Horizontal reduction genioplasty is also most easily accomplished by simple bony reduction of the anterior prominence, but this method is again less than satisfactory except in the case of minor adjustments. The problem appears to be that after the soft-tissues have been detached, the bone reduced, and the soft-tissues replaced, the natural elasticity of the soft-tissue integument tends to lead to retention of the original shape. A dead space is left where the bone has been reduced, and this fills with blood clot which soon becomes organised to form new fibrous tissue. Thus the total chin thickness is little altered, despite a reduction in the bony contribution.

The best way of reducing this effect is seen in the series **824** to **828**. The mandible is degloved only to the level necessary to accomplish a sharply angled wedge excision in the subapical region (**824** and **825**). The instrument indicates the point of the bony chin. The upper limit of the wedge can be seen. The saw is used and angled down towards the lower border at 45° to make both upper and lower cuts (**826**) and when the wedge is excised the sloping upper surface is clearly seen (**827**). The lower border, with its soft-tissues still firmly attached, is then wired into position with backward displacement (**828**). This prevents the development of any dead space and is adequate for the majority of cases.

The illustrative case is typical and the tracing shows a correction at the soft-tissue pogonion of two fifths of the correction at the pogonion itself. This is probably the maximum attainable in backward displacement of the chin, in contrast to the 1:1 movement in advancement genioplasty. The patient shown (**829** preoperatively, **830** postoperatively) is a Class 2 Div 1 case with concomitant progenia, having a total chin thickness of 25mm anterior to the line NB projected inferiorly. Treatment could be by mandibular advancement (bilateral FSS) plus reduction genioplasty, or by total subapical mandibular osteotomy. The former was chosen as the simpler option, although in retrospect the latter would have allowed improvement in the vertical height of the mandibular body, with benefit.

832

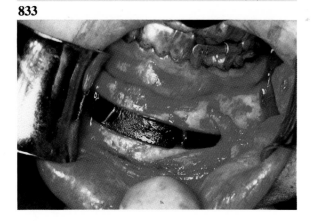

insert bone
or proplast

833

832 to 838 **Vertical augmentation genioplasty.**
Proplast implant (**833**); correction of Class 2 Div 1 case
(**834** to **838**).

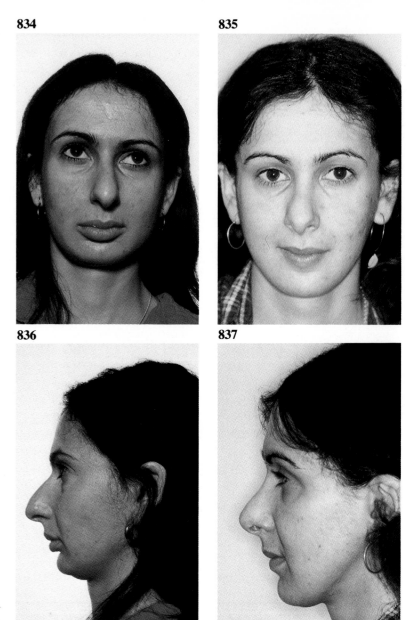

834

835

836

837

Augmentation genioplasty may also be required in the horizontal plane (advancement genioplasty, anterior augmentation genioplasty) or the vertical plane (vertical augmentation genioplasty). The indication for increase in vertical height of the subapical bone will be discussed in the section on vertical dysplasia (Section 5) but in general if the ALDH is below the indicated normal when the linear and angular measurements for the whole face are compared, increase in subapical bone height is indicated. This is done (**832**) by making an oblique cut below the apices of the anterior teeth, and carrying it to the lower border (at a distance indicated by the case assessment) below the mental foramina. The anterior lower border is angled down and bone or proplast is inserted to make up the required increase in vertical height (**833**). This is most often indicated in Class 2 Div 1 cases and an example is shown, corrected by proplast implant. Proplast is excellent for this purpose (**834** to **838**).

838

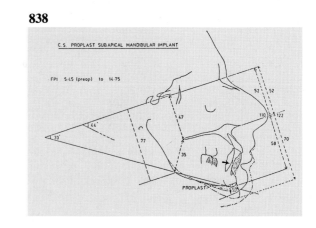

C. S. PROPLAST SUBAPICAL MANDIBULAR IMPLANT

FPI 5.45 (preop) to 14.75

PROPLAST

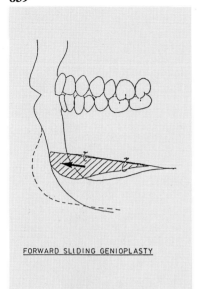

839 to 843 **Advancement genioplasty: 840,** wiring of lingual plate to labial plate; **841,** packing with cancellous chips; **842** and **843,** profile changes (with mandibular advancement).

FORWARD SLIDING GENIOPLASTY

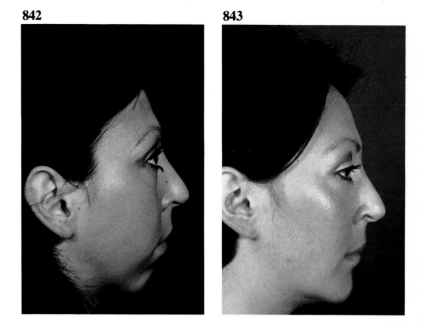

842

843

840

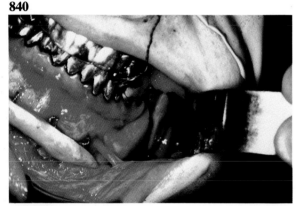

841

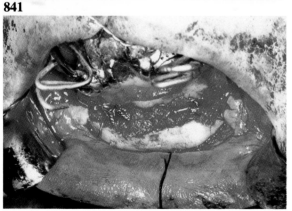

Horizontal augmentation of the chin is achieved by **advancement genioplasty** according to the method of Obwegeser (1971), except that a soft-tissue pedicle is maintained to the lower border fragment. The lower border is sectioned as described for vertical augmentation genioplasty and advanced until the lingual plate lies underneath the labial plate of the subapical region (**839**) to which it is wired in 3 or 4 places (**840**). Contouring at the distal end of the segment is often necessary to obtain a smooth lower border and bone may be added if desired, usually by packing cancellous chips around the advanced edge (**841**). Bone grafting is rarely necessary for single advancements as there is soon good adaptation; the author only uses it if the hip is open for other reasons.

The direction of the cut may be angled to allow the anterior chin to slide upwards or downwards during advancement, according to the case. The midline is sometimes divided to improve transverse adaption, but the method of Converse (1952) whereby the lower border is adapted to the anterior part of the subapical bone is never used; it is preferable to perform an anterior mandibuloplasty in almost every case where this technique is suggested, or alternatively to use the simple forward sliding genioplasty with iliac bone grafting in addition. The problem rarely arises after full assessment. A typical case involving also mandibular advancement is shown (**842** and **843**).

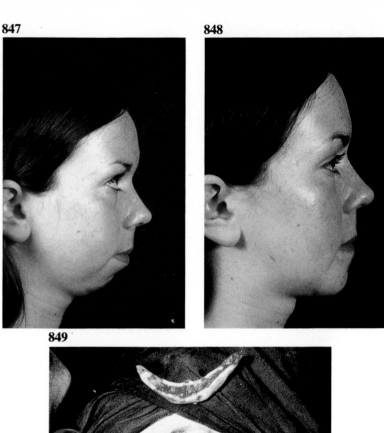

844

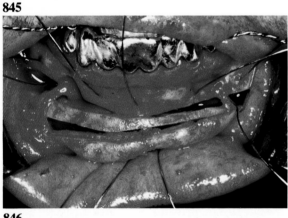

844 to 850 Double sliding genioplasty. Surgical technique (**845** and **846**); correction of severe retrogenia (**847** and **848**); detachment of soft-tissue from lower border segment (**849**); follow up radiographs showing marked resorption of the chin (**850**).

? Bone chips

847

848

845

846

849

850

In severe retrogenia a double layer forward slide is necessary (**844**), bringing the two layers of subapical bone forward like two drawers opening under each other, the lower coming forward further than the upper. The cuts are laborious and must be made with a saw in order to preserve vertical bone. Bone grafting is useful here in order to obtain good contour

and the mental nerves must be watched carefully to prevent damage from the distal ends of the sections during manipulation (**845**). The two layers are wired firmly (**846**) and bone is packed around the interstices after fixation. In this way quite severe retrogenia can be corrected.

The case shown (**847** and **848**) is interesting for several reasons. Double forward sliding (advancement) genioplasty was combined with mandibular advancement. However, at that time (1973) the author followed the technique of detaching all soft-tissue from the lower border segment, thus creating a free bone graft (**849**) and subsequent follow up radiographs have shown marked resorption of the chin with loss of contour (**850**).

This has been our experience, and a dilemma is produced by the conflicting requirements of blood supply (inhibiting resorption by maintaining a pedicle) and the tension introduced by stretching a pedicle forwards. In these cases we perform the operation without detaching the soft-tissues but with a division of the anterior bellies of the digastric about 1 cm from their attachment to the back of the segment. This has been stable in our hands. Incidentally the radiographs (**850**) also show the now outdated technique of over-correction in mandibular advancement.

Indications and results

The chin is augmented if there is disproportionate deficiency on radiography, supported by clinical observation of the labiomental groove. Where total chin thickness exceeds 18 mm anterior to NB projected inferiorly, horizontal reduction genioplasty is considered. Where reduction of ALFH can be traced to deficient ALDH, vertical augmentation genioplasty is considered. Where total chin thickness drops below 14 mm advancement genioplasty is considered. Where vertical height in the subapical area appears excessive, vertical reduction genioplasty is considered. In all cases clinical assessment overrides cephalometric measurement as a criterion of need; and the contour of the chin in profile as well as the shape in full face view are used to guide the details of technique.

Advancement of the pogonion results in a 1:1 advancement of the soft-tissue pogonion while about two fifths of the posterior movement achieved by the technique described is accomplished in horizontal reduction genioplasty.

Corrective surgery of the maxilla

Osteotomies of the maxilla are traditionally described by comparison with the common fracture patterns of the mid-third of the facial skeleton, named after the work of Réné Le Fort (1900). Hence the Le Fort 1, Le Fort 2 and Le Fort 3 fractures which are illustrated here indicate levels at which the maxilla may be sectioned electively from the rest of the skull (**851**).

The fractures occur at the lines of weakness least able to resist anteroposterior or oblique forces applied to the face. Thus the low level fracture (Le Fort 1) results from trauma localised over the lower maxilla, the intermediate fracture (Le Fort 2) reflects more widespread mid-facial trauma, and the total maxillary fracture (Le Fort 3) results from the most broadly applied facial force. At roughly corresponding levels therefore the Le Fort 1, 2 and 3 maxillary osteotomies are named.

However, there are several important differences between the fractures and the osteotomies. First, the fractures pass across the pterygoid plates, while the osteotomies aim to separate the maxillae anteriorly from the pterygoid plates posteriorly. Second, there is no reason to select the lines of weakness when making osteotomy cuts; indeed this may result in sectioning very thin bone when it is more desirable to divide through thicker sections for the placement of fixation wires, or the attachment of bone grafts. Finally there is a danger of thinking in narrow and restricted terms of the classical lines of fracture, whereas the abnormality being corrected may indicate the desirability of tailoring the osteotomy to the individual patient in a way quite different to any fracture pattern. In fact maxillary osteotomies can be devised along widely varying lines, which may be symmetrical or asymmetrical, unilateral or bilateral.

Once the maxilla has been separated from the rest of the skull it may be brought forwards, or inferiorly repositioned to lengthen the mid-face. If appropriate sections are removed, it may be elevated to shorten the mid-face. Shortening is really only practicable at the Le Fort 1 level by removing a section of bone from the maxillary antral walls and the nasal septum; lengthening can be achieved at all three levels, with interpositional bone grafting.

851

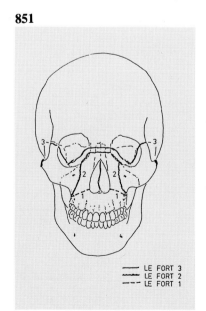

851 Le Fort lines of facial skeletal weakness: fracture patterns.

The surgical options in the maxilla may be divided into two groups – total maxillary osteotomies and segmental alveolar osteotomies. Broadly speaking the following procedures must be described:

(a) Total maxillary osteotomies
    1. Le Fort 1 procedures
    2. Le Fort 2 procedures
    3. Le Fort 3 procedures
(b) Segmental alveolar maxillary osteotomies
    1. Anterior segmental osteotomies or ostectomies
    2. Posterior segmental osteotomies or ostectomies
    3. Combined anterior and posterior procedures.

Total maxillary osteotomies

These, while differing in the upper part of the mid-face, share many points of principle and technique. All are used to advance the mid-face leaving the *pterygoid columns* (the medial and lateral pterygoid plates) intact on the rest of the skull *(cranial residue)*.

This is accomplished by carrying the osteotomy line posteriorly on the lateral wall of the maxilla to a point just above the pterygomaxillary 'suture' (ie the conjoined pterygoid plates posteriorly with the maxillary bloc, which includes most of the palatine bone, anteriorly – a topographical 'suture' rather than a strictly osteological one). Curved osteotomes are then used to separate the maxillary bloc anteriorly from the pterygoid columns posteriorly. This *pterygomaxillary dysjunction* (**852**) is common to all total maxillary osteotomies, and is discussed in detail on pp. 233 to 236.

The Le Fort 1 osteotomy

This sections the mid-face through the walls of the maxillary sinuses, the lateral nasal walls, and the nasal septum at a level just superior to the apices of the maxillary teeth.

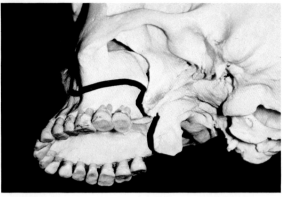

852   Pterygomaxillary dysjunction.

853

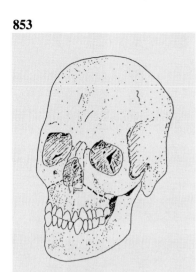

LE FORT 1 - CUTS

854

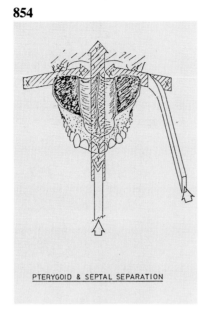

PTERYGOID & SEPTAL SEPARATION

Starting at the inferolateral margin of the pyriform aperture of the nose it traverses the anterolateral and posterolateral walls of the maxillary antrum about 3 mm or 4 mm above the apices of the canine, premolar and molar teeth (**853**). It passes across the canine fossa to the base of the zygomatic buttress and curves around and above the maxillary tuberosity to the lowest part of the pterygomaxillary fissure, whence it crosses the posterior wall of the antrum at the same level. It then turns forwards through the lateral wall of the nose below the inferior turbinate bone, to join the point of origin (**854**). This cut is made bilaterally.

The pterygoid plates are next separated from the posterior aspects of the maxillary tuberosities (X to X^1 in **854**) and the nasal septum is detached from the superior aspect of the hard palate by dividing it along its length with a chisel (Y to Y^1 in **854**). The dentoalveolar part of the maxillae and the hard palate are now free from the cranial residue, and may be repositioned anteriorly (**855**), or inferiorly, or rotated transversely. Further cuts are necessary for other repositioning requirements and these will be discussed at a later stage.

855

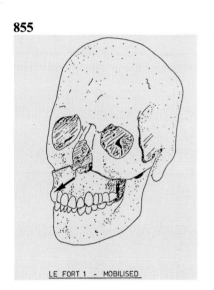

LE FORT 1 - MOBILISED

853 to 855 Le Fort 1 osteotomy.

856

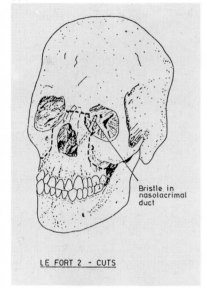

LE FORT 2 - CUTS

857

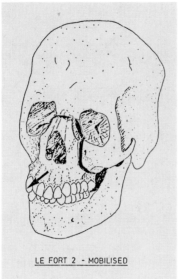

Bristle in
nasolacrimal
duct

LE FORT 2 - MOBILISED

858

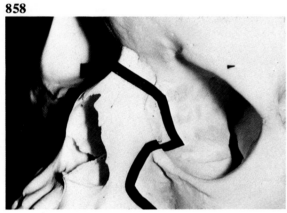

859

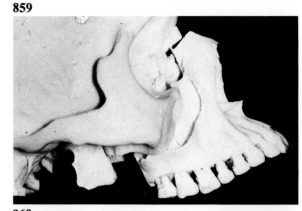

860

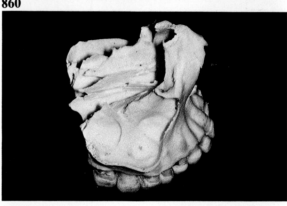

861

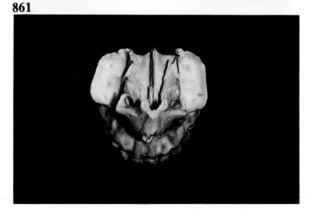

The Le Fort 2 osteotomy

This (**856** and **857**) is a pyramidal osteotomy which is identical to the Le Fort 1 procedure from the pterygoid column forward to the zygomatic buttress. It then passes, not to the pyriform aperture of the nose, but superiorly towards the orbit.

It is kept anteromedial to the infraorbital foramen to cross the inferior orbital margin at a point halfway between the lacrimal duct medially and the infraorbital canal laterally (**858**). The osteotomy then passes posteriorly along the orbital floor at right angles to the orbital rim to gain the area behind the lacrimal groove and its contained lacrimal sac. The cut then turns medially to pass behind and parallel to the posterior lacrimal crest as far as the upper part of the lacrimal groove.

It then turns forwards across the apex of the lacrimal groove to emerge from the orbit medially, just below the midpoint of the medial canthal attachment. The frontal process of the maxilla is then crossed and the cut becomes continuous with the osteotomy of the other side across the nasal bones. The nasal septum is divided at a higher level than in the Le Fort 1 osteotomy, passing from the nasal bones anteriorly in a downwards and backwards direction to the posterior part of the septum just above the posterior nasal spine (**860**). The lateral nasal walls are fractured during mobilisation of the maxilla at levels corresponding to the septal cut. An alternative way of dealing with the septum, especially in the presence of septal deviation, is by formal submucous resection (SMR).

The mobilised maxillary bloc is shown on a dried skull (**859**), and the part of the maxillae mobilised is shown from the side (**860**) and from above (**861**) to demonstrate the lines of section and the varying depth of bone at the various osteotomy sites.

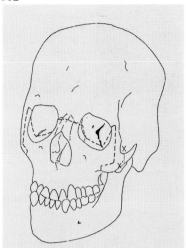

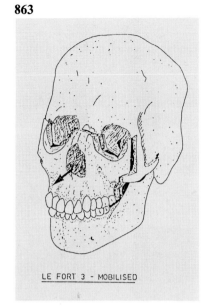

862 and 863   Le Fort 3 osteotomy.

The Le Fort 3 osteotomy

This (**862** and **863**) lies at the interface of orthognathic and craniofacial surgery, the latter lying outside the scope of this book. The varieties of craniofacial problems to which the Le Fort 3 procedure and its many variants can be applied in combination with surgery of the cranial vault constitute a separate study, but there are many important areas of overlap with subcranial orthognathic surgery where the mid-face is concerned. The descriptions in this volume will be confined to the application of the subcranial Le Fort 3 to the correction of symmetrical mid-facial recession affecting the zygomatico-maxillary and orbital regions, but excluding hypertelorism and deformities of the cranial vault and cranial base. All these conditions (including those scheduled for subcranial Le Fort 3 osteotomy) require detailed analysis by experienced cranio-facial teams if associated anomalies and potential operative problems are to be identified and evaluated. Several different disciplines contribute usefully to the craniofacial team.

The basic osteotomy as orginally described by Tessier (1971) was designed to achieve anteroposterior movement of the whole facial mass, establishing normal dental occlusion and increasing orbital capacity, enlarging both the height and depth of the orbits. It is (in Tessier's words) 'part of a *system* focused upon the orbit'. It aims to separate the facial mass from the cranial base along the inter-frontofacial and inter-pterygo-maxillary planes (**862**). To do this the osteotomy traverses, on each side, the medial orbital wall, the orbital floor, and the lateral orbital wall to reach the frontozygomatic suture region.

The frontal process of the zygomatic bone is then split sagittally (effectively splitting the lateral wall of the orbit) and the cut is continued inferiorly to complete division of the zygoma. The two sides are connected, centrally through the frontonasal area, as in the Le Fort 2 osteotomy. Pterygo-maxillary and septal separation are then completed as for the Le Fort 2 operation and the central facial block is mobilised (**863**). A common alternative is to complete the lateral orbital wall cuts through the full thickness of the zygomatic bone at its junction with the sphenoid, emerging from the orbit at the frontozygomatic suture region. A separate section is then required through the arch of the zygoma (usually sited X to X^1 in **862**) to complete separation from the cranial residue.

Surgical technique of total maxillary osteotomies

Regardless of level and extent the basic technique is common to all total maxillary osteotomies, although the operative work and potential complications increase as a wider facial area is involved. The technical stages may be divided into four areas:
1. The osteotomy cuts and pterygomaxillary dysjunction
2. Mobilisation and advancement
3. Fixation
4. Bone grafting

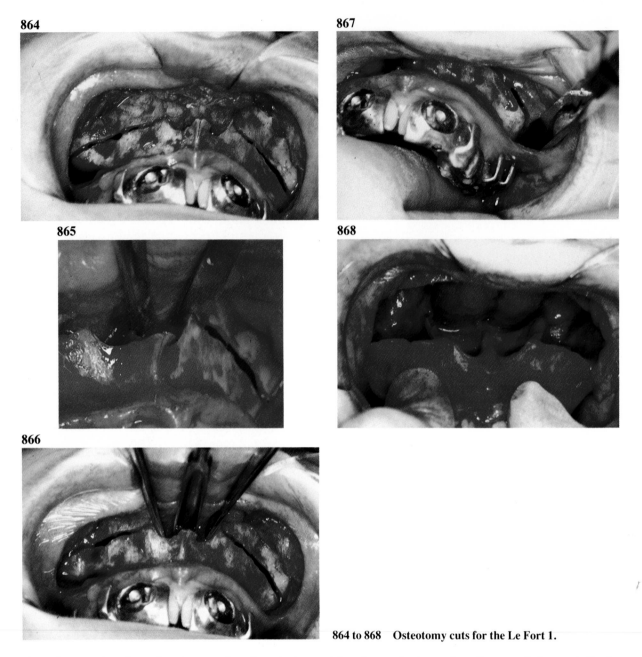

864   **867**

865   **868**

866

864 to 868   Osteotomy cuts for the Le Fort 1.

It is proposed to discuss the three levels together in relation to these headings, with special attention to areas which relate specifically to particular levels.

Osteotomy cuts for the Le Fort 1 are made after exposure of the lower maxilla intraorally, as described on pp. 150 to 152. In uncomplicated, non-cleft palate patients the horseshoe incision (**552**) gives the best access and control, although many surgeons still prefer divided vestibular (**553**) or multiple vertical incisions (**554**). The horseshoe incision is mandatory for the down-fracture technique to be described, giving access to the upper surface of the palate for combined anterior and posterior segmental modifications or for repositioning the maxilla superiorly. Divided vertical incisions are necessary if the palatal

blood supply is to be disrupted (especially by raising palatal flaps), and certain procedures carried out on cleft palate patients (see Section 5) require this approach.

The lateral bone cuts are easily made with surgical burs or saw (**864**). The nasal spine is then carefully dissected free and the pyriform aperture of the nose defined subperiosteally. The nasal mucosa can then be raised from the palate, nasal septum and lateral nasal wall below the inferior conchae. This is done as far back as possible so that the whole of the mucosa of the nasal floor on each side is draped from the septum to the conchae, if possible without a split. With a Howarth's nasal raspatory in place to protect the mucosa, the lateral nasal wall is sectioned *anteriorly* with a bur or osteotome through the

228

anterior part of the lateral cut (**865**). Howarth's raspatories are then placed on each side of the nasal septum to protect the mucosa and a notched nasal chisel is driven back to separate the base of the septum from the upper surface of the palate (**866**). The depth may be assessed directly with a finger curved round the back of the soft palate, palpating the advancing chisel; or the depth may be estimated on the chisel by comparison with the intraoral palatal depth.

Pterygomaxillary dysjunction (see **890**, **891** and **892**) is performed with a curved chisel on each side (**867**). At this stage the maxilla may be started on the first stage of mobilisation by downward traction (often the fingers are adequate), and as it hinges down (**868**) the opening anterior osteotomy lines improve access posteriorly for completion of soft-tissue detachment from the nasal floor, and for final sectioning of the lateral nasal walls with an osteotome as far as the posterior antral walls. If the maxilla does not begin to hinge down under finger pressure at this stage, the insertion of a small osteotome along the line of the lateral nasal wall cut, which can then be gently driven posteriorly, invariably starts the downfracture movement. This completes the cuts shown in **853**, **854** and **855**.

Osteotomy cuts for the Le Fort 2 are made through two intraoral vestibular incisions, from the upper canines to the second molars; and through two paranasal incisions as shown in **603** and **604**. Preliminary temporary tarsorraphies are undertaken (**869**).

Paranasal exposure of the nasal bones and upper maxillae, together with the medial orbit, is completed (**870**) and the skin is raised subperiosteally over the glabellar region. A small incision is usually made above the nasal bridge (**610**) to assist periosteal elevation over the nasal bones and the glabellar region generally, and later for access in the placement of bone grafts in the same region. The anterior and posterior lacrimal crests, the lacrimal duct and the medial part of the orbital floor are now fully exposed on each side.

With a surgical fissure bur a cut is started from the orbital rim back into the orbital floor until the lacrimal apparatus has been passed on its lateral side (**871** and **872**). The medial orbital wall is sectioned across the apex of the lacrimal groove on each side, taking care not to strip more than the minimum amount of the medial canthal attachment necessary to provide proper protection of the soft-tissues during bone cutting (**871** and **873**). The lacrimal duct is drawn laterally so that the two cuts (medial wall and floor) can be joined together with an osteotome behind the posterior lacrimal crest. The instrument is directed downwards behind and parallel to the posterior lacrimal crest (**871**). This must be checked for completeness, because jagged spicules of bone may otherwise fragment during mobilisation of the maxilla, damaging the lacrimal duct or sac.

869

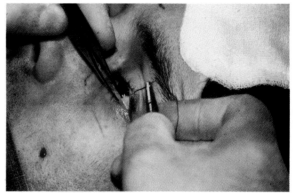

870

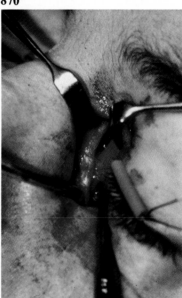

871

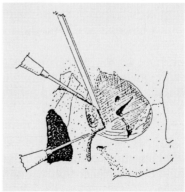

869 to 877   Osteotomy cuts for the Le Fort 2.

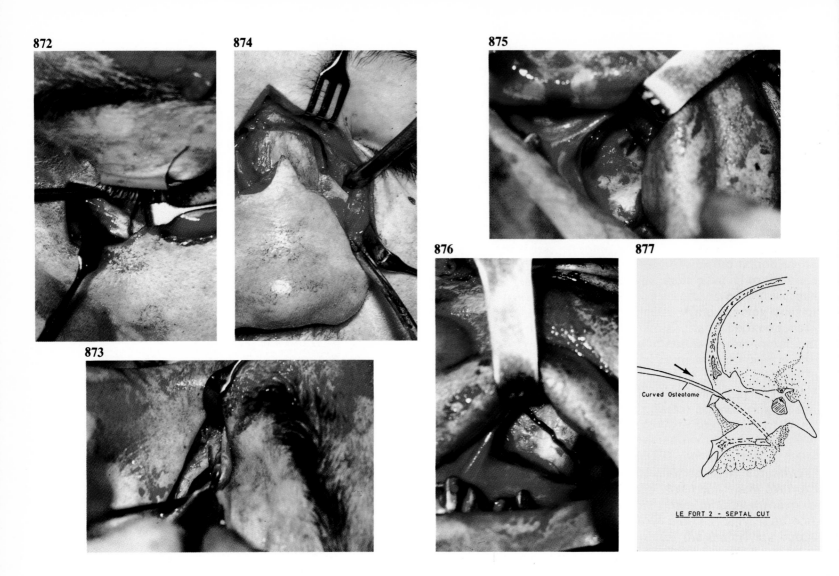

872

874

873

875

876

877

Curved Osteotome

LE FORT 2 - SEPTAL CUT

Finally a channelled retractor (such as the Seldin Pyriform Rim retractor) is passed under the soft-tissues of the nasal bridge, and the cuts in the right and left medial orbital walls are connected with a bur or saw beneath its protection. Only the horseshoe-shaped section of bone at the nasal bridge (**861**) has to be cut and deeper penetration below the cribriform plate is unnecessary. Preoperative radiography of this region is essential to determine that the cribriform plate is at the normal level (or to establish any abnormality so that avoiding action can be taken) and that no other abnormalities of the anterior cranial floor are present. Sectioning into the nose usually provokes brisk haemorrhage from the torn nasal mucosa, but this settles quickly either spontaneously or with light packing.

The completed naso-orbital cuts are shown in **874** through a V–Y incision, with the lacrimal duct displayed. It must be emphasised that this incision is hardly ever used, and is chosen here for demonstration purposes from an early case. Although these bony cuts are difficult to display through paranasal incisions, the mobility of the skin in this region makes it a simple matter to complete the osteotomies through them. The anterior maxillary cuts are next started from the same access, continuing the line of the osteotomy from the inferior orbital rim downwards, keeping medial to the infraorbital foramen.

Attention is then directed to the intraoral incisions, the tissues being retracted upwards with a Hajek's retractor until the bottom of the cut made so far comes into view (**875**). This is extended around the zygomatic buttress to the pterygoid region (**876**). Pterygomaxillary dysjunction is performed as for the Le Fort 1. A curved osteotome is introduced through the glabellar incision (or by lateral displacement of the nasal bridge skin) into the nasal bone cut, and directed backwards and downwards towards the posterior nasal spine to complete division of the nasal septum with a few sharp taps (**877**). No attempt is made to protect the nasal mucosa, and this has never been the cause of any complication. Alternatively a formal submucous resection may be undertaken, usually at the outset of the operation.

Osteotomy cuts for the Le Fort 3 are accomplished via a bifrontal flap (fully described on pp. 169 and 170) in the upper part; this is usually combined with separate incisions for access to the orbital floor, and intraoral vestibular incisions to allow pterygomaxillary dysjunction. It is *possible* to complete all the cuts from a fully extended bifrontal flap, including the orbital floors and the pterygomaxillary dysjunction, but this can lead to difficulties, especially at the later stages of bone grafting. The author's preference is for a bifrontal flap access combined with subciliary and small intraoral vestibular incisions in the second molar regions of the maxilla.

As previously described, the whole of the frontal area, the orbital roofs, walls and floors, and the whole of the infra-temporal aspect of the lateral orbital walls together with the zygomatic bone in its entirety must be exposed subperiosteally for the cuts to be completed. The special advantage of the bifrontal flap exposure (**878**), by comparison with multiple small periorbital incisions, is the opportunity it affords for right/left comparison during the reconstructive phase. Some operators prefer to use the transconjunctival approach to the orbital floor.

The osteotomy lines already described (**862** and **863**) can all be performed easily once the exposure is complete. In the simpler variation (**884**) (the sagittal split of the orbital walls will be described separately) a cut is started at the frontozygomatic suture region through the lateral orbital wall in its full depth (**879**). The orbital contents are retracted during this cut so that the full extent of the orbital wall is visualised, and the tip of the bur observed intraorbitally to ensure that the middle cranial fossa is not entered inadvertently. It is important to remember that in the craniostenotic syndromes for which this operation is most often indicated the orbit is very shallow anteroposteriorly. The lateral wall may be little more than a rim applied to the edge of the orbit, and the unwary operator can easily allow the bur to wander into the cranial cavity if it is not kept under continual observation throughout its length. The cut is continued down to the inferior orbital fissure (**880**).

The zygomatic arch is next divided at the point shown (**881**) to allow fixation of an interpositional bone graft on the two cut ends of the arch. The nasofrontal cut is then made, great care being taken to evaluate the position of the cribriform plate and to exclude intracranial abnormality in the anterior cranial fossa and floor. Preoperative tomography of this region should always have been undertaken, and the existence of any intra-cranial abnormality is an absolute indication for a transcranial

878

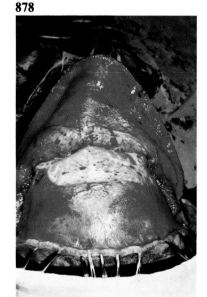

879

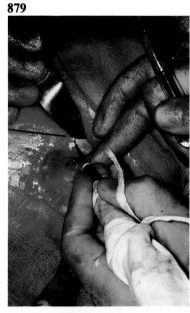

880

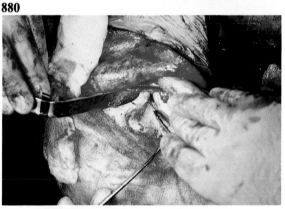

881

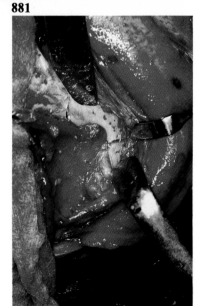

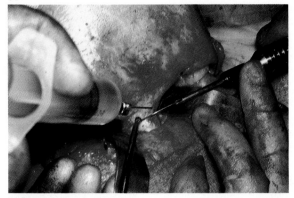

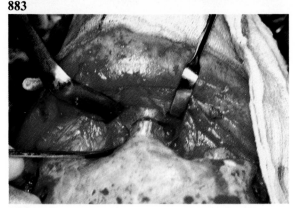

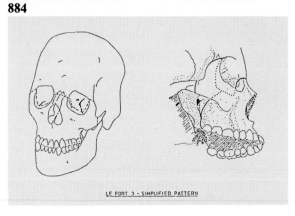

LE FORT 3 - SIMPLIFIED PATTERN

878 to 884   Osteotomy cuts for the Le Fort 3. (**878** and **883** are viewed from above looking down over the supraorbital ridges. **879, 880** and **881** are viewed from above on the right side. **882** is viewed from the front, right side.)

approach to the anterior cranial floor. The saw is angled downwards and backwards through the nasofrontal region as shown (**882**). The cut is then carried down the medial orbital wall (**883**) posterior to the lacrimal groove and then forwards and laterally to the inferior orbital fissure across the orbital floor.

If preferred the cut can run anterior to the fissure where there is a sufficient depth of bone, preserving the infraorbital nerve. This is a variable area anatomically; sometimes the fissure gives way to a groove along which the nerve passes to exit through the foramen below the orbital rim. Once the medial and lateral orbital cuts are connected (directly or via the inferior orbital fissure) the upper dissection is completed. A curved Tessier pattern osteotome is used to separate the pterygoid plates from the maxilla via the intraoral vestibular incision, and the nasal septum is divided as in the Le Fort 2 procedure. The maxilla can then be mobilised. This completes the cuts shown in **884**.

Sagittal splitting of the lateral orbital wall combined with a step osteotomy of the zygoma (**885**) was introduced by Tessier in the early days of the Le Fort 3 procedure. The lateral wall of the orbit is only partially sectioned from the orbital side and then continued vertically down through the frontal process of the zygoma to its mid-body; from here it is carried forwards and downwards as shown (**886**) to form a step anterior to the attachments of the masseter muscle.

The vertical cut through the frontal process of the zygoma is best made with a saw, angled back into the orbit to achieve the desired sagittal section of the lateral wall (**887**). The main advantage of this is that a greater surface is made available for interpositional bone grafting at an area critically important in maintaining the forward position of the advanced mid-face. The step is a logical extension of this to avoid backward displacing forces.

The simpler method described (**878** to **884**), supported by rigid malar arch grafting (see **917**) is, however, quite adequate and much simpler to perform.

Pterygomaxillary dysjunction is the separation of the pterygoid column from the maxillary bloc, and is an important part of all total maxillary osteotomies as well as posterior segmental alveolar maxillary procedures. It is necessary to appreciate the normal anatomy of the region and the possibilities for abnormality in the patients being treated.

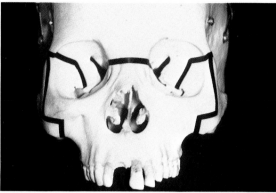

885

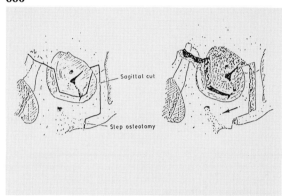

886

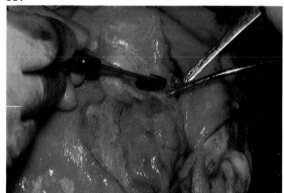

887

885 to 887 **Sagittal splitting** of the lateral orbital wall combined with a **step osteotomy** of the zygoma.

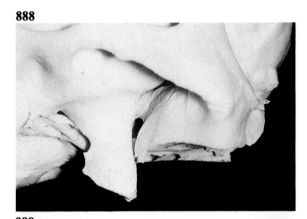

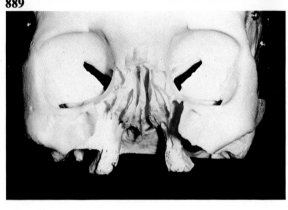

888 and 889   The pterygoid column from the side (**888**) and from the front (**889**).

In the non-cleft palate group the area of pterygomaxillary abutment is a small discrete one, shown in **888** and **889** where the maxillary bloc has been removed from a dried skull after Le Fort 2 pattern osteotomy lines have been completed. The pterygoid column can be seen from the side (**888**) and from the front (**889**). Separation in the non-cleft patient is easy and thus leaves a solid wall of bone posteriorly on the pterygoid column, and a less solid but definite bony surface on the back of the maxillary bloc. It avoids surgical entry into the area behind the pterygoid laminae, which gives attachment to the pterygoid muscles and which is highly vascular. There is no need to enter the pterygomaxillary fissure at all deeply, the dysjunction occurring inferolaterally to the main fissure.

Over-enthusiastic chiselling, or too superomedial a direction of the chisel, can provoke troublesome haemorrhage from the pterygoid plexus of veins or one of the vessels normally contained within the fissure. Division of the pterygoid plates (as in a fracture) increases the risk of haemorrhage considerably; post-traumatic maxillary osteotomies tend to bleed in the pterygoid region due to the tendency to re-open this area.

The intact pterygoid column provides a base against which a bone graft may be placed if so desired. Additionally the intact muscle attachments probably help to minimise postoperative speech disturbances by maintaining muscle function in the area more adequately. These are all strong reasons for rejecting posterior repositioning of the maxilla at the Le Fort 1 level (advocated by some operators) for the correction of maxillary protrusion. Where such a procedure is indicated it should be done by anterior segmental surgery, or by removing a section of the maxilla anterior to the interpterygomaxillary plane.

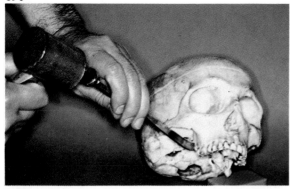

890

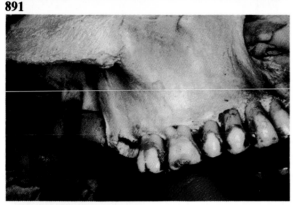

891

892

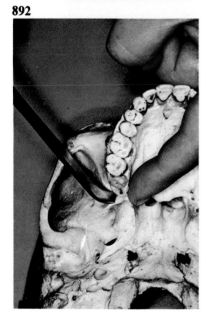

890 to 892 Pterygomaxillary dysjunction: method.

In cleft palate patients, and in some with very severe maxillary hypoplasia, the area of contact tends to be flatter and to extend more widely, placed more medially and rather higher up than normal. This is more difficult to locate accurately, and harder to separate cleanly, with a tendency to leave a thin bony wall on the maxilla as the only anterior boundary to the space between maxilla and pterygoid column. This thin bone may disintegrate under the chisel, or the chisel may pass in front of it into the antrum, thus converting the space in front of the pterygoid column into a posterior extension of the antrum. This situation is unsuitable for placement of a 'retromaxillary' bone graft. The same occurs when the maxilla is inferiorly repositioned and a space is developed where the anterior wall of the space would otherwise lie.

Pterygomaxillary dysjunction – method: A thin curved chisel is selected, the width of which is approximately the same as the apparent height of the pterygomaxillary area of contact (**890**). This is inserted in the pterygomaxillary groove at the bottom of the contact area and directed palatally and slightly upwards towards a guard finger placed on the palatal aspect over the periosteum (**891** and **892**). This finger can usually detect the pterygoid hamulus distally and the inner aspect of the maxillary tuberosity medially; proprioceptive awareness enables the chisel to be directed accurately between the two, and as it is malletted firmly into the groove it can be felt penetrating between hamulus and tuberosity below the palatal mucoperiosteum.

In the cleft patient the chisel usually requires to be directed more superiorly and guided further round the back of the tuberosity. As soon as the chisel is palpated beneath the palatal mucoperiosteum it should be withdrawn.

893

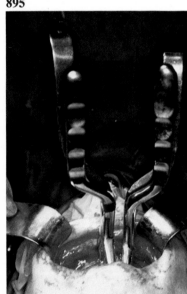

894

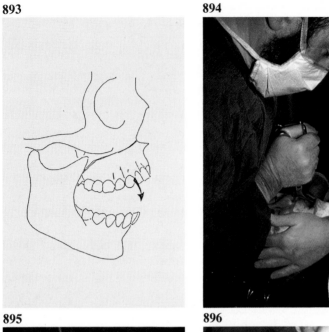

895

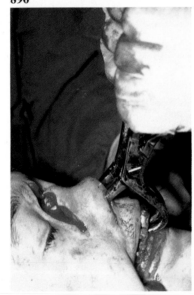

896

893 to 896   Maxillary mobilisation: Stage 1, dysjunction. Le Fort 1 (**895**);
Le Fort 2 and 3 (**896**).

Maxillary Mobilisation

Adequate mobilisation of the maxilla is the most important stage of mid-facial osteotomy surgery. The Le Fort 1 maxilla is the most easily mobilised and must be capable of repositioning with finger pressure alone after it is fully mobile. Considerable force may be necessary to mobilise Le Fort 2 or Le Fort 3 maxillae and it is rarely possible to achieve sufficient freedom to position the bloc by finger pressure alone.

Mobilisation should be thought of in three distinct stages, following each other in sequence:

Stage 1 – Stage of dysjunction
Stage 2 – Stage of detachment
Stage 3 – Stage of advancement

Stage of dysjunction (**893**). Objective – to complete the bony separation of the maxillary segment from the cranial residue. After the appropriate bony cuts have been made there always remain some attachments of maxilla to skull, usually along the lateral nasal walls or in the posterior antral walls. The object of the first movement of mobilisation is to sever these remaining attachments by fracture, this being achieved by displacing the maxilla in a firm, definite and purposive movement downwards as indicated, whilst an assistant holds the cranial vault firmly (**893** and **894**).

In the Le Fort 1 this can be accomplished by grasping the maxilla in the fingers and pressing firmly down towards the neck, assisted by the use of a small osteotome along the lateral nasal walls. If this fails, then Rowe's maxillary disimpaction forceps are inserted with the nasal blades inside the mouth passing beneath the nasal mucosa through the vestibular incision (**895**).

In Le Fort 2 or 3 osteotomies the nasal blades are inserted through the nostrils above the nasal mucosa (**896**), and during the downward movement the osteotomy lines are checked at the orbital and nasofrontal sites to confirm that the whole maxillary bloc is moving as one. It is important to detect any unwanted dysjunction between left and right sides (at the nasal bridge, and especially in cleft cases) and between the malar and maxillary components (in Le Fort 3 cases). Any incomplete cuts must be finalised with small osteotomes, and these can be used in the upper part of the mid-face to assist the dysjunction. Once full downward separation has occurred the second stage is commenced.

897

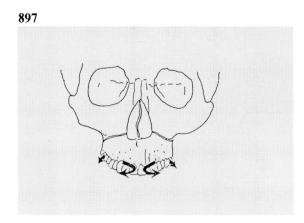

897   Maxillary mobilisation: Stage 2, detachment.

898

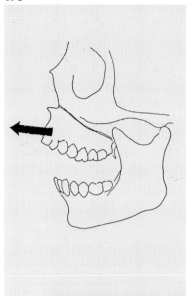

898 to 900   Maxillary mobilisation: Stage 3, advancement.

Stage of detachment (**897**). Objective – to separate the restraining soft-tissue attachments which prevent movement of the maxilla, while protecting those upon which the blood supply and innervation depend. In practice this means separating the tighter periosteal attachments in the deeper parts of the face which bind the maxilla to the rest of the skull after the bony separation is complete. The Rowe's forceps are left in place (or applied if not used in Stage 1) and a vigorous figure-of-eight movement applied to the maxillary block. A true figure-of-eight is achieved with Le Fort 1 maxillae, and the final separation at the pterygomaxillary region will be felt first on one side then on the other. A more restricted movement occurs with Le Fort 2 and 3 maxillae, but vigorous mobilisation is required. When the maxilla moves freely, the third stage is commenced.

Stage of advancement (**898**). Objective – to advance the mobilised maxilla to the predetermined position. While it is possible to pull the maxilla forwards with the same forceps used in Stage 2, the shape of the palate is not well adapted to forward traction while in the grip of metal forceps (even if protected). Much better is a positive force applied from behind the maxilla, a *vis-a-tergo*. Tessier's maxillary mobilisers (**899**) are recommended. The beaks are inserted behind the tuberosities anterior to the pterygoid columns, their position being confirmed with a palpating finger as for the osteotome during pterygomaxillary dysjunction. The head is steadied and the two instruments are drawn forward with controlled force, alternating the pressure between the right and left sides (**900**). Care must be taken that the beaks are applied to a firm bony surface, and that there is no bony obstruction to forward movement. The procedure is identical for all levels of osteotomy, and the mobilisation should continue to the maximum attainable, not only until the planned position can just be reached.

899

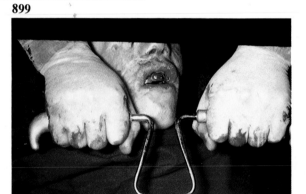

900

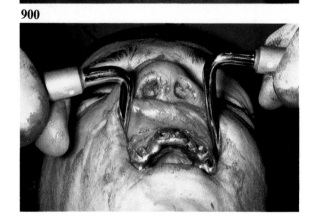

Fixation

The repositioned maxilla must be held in the planned position in relation to the lower dentition and in relation to the rest of the facial skeleton. The former is secured by intermaxillary fixation by any preferred method (interdental wiring, arch wiring, occlusal wafers, orthodontic banding or cast cap splints).

The choice of fixation to secure the maxilla in relation to the rest of the skull lies between (a) Internal skeletal suspension, (b) Extraskeletal fixation, either craniomaxillary or craniomandibular, and (c) no fixation at all. Solid bone grafts at sites where there is substantial bony support for the grafts are also held to provide fixation during the healing period. While the methods have their parallel in fracture work, there are significant differences also. In orthognathic surgery the bony fragments are to be placed in an 'unnatural' soft-tissue relationship and the pressures of these tissues tend to displace during bony union, whereas in the fracture case the tissues are in their pretraumatic relationship and displacement is much less of a problem after the initial stages of healing.

Significant relapsing changes can occur in the bony bases even while fixation is in place. In the author's experience the use of IMF *alone* delays union of the maxilla which can then take up to 3 months. When used in conjunction with functional orthodontic treatment good results are obtained in some hands, and maybe there is a future for this combination. Otherwise craniomaxillary fixation supplemented by intermaxillary and direct wiring is recommended for Le Fort 1 and 2 procedures as first choice, internal suspension being used for straightforward Le Fort 1 osteotomy cases with good postoperative occlusal interdigitation.

For Le Fort 3 cases there is much less need for extracranial support because of the extensive bone grafting; the latter with good interosseous wiring, combined with intermaxillary fixation is all that is necessary. Certain cleft palate patients do well on craniomandibular fixation, the maxillary segments being brought into correct relation with the mandibular segments by elastic traction, followed by wiring.

The duration of fixation depends on the procedure undertaken. The author tries to persuade patients to maintain their fixation for as long as they can tolerate it, up to 12 weeks; there is little doubt that longer fixation makes for greater stability. In practice only those types of case where stability is known to be a problem require the full 12 weeks and these include (a) Cleft palate cases undergoing maxillary advancement, (b) Those involving simultaneous mandibular advancement, especially by sagittal splitting methods, (c) Mid-facial lengthening, usually by inferior repositioning of the Le Fort 1 maxilla.

All maxillary osteotomies are kept in fixation for a minimum of 5 weeks, and Le Fort 2 cases rather longer. External fixation is removed from these at 6 weeks if the maxilla is clinically firm, and then intermaxillary fixation is removed 2 weeks later. Adult or adolescent Le Fort 3 cases unite quite quickly, but

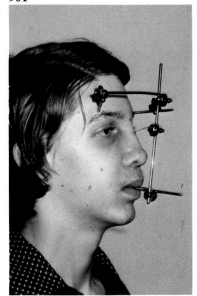

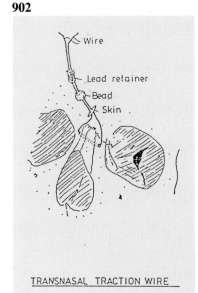

TRANSNASAL TRACTION WIRE

IMF is left for at least 6 weeks, followed by intermittent elastic traction (usually night traction). A useful construction where splints are used is to solder two projections onto the upper and lower splints in the canine regions, which match 'flat surface to flat surface' in the planned position. This is useful to locate the maxilla at operation and helps to maintain stability during early jaw mobilisation. The device is illustrated in **904** and **905**.

Direct craniomaxillary fixation has several advantages (**901**). First, the maxilla may be placed in its definitive position while bone grafts are tailored into the defects, overlaps, etc, with no danger of being disturbed during removal of packs, pharyngeal toilet, or early postoperative management (eg extubation, vomiting). This is especially useful in Le Fort 2 cases where careful bone grafting of the upper-face is necessary.

Second, the extraskeletal apparatus allows the use of direct traction on the upper parts of Le Fort 2 maxillary blocks. It is useful to drill a hole through the nasal bones and pass a wire from side to side, then bringing it below the skin to the midpoint of the nasal bridge, through a puncture in the midline and thence to the craniomaxillary bars (**901** and **902**). The wires are kept together in the midline by a crushed lead bead. This keeps the upper part of the bloc in position while bone grafting is placed and for the first 14 days of early consolidation.

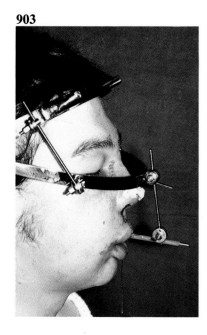

903

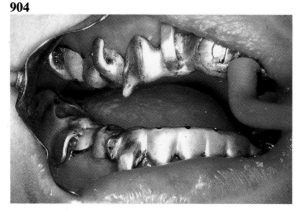

904

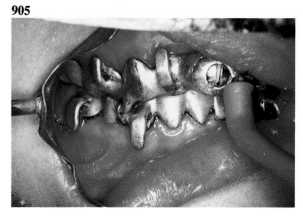

905

901 to 905   Direct craniomaxillary fixation.

Third, craniomaxillary fixation provides a mechanism for monitoring changes in the vertical height of the mid-face. Advancement of the mid-third (especially in the upper-face) has a tendency to increase vertical height unless the situation is carefully watched and measured. This is of course deliberately used to increase or decrease vertical height where indicated; in Le Fort 1 procedures the changes are readily observed at the osteotomy sites, but in Le Fort 2 cases an external reference is useful. Vertical bars can be marked to provide such a reference.

Fourth, craniomaxillary fixation is mandatory in bimaxillary cases in order to ensure that the planned proportion of movement is maintained as between maxilla and mandible. Internal suspension cannot secure this.

Finally it is often useful to be able to 'hold' the maxilla in a partially mobilised position while soft-tissue tethering is attended to – for example in the scarred area behind the palate in a secondary cleft palate case. The main disadvantage of extraskeletal fixation lies in its bulk, and inconvenience during the period of fixation. The most suitable form of fixation is the use of two supraorbital pins to which the maxillary block can be fixed (**901**) although haloframes can be used, if desired, with a visor attachment to provide another good method of direct mid-facial traction (**903**).

External craniomaxillary fixation is not recommended for Le Fort 3 cases where it interferes with finalisation of surgery and is unnecessary in view of the large areas of interpositional bone grafting. The locating 'ears' used on splints to position the advanced maxilla at the occlusal level in the planned position in relation to the mandible are shown at **904** (mouth open after IMF removed) and **905** (in the closed position). The anterior-facing flat surface of the mandibular 'ear' lies against the posteriorly-facing flat surface of the maxillary counterpart when the maxilla is in the planned position.

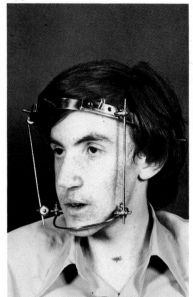

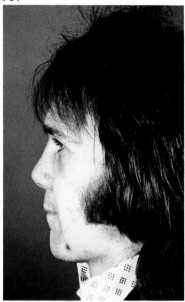

Craniomandibular fixation using the four-pin facial frame (**906**) is not recommended as a routine, mainly because it is not as flexible a method as direct craniomaxillary fixation and because it has a tendency to leave depressed scars at the sites of the mandibular pins (**907**). Where the maxillary segments of difficult secondary cleft palate cases cannot be brought into the required position at operation, the method is sometimes useful as a means of applying elastic traction to, eg, the lesser segment postoperatively.

Internal skeletal suspension in one or other of its many forms is widely employed for fixation, and has the great advantage of simplicity. The simple method of zygomatic arch suspension, either to an upper splint secured in intermaxillary fixation alone, or with the additional support of circumferential mandibular wiring, as shown on the model (**908**), provides excellent support. It is contra-indicated where the maxilla has been repositioned inferiorly with interpositional bone grafting (see pp. 251 to 252), and in the author's view should not be used where bimaxillary procedures have been undertaken. Where the bone cuts have crossed reasonably thick bony margins direct interosseous wiring greatly stabilises and supplements the method.

There are many different variations, each with their advocates. Some are illustrated (**909**), and include inferior orbital rim suspension, Epkers 'Sling' suspension, and pyriform rim suspension. Choice of method is largely one of personal preference.

908

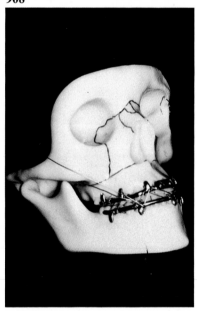

909

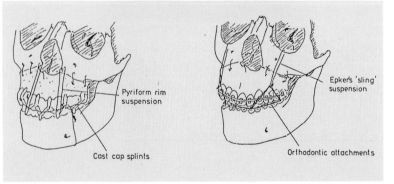

906 and 907 Craniomandibular fixation: the four-pin facial frame (**906**); scars at the sites of the mandibular pins (**907**).

908 and 909 Internal skeletal suspension.

Bone Grafting

The use of autogenous bone grafts to bridge osteotomy gaps and to promote early consolidation is routinely used by most operators, although there are some who do not bone graft the standard advancement Le Fort 1 osteotomy, and others who prefer to use lyophilized bone from bone banks (Sailer, 1976, 1980, Marx *et al*, 1981).

The donor site for autogenous bone will usually be the hip *(ilium)* or the rib. The latter is best in young children, but has a strong tendency to resorb in older patients. Where solid struts are needed the cortical bone of the ilium is best, but for most purposes it is desirable to obtain cancellous bone. The cells of the graft are important in the early development of osteogenesis.

In an excellent study of this aspect of bone grafting, Craig Gray and Elves (1979) conclude that 'the living cells of a bone graft play an important part in producing the early new bone in and around the graft. The endosteal and intrahaversian osteoblasts produce about 60% of the new bone, including a possible contribution by stromal cells of the marrow, and the periosteal cells are responsible for approximately 30% of the osteogenesis. There is little or no contribution to osteogenesis by graft osteocytes or by the free hemopoietic cells of the marrow. The endosteal osteoblasts of cortical bone are easily removed when marrow is gently washed out of the medullary cavity.'

In a subsequent paper (Gray and Elves, 1981) these authors further conclude that the size of individual grafts is important, and that the smallest dimension should not exceed 5mm, the best shape being a flat slab or strip of bone. Immersion in saline was found to be detrimental to cell survival, whereas exposure to moist air for up to 3 hours after harvesting from the donor site was safe; antibiotics in powder form were absolutely detrimental to cell vitality and vigour. They therefore recommend storage of grafts for not more than 3 hours in a closed container covered by a swab moistened with normal saline (but not immersed).

The author favours autogenous grafts wherever possible, using Flint's technique (Flint 1964) for obtaining small pieces of cancellous bone when the requirement is for rapid bone union, and cortico-cancellous strips for maintenance of space during union. Fillets of bone (**1127** to **1132**) are good in the closure of defects, and split ribs are useful for contouring and for the provision of narrow sheets of bone to overlie defects in, for example, the orbital walls.

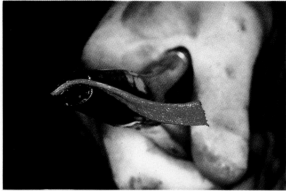

911

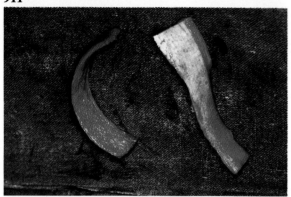

912

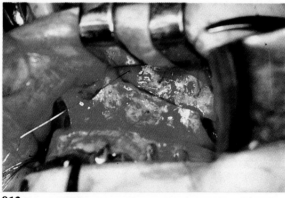

913

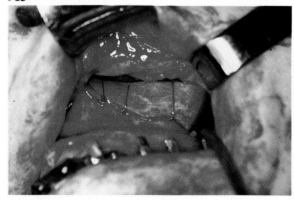

Split rib grafts are very useful over the lateral maxillary cuts when there is no need for interpositional grafting. The rib is split longitudinally with a broad osteotome, and then Tessier's bone bending forceps are used along the length of the split rib, first one way and then after reversal of the rib, until the bone has become pliable and can be bent or twisted to any desired shape (**910** and **911**).

After the maxilla has been advanced fine soft wire (32 gauge stainless steel, for example) is passed through two or three holes drilled above and below the lateral osteotomy line. It is sensible to place these before the craniomaxillary fixation is applied as the mobility of the maxilla aids passage of the wires (**912**).

The split rib is then applied to the maxilla after cranio-maxillary fixation has been secured, and the malleability of the rib allows symmetry between right and left with good adaptation (**913**). The rib then provides a smooth contour where there was previously a step and is secured with light twisting of the retaining wires. The main value of this exercise is the smooth cheek contour achieved (cf. the cheeks in profile and full face of Figures **928** to **931** with Figures **925** and **926**, and **250** and **251**. The first was rib grafted the second not, and the difference is typical).

Split rib is also useful in the orbits to cover medial wall and floor defects in Le Fort 3 osteotomies. It is not useful in the pterygomaxillary gap, and its use may be conditioned by the operator's view of the importance of bone grafting the gap behind the maxilla. The same technique is used in the Le Fort 2 at the level of the maxillary antra, with extra pieces of split rib placed laterally to the pyriform aperture of the nose after the orbital margin has been grafted with cancellous bone from the hip. This extra piece of split rib can be retained with its lower edge tucked underneath the main lateral graft.

Bone grafting the pterygomaxillary gap (**914**) is one of the most controversial aspects of maxillary osteotomies. There are those who insist that it is essential to insert a solid piece of bone between the maxilla and pterygoid column in order to prop the maxilla forwards and it is claimed that this is essential for stability. Evidence is adduced on the basis of comparisons between bone grafted and non-bone grafted cases. Unfortunately bone grafted cases are also always grafted along the anterolateral maxillary walls as well, and it is not possible to prove that the *posterior* graft is the critical technical manoeuvre.

The author does not believe that the posterior bone graft is necessary, and in many cases (where the pterygomaxillary gap

910 to 913   Split rib grafts.

has no anterior wall – see previous discussion) the gap is not suitable to take a piece of tightly wedged bone. Attempts to graft this type of case result in the bone entering the antrum. Proper mobilisation and lateral bone grafting results in stable maxillary advancements. Hence in Le Fort 1 cases no attempt is made to graft posteriorly, if rib has been used for contouring and grafting the lateral wall. If hip bone has already been taken (for example when lengthening the face, performing a Le Fort 2 or 3 osteotomy, or for cleft palate closure) and if the pterygomaxillary gap has good anterior and posterior walls, then a piece is inserted. It is conceded that in Le Fort 3 cases the pterygomaxillary graft is useful in propping the lower maxilla forwards, there being no lateral grafting at that level, while higher up the face the grafts are extensive.

It is also theoretically important to eliminate dead space in the pterygomaxillary gap if there is no good communication with the antrum. Otherwise the gap will fill with blood clot, become organised, and there is a danger of fibrotic contraction, a possible relapsing force. Hence the author's practice is to insert a finger into the gap at the stage of definitive fixation; if the gap opens into the antrum anteriorly, nothing more is done there, but if there is a defined space with an anterior wall then a piece of bone is tucked in to eliminate the space – hip if available, bits of excess rib if not.

In the Le Fort 2 operation the lateral maxillary walls are grafted with split rib as described, but the nose, anterior orbitomaxillary cuts, and sometimes lateral inferior orbital rim require corticocancellous or cancellous bone from the ilium.

In Le Fort 2 cases bone grafting is required (**915**) at the nasal bridge and the medial orbital wall, the orbital floor and inferior orbital rim, and down the anterior surface of the maxilla, in addition to the lateral grafting already described (for which split rib is best). There is often a need for a nasal strut along the dorsum of the nose as well (**916**). Corticocancellous or cancellous bone from the ilium is used at the nasal bridge, inferior orbital margin and anterior maxilla; either a flake of cancellous bone or a piece of moulded split rib is used in the orbital wall and floor. A solid corticocancellous strut is used in the nasal dorsum if needed. **916** shows again the rarely used V-Y incision for demonstration purposes.

It is preferable *not* to use wire in the nasal and orbital region if the grafts can be wedged into place without it, as there is a high risk of late infection associated with wiring in these sites. When paranasal incisions are used the grafts can usually be self-retained without wire. It is important to insert a solid piece of bone in the nasofrontal osteotomy site if there is a gap after repositioning the maxilla, ie if the maxilla has been displaced inferiorly. Usually both rib and hip are used in Le Fort 2 cases. Although two sites, each donor site is thus kept much smaller with less local morbidity, and the most appropriate bone for the purpose is available. Only when there is good lateral wall contour after maxillary repositioning is the ilium used alone.

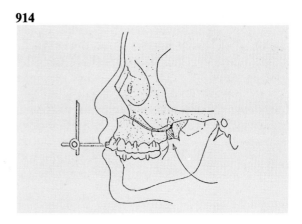

914

914   Pterygomaxillary bone graft.

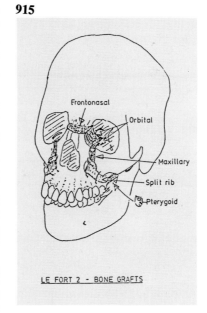

915

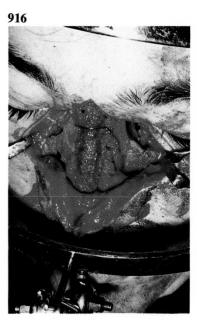

916

915 and 916   Bone grafting in Le Fort 2 cases.

243

Bone grafting in Le Fort 3 cases (**917** to **923**) is essential to build up the many deficient areas around the orbits and frontal region, as well as the zygomatic arches (**917**). It is advisable to graft the pterygomaxillary gap as well, there being no lateral maxillary grafts at a low level.

Large amounts of bone are required, taken from the ilium (in children it is often necessary to open both sides for donor bone) and from the ribs, two or three being taken. It is an advantage if lyophilized ribs are available when multiple onlay rib grafts are needed in the supraorbital region (see **997** to **1003**).

The areas which must be grafted are: (a) The lateral orbital walls, where it is usually possible to place substantial sheets of corticocancellous bone, wiring them in firmly and thus stabilising the position of the advanced upper mid-face (**918**). The interpositional graft in the sagittal split technique (**919**) is even more stable. (b) The zygomatic arch or body (**917** for the sagittal split and step, inset **917**, and **920** for the simplified cut). (c) The pterygoid region in the pterygomaxillary space. (d) The frontonasal region (**921**) and the orbital walls (**917**). The frontozygomatic angle is contoured with bone (**922**).

918

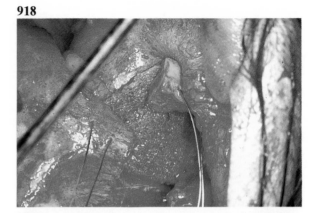

919

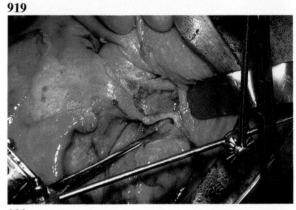

920

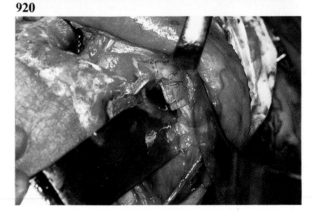

917

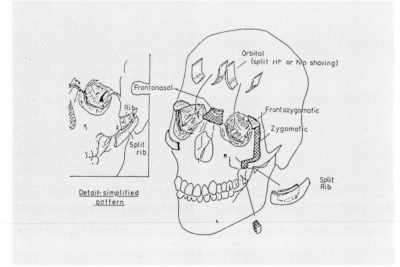

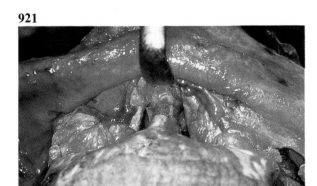

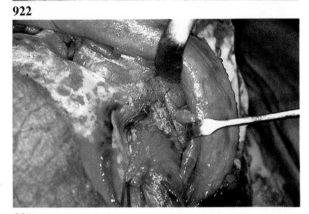

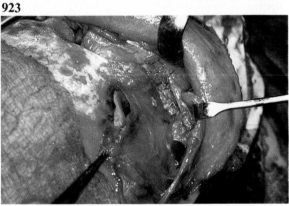

917 to 923   Bone grafting in Le Fort 3 cases.

Most grafts are wired into place, except those around the nasal bones. The lateral maxillary walls are thin and softened wire is used, making the best use of the thickest available bone in the maxillary walls. More solid areas will take thicker (0.35 mm diameter tempered S/S wire) and the grafts may be more tightly secured. Suturing must be done with care, especially in the mouth. Horizontal mattress sutures have been found best for the intraoral incisions, taking care that the mucosa is not trapped beneath the bone grafts. Paramedian and para-nasal incisions are closed in two layers, the knots being deep in the subdermal layer.

In Le Fort 3 cases where the medial canthal ligaments have been separated from bone they are picked up with chromic catgut or fine wire sutures and sutured to each other trans-nasally. Bony holes must be made through the nasal bones to achieve this. The temporalis muscle is rotated forwards to abut on the new position of the lateral orbital rim (**923**), and the lateral canthal tissues are sutured to the temporalis fascia to hitch them up laterally. Drains are inserted under the bifrontal flap and kept under suction for 48 hours.

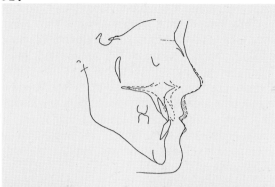

924

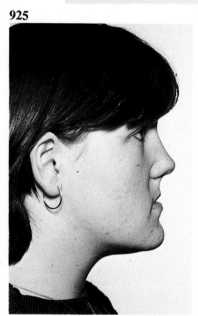

925

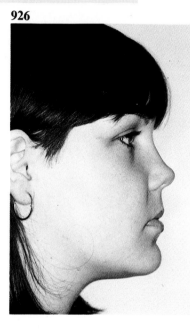

926

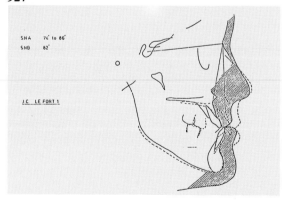

927

924 to 927 **Profile changes** following Le Fort 1 advancement.

Results – Le Fort 1 osteotomy. With proper case selection maxillary advancement at the Le Fort 1 level produces some of the most pleasing improvements in facial aesthetics. The specific profile changes are illustrated (**924**), and the full face changes can be seen in the next case (**928** to **934**). (See also **250** and **251** for a full face view of case **925** and **926**).

*Profile changes in Le Fort 1 advancement (**924**):*

1. The nasal tip is advanced by one third of the maxillary advancement, with slight elevation of the tip. If the anterior movement of the A point is measured (parallel to the Frankfort plane) the nasal tip will move about one third of that distance.
2. The nasolabial angle is decreased, and the upper lip flattens, slightly lengthens, and its vermillion exposure is increased. The lip is 'thinned' when seen in profile.
3. The vermilion/skin junction moves with the incisor tip to about 60% of the tooth movement. This is, however, one of the least predictable changes, and there is some inconsistency in lip posture in many patients. This in particular *does not* apply to the repaired hare lip (see p. 299).
4. The stomion is lowered and advanced.
5. The lower lip may be shortened, everted and the vermilion exposure is decreased. The degree of eversion is very variable, and will be cancelled out if the maxilla is raised at the same time (**1088**, ii) with resultant elevation of the mandibular incisor segment. Equally it is increased if the maxilla is lowered (**1088**, iii; **925**, **926** and **927**). Similarly simultaneous mandibular retrusion cancels the effect of the maxillary advancement on the lower lip, (**1088**, iv – cleft palate case also with rhinoplasty). The result of lower lip eversion is to increase the concavity of the labiomental groove, the extent reflecting the combination of factors indicated above.

The effects of simple Le Fort 1 maxillary advancement are well illustrated by the case shown (**928** to **934**). In full face (**928** and **929**) note the increase in width of the alar flare (and the preoperative narrowness, indicative of supra-apical maxillary hypoplasia).

The para-alar hollowness is eliminated, the lips become more balanced with equal exposure of vermilion borders in both upper and lower lips. The rounding of the cheeks in profile is improved not only by the advancement but also by the use of rib grafts (cf. **926** where no grafting was employed). The profile changes already described are clearly seen (**930**, **931** and **934**). Postoperative stability in Le Fort 1 advancements is good provided that the maxilla is properly mobilised. If cuspal interdigitation is good in the planned position then no over-correction is necessary; if it is not so good the maxilla should be advanced 2mm to 4mm in excess of requirements and controlled orthodontically into the planned position after removal of fixation, because there is then a tendency for slight relapse during the first 6 months after operation.

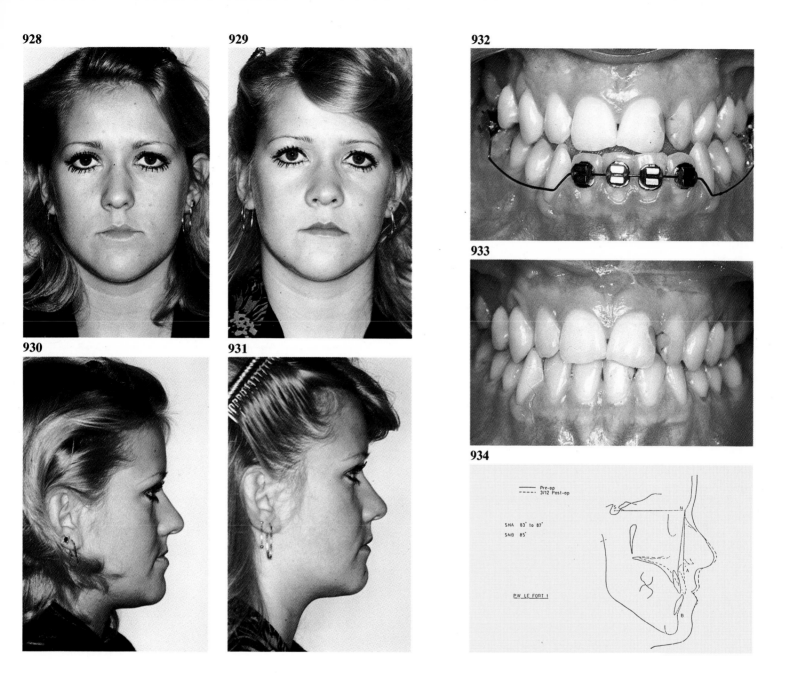

928 to 934 **Full face, profile and occlusal changes** following Le Fort 1 advancement (**928, 930, 932**, before operation).

Variations of the Le Fort 1 osteotomy

The Le Fort 1 procedure is exceedingly flexible, and when undertaken by the downfracturing technique a number of variations are available to deal with specific clinical abnormalities. The following will be described at this stage:

(a) The Le Fort 1 with midline narrowing.
(b) The Le Fort 1 with midline widening.
(c) The Le Fort 1 with reduction in vertical maxillary height (superior repositioning).
(d) The Le Fort 1 with increase in vertical maxillary height (inferior repositioning).

In addition the Küfner procedure is a compromise between Le Fort 1 and Le Fort 2 levels (described under variations in the Le Fort 2, p. 256); transverse rotation may be carried out as necessary to centralise the midline of the maxilla; the occlusal plane may be levelled to correct asymmetrical discrepancy between the right and left maxillary height (pp. 312 and 313); and combined segmental procedures may be carried out after downfracturing at the Le Fort 1 level (p. 272).

Variation 1 – Le Fort 1 with midline narrowing. The indications for contracting the transverse width of the maxilla are: (1) A central diastema requiring closure – the technique is seen in **935** and an example in **936** (preoperatively) and **937** (after excision of a central strip of palatal bone), and (2) Where maxillary advancement will result in a unilateral or bilateral excess buccal bite. The latter type of case arises where the preoperative occlusion exhibits no crossbite before maxillary advancement (**939**).

Again working from above the downfractured maxilla a preplanned wedge of bone can be removed (**938**) using a preformed metal template, seen to the patient's right in the operative picture for comparison with the ostectomy performed to the left of the midline. The maintained posterior occlusion after maxillary advancement is seen in **940**. It is better to remove segments from one side of the midline, but if this is not possible it is advisable to split the maxilla with an osteotome through the midline alveolar suture after cutting all the maxillary osteotomy lines, but before downfracturing the bone. This simplifies division of the alveolus, especially where no bone is to be removed from the anterior alveolus itself.

935

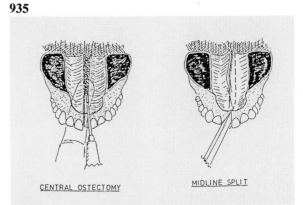

936

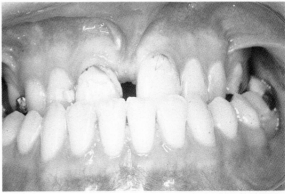

937

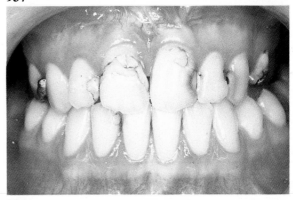

938

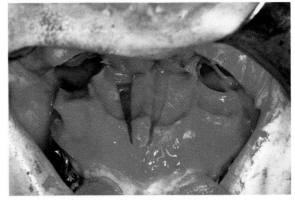

939

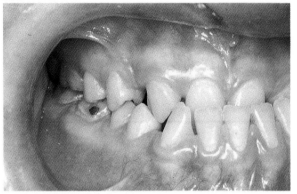

940

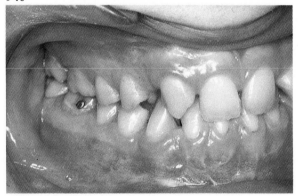

941

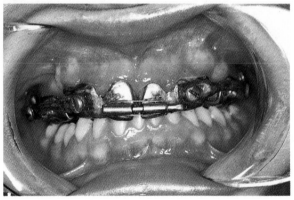

935 to 941   Le Fort 1 with midline narrowing.

Variation 2 – Le Fort 1 with midline expansion. In general it is preferable to expand the maxilla orthodontically, either by standard appliances or by rapid maxillary expansion. If necessary this can be accelerated by preorthodontic surgery, cutting the lateral, nasal and pterygoid Le Fort 1 cuts and splitting the maxilla through the palate with an osteotome (but not down-fracturing), prior to fitting the expansion appliance. However, moderate expansion can be achieved at operation (**935**) by splitting the maxilla either along the centre of the palate or to one side of the centre. There is a danger to the viability of the central palatal bone if this requires much detachment of mucoperiosteum from the oral surface to allow the expansion to take place; in these circumstances it is better to make lateral cuts as indicated in the section on combined segmental surgery (see p. 272).

Whenever the midline is split, both in total and in anterior segmental maxillary surgery, it is important to ensure that the two sides of the maxilla are correctly related between the central incisors. One method of ensuring this is shown in **941**. A pin and tube ensures vertical stability during healing, while a wire ligature passed round the projecting ends of the pin and tightened keeps the two sides together in the transverse relationship.

942

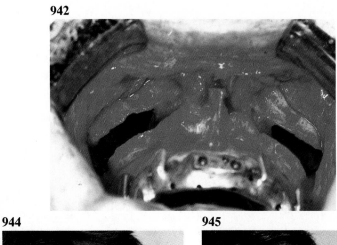

943

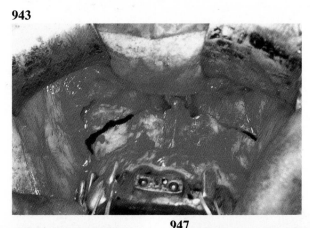

944

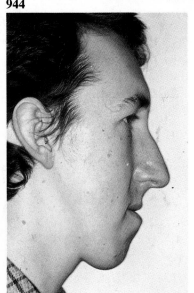

945

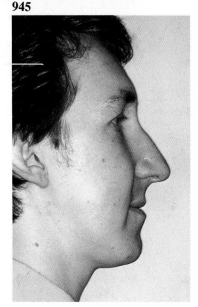

946

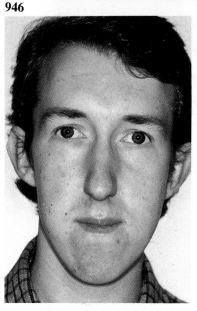

947

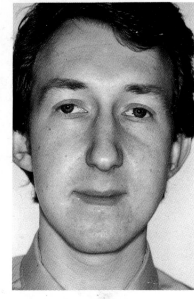

Variation 3 – The Le Fort 1 with superior repositioning. This is most commonly indicated in the correction of long faces, of which the excessive height of the maxilla (anteriorly, posteriorly or both) is usually only one component feature of the deformity (see p. 108); these cases are thus most often in need of mandibular surgery as well as maxillary repositioning.

Correction of excessive maxillary height is technically simple. The amount of bone to be removed is planned on the models and lateral cephalograms, and either a malleable metal template or a series of measurements prepared. At operation the template is adapted to the lateral maxillary wall and marked out, or the measurements are transferred with calipers. The planned segment of the lateral wall is then removed (**942**). The remaining Le Fort 1 cuts are completed in the usual way and the maxilla is downfractured. Equivalent sections of the lateral nasal walls, the posterior walls of the antra and the nasal septum are removed with ease after the downfracture. The superior aspect of the palate is grooved to locate the nasal

942 to 948   Le Fort 1 with superior repositioning.

948

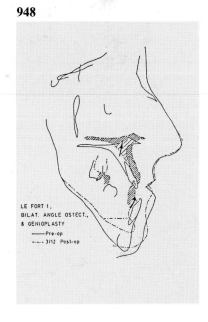

LE FORT 1,
BILAT. ANGLE OSTECT.,
& GENIOPLASTY
—— Pre-op
----- 3/12 Post-op

250

septum after superior repositioning (**943**) and all interferences with easy upward displacement of the maxilla are removed after inspection.

The inferior turbinates sometimes obstruct and can be trimmed through the nasal vestibule with a pair of scissors. If the obstruction is towards the back of the nose, the floor of the nose should be opened from below and the turbinates trimmed posteriorly, after which the nasal floor is repaired with 4/0 catgut. Only for patients living in arid desert conditions is it necessary to resect the bony turbinates subperiosteally, trim the soft-tissue excess and repair the turbinate mucosa, as these patients may develop *rhinitis sicca*. Provided there is not a great deal of concomitant maxillary advancement, or mandibular surgery, fixation is by internal suspension wiring. The

952

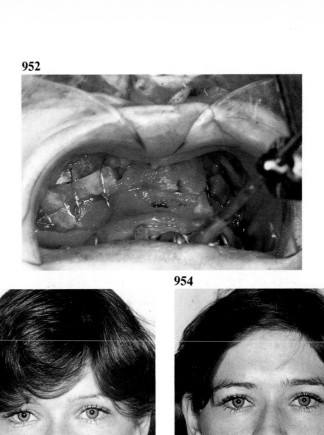

949

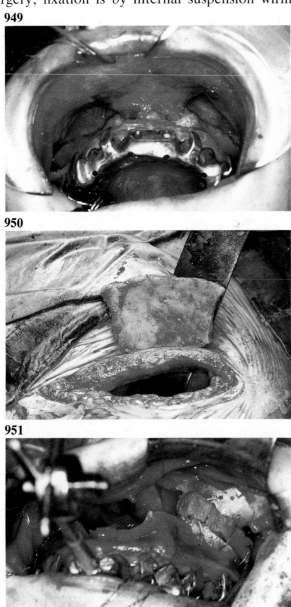

950

951

953   **954**

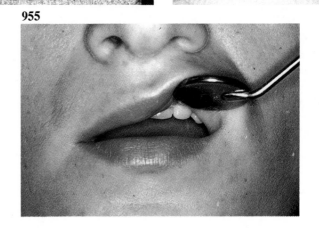

955

949 to 957   Le Fort 1 with inferior repositioning.

956

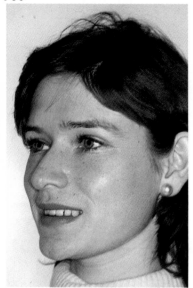

957

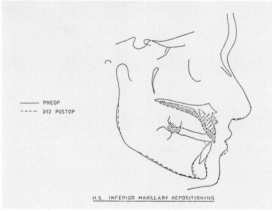

H.S. INFERIOR MAXILLARY REPOSITIONING

— PREOP
---- 3/12 POSTOP

Variation 4 – The Le Fort 1 with inferior repositioning. The technique of maxillary lengthening by inferior repositioning is the same as the standard Le Fort 1 operation until the stages of mobilisation are complete. When the maxilla is exposed with a horseshoe incision (**949**) the shortness of the maxilla is immediately apparent, with very little supra-apical bone and the pyriform rim of the nose at a low level. The infraorbital nerve and orbital rim are also more quickly exposed as subperiosteal dissection proceeds in an upward direction. Care is taken to preserve the nasal floor mucosa intact, because it is better protection for the bone grafts near the anterior nasal spine.

positioning of the maxilla must be determined anteriorly by the lip to incisor relationship. The case illustrated shows a typical correction of the long face, following the method of Bell *et al* (1977). It is interesting to observe how little the nasal tip has altered in this case (**944** to **948**).

958   **959**

960   **961**

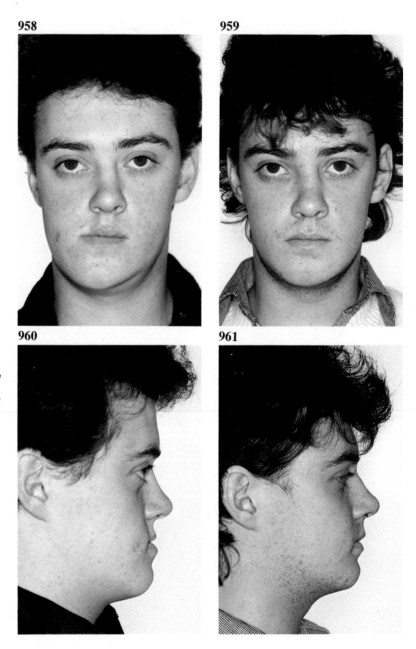

962

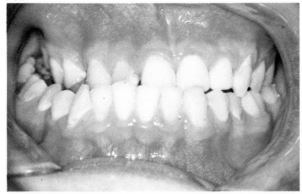

963

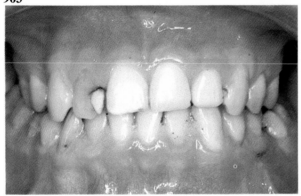

964

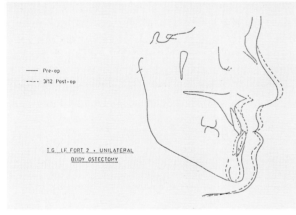

— Pre-op
---- 3/12 Post-op

I.G. LE FORT 2 + UNILATERAL
BODY OSTECTOMY

958 to 964 **Full face, profile and occlusal changes** in a patient treated by Le Fort 2 osteotomy and unilateral mandibular set-back (**958, 960, 962**, before operation).

A full thickness block of bone is taken from the ilium, preserving the crest (**950**) and the maxilla is positioned in the planned relationship to the rest of the skull, using extraskeletal fixation and preplanned templates. Bony segments are cut slightly in excess of the desired height, hollowed out slightly to accommodate the cut antral walls, and secured with wires in the lateral maxillae (**951**). The spacing is checked, and if correct the large dead space in the anterior part of the maxilla, between the old anterior nasal spine and the anterior part of the nasal floor, is carefully grafted, attempting to recreate an anterior spine at a higher level (**952**).

Typical results are shown (**953** to **957**) in a case of short face syndrome (see pp. 110 and 111), where the maxilla has been brought down into the excessive freeway space, thus bringing the anterior teeth into a pleasing relationship with the upper lip (**956**), whereas previously the teeth could not be seen without raising the lip deliberately (**955**). With the teeth together (**953** and **954**) the overclosure is eliminated, but at rest there is little difference in either full face or profile views (not illustrated).

Results – Le Fort 2 osteotomy. The commonest indication for this operation is nasomaxillary hypoplasia in the cleft palate group, and it will be discussed again in that context in Section 5. Other cases of nasomaxillary hypoplasia, including the so-called Binder's Syndrome (see p. 113) yield pleasing results, which often require simultaneous or subsequent rhinoplasty to realise their full effect. The operation is probably more stable than the Le Fort 1, especially in the cleft palate group, given the same occlusal relationships. The profile and full face changes are illustrated in the case shown in **958** to **964**, typically requiring simultaneous mandibular surgery (here a unilateral body ostectomy to correct mandibular asymmetry).

Profile changes in Le Fort 2 advancement (**964**):
1. The changes are the same as the Le Fort 1 changes apart from the nasal contour.
2. The nasal tip is advanced by two thirds of the maxillary advancement, with less tendency to lip elevation unless the whole maxilla is rotated forwards and upwards from the nasal bridge osteotomy site. This usually requires a mandibular split to correct the occlusal plane.
3. The pattern of change extends further towards the nasal bridge, and is under the control of the operator by varying the extent of bone grafting at the bridge and along the dorsum of the nose.

In full face view the main difference from the Le Fort 1 is seen in the infraorbital region where there is increased infraorbital projection, decreased scleral exposure (often, as here, best appreciated in the lateral view) and more balanced contour to the cheeks and para-alar regions. The nasal and labial effects are the same as the Le Fort 1 effects. This patient has a degree of nasal asymmetry, not corrected at this operation. Where there is recession of the nasal base but a normal incisor relationship it is useful to bring the whole maxilla forwards and allow consolidation; subsequently the premaxilla can be set-back again by premaxillary ostectomy to restore the occlusion. The technique is discussed in depth by Henderson (1980) and by Henderson and Jackson (1973).

In the case illustrated the effect of the slight mandibular set-back reduces the effect of the maxillary advancement on the lower lip (**964**).

Variations of the Le Fort 2 osteotomy

There is less scope for flexibility at the occlusal level when undertaking a Le Fort 2 procedure. Very slight maxillary expansion is possible in cleft cases, but this acts from the nasal bridge as a fulcrum and rotates the crowns further buccally than the apices. The maxilla cannot be shortened during Le Fort 2 osteotomy. If either shortening or transverse arch alteration are needed, these must be undertaken at the Le Fort 1 level, or orthodontically in the case of maxillary expansion. The main variations which can be undertaken are as follows:

(a) The Le Fort 2 with increase in maxillary height (inferior repositioning).
(b) The naso-orbito-maxillary advancement of Converse.
(c) The Küfner procedure, for advancement of the maxilla and infraorbital rim without the nasal bridge (Küfner, 1971).
(d) Lateral extensions of the osteotomy to include greater movement of the orbital floor, rim and even lateral wall. Eventually this variation shades into the full subcranial Le Fort 3.
(e) Combination osteotomies to include malar bone shifts, separately cut and independently moved.

Steinhauser (1980) gives a useful discussion of Le Fort 2 variations.

Variation 1 – The Le Fort 2 with inferior repositioning. The mobilised Le Fort 2 maxilla can be positioned so that the vertical height of the mid-face is increased by a preplanned amount, and this can be useful in cleft palate cases where there has been shortening of the maxilla during growth. Mid-facial retrusion is often associated with vertical deficiency, as in the non-cleft case (**965** to **969**), and this contributes to nasal short-ness where there is an element of nasomaxillary hypoplasia. Inferior repositioning of the maxilla makes a useful contribution to nasal correction in such cases.

The tracing shows the resultant change in profile – the maxilla has been brought forwards and downwards, and the

965

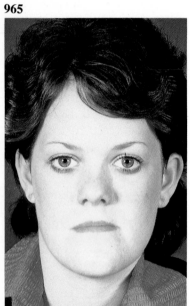

966

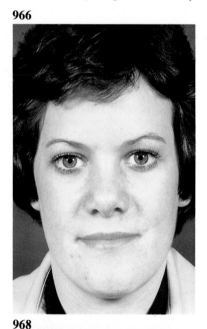

967

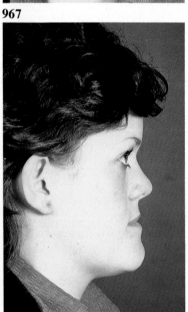

968

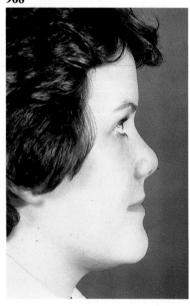

969

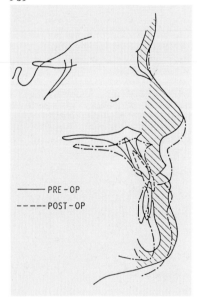

PRE-OP
POST-OP

965 to 969 Le Fort 2 with inferior repositioning. Full face and profile changes.

254

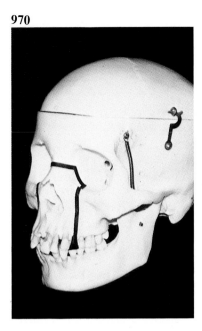

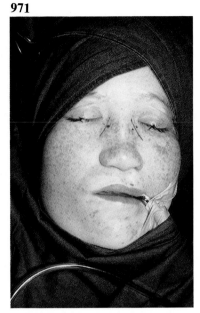

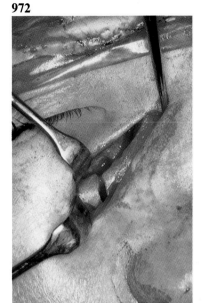

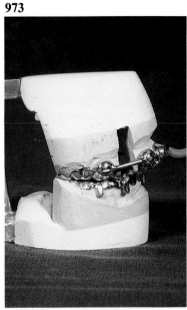

974

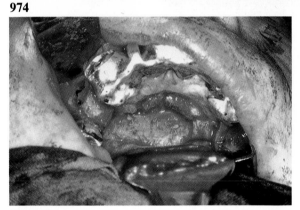

975

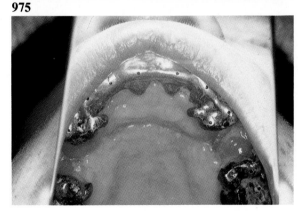

tissue redistributed to obtain maximum nasal elongation. The practical points to watch are: (a) Vigorous elevation of the skin and periosteum in the glabellar region is needed to allow sufficient mobility for some transfer to take place as the nose moves down. Care needs to be taken where the eyebrows are prominent and nearly meet centrally, as the central parts may be drawn inferiorly in an ugly fashion. (b) Some medial canthal attachment must be maintained to bone above the osteotomy or the medial canthus will be drawn downwards with the maxilla. If there is much movement the osteotomy should be cut anterior to the lacrimal apparatus, preferably from above, using a 'flying bird' incision (**608**). (c) Extraskeletal fixation should be used, and solid bone grafting is important in the nasal bridge.

Variation 2 – Le Fort 2 pyramidal naso-orbital osteotomy. This was historically the precursor of the full Le Fort 2, and was described by Converse *et al* (1970).

The operation is limited to the anterior maxilla, combining the upper part of the Le Fort 2 procedure already described with an anterior maxillary osteotomy performed in the manner of Wunderer's technique (**970**). The anterior mid-face is thus moved forwards *en bloc*, leaving the posterior dentition and occlusion intact. It is thus one method of advancing the mid-face while avoiding a difficult posterior occlusion, where the posterior arches are in good relationship preoperatively. It is contra-indicated in cleft palate cases.

The upper access is via two paranasal incisions, there being no reason why oral intubation should not be employed throughout (**971**). The nasal and orbital cuts are completed as for the Le Fort 2 (**972**). The premaxilla is sectioned, preferably between the premolars, and a cut made across the palate after reflection of a palatal flap as for the Wunderer technique. The

970 to 975 Le Fort 2 pyramidal naso-orbital osteotomy.

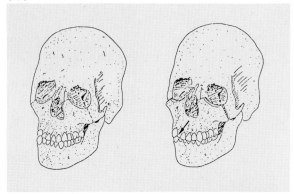

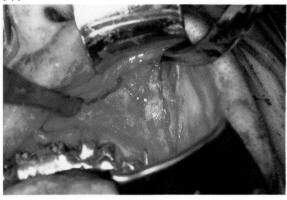

976 Le Fort 2: Küfner modification.

977 Le Fort 1 with wing extension.

upper and lower osteotomies are joined, without entering the pyriform aperture (**970**), the nasal septum is separated as for the Wunderer osteotomy, and the premaxilla, nasal base and nasal bridge are displaced forwards by the planned amount, and held by a rigid connecting bar across the premolar gap (**973**). The palatal, lateral and naso-orbital spaces are bone grafted (**974** for the palatal grafts) and the incisions closed. The secondary defect in the palate epithelialises in 2 to 3 weeks (**975**).

Variation 3 – The Le Fort 2 modified by Küfner. This technique was described by Küfner in 1971, who had already performed over 60 operations using the method. The cuts (**976**) do not involve the nasal bridge and run anterior to the lacrimal apparatus. Laterally the osteotomy is extended onto the zygoma and thence is carried down the posterolateral aspect of the maxilla to the pterygoid region. Medially the upper part of the pyriform aperture is entered. Pterygoid dysjunction and nasal septal separation are then completed. The operation is indicated when the nasal bridge and projection are both good, but the infraorbital region and dentoalveolus are retruded, with mild zygomatic flattening.

Access is difficult without a large incision, and the subciliary access is recommended. Steinhauser uses a transconjunctival approach with an extended cantho-conjunctival incision (1980). The author finds this osteotomy difficult to perform well without scarring or other postoperative problems (disturbance of lacrimation, ectropion) and mobilisation is difficult. However, the procedure is very logical in the circumstances described. The author prefers Le Fort 1 with a more limited wing extension (**977**) combined with Proplast 2 malar augmentation (see p. 258).

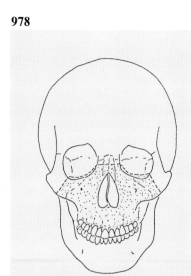

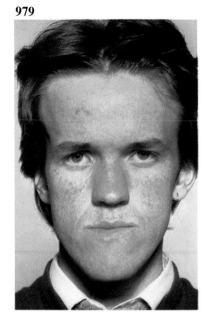

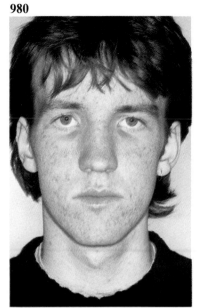

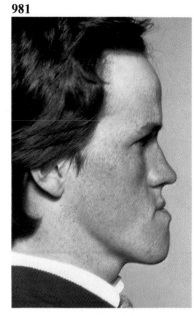

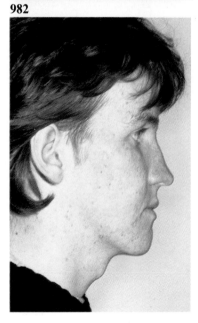

982

Variation 4 – The Le Fort 2 laterally extended. The cuts along the orbital floor may be extended laterally to include increasing areas of the inferior orbital rim and malar bodies, according to the clinical assessment of the extent of hypoplasia (**978**). Full lateral extension turns the procedure into a subcranial Le Fort 3. In order to perform these extended Le Fort 2 osteotomies a subciliary incision is needed. Alternatively a standard Le Fort 2 osteotomy can be supplemented by preformed Proplast 2 onlays (see **984** to **989**) and this is a simple way of achieving pleasing contour.

The case illustrated was undertaken in this way (**979** to **982**), with a concomitant mandibular set-back. The malar contour and infraorbital correction is quite adequate, and this method is highly recommended. There seems to be no problem with simultaneous alloplastic onlaying provided that the proplast is not placed near the oral mucosa and is well covered during closure.

978 Le Fort 2 laterally extended.

979 to 982 **Le Fort 2, supplemented by preformed Proplast 2 onlays**, with mandibular set-back; full face and profile changes. (**979** and **981** preoperative.)

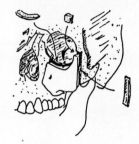

983

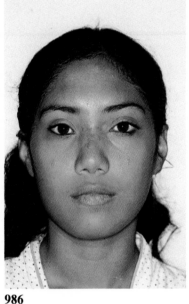

984

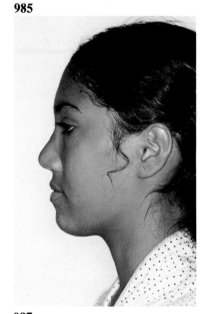

985

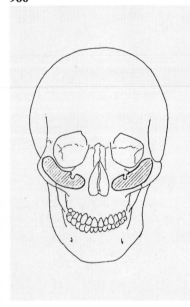

986

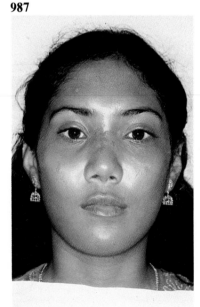

987

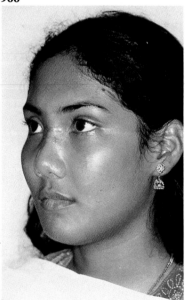

988

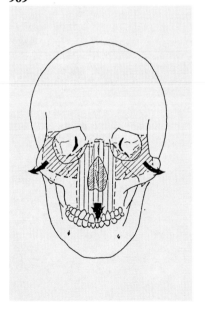

989

Malar augmentation

Combination osteotomies about the mid-face have been described to relocate almost every part of the underlying skeleton, the only limitation being the ingenuity of the operator. All these variations follow the principles of access and design already described. The correction of *malar underdevelopment* or longstanding post-traumatic *depression* is sometimes indicated, either as a part of wider facial dysharmony, or as an isolated (unilateral or bilateral) problem. The malar complex may require to be brought forwards and laterally in these cases, and for this reason advancement *en bloc* with the rest of the mid-third may not achieve adequate lateral expansion. Isolated malar depression may be corrected by malar osteotomy (**983**), with bone grafting in the osteotomy sites as indicated, or by alloplastic onlay.

The case illustrated (**984** and **985**) shows post-traumatic inhibition of malar development following injury in early childhood, evidenced by the nasal scarring. This type of case is very satisfactorily treated by preformed *Proplast 2 onlays*, placed either subperiosteally or supraperiosteally from either an intraoral or extraoral access (**986**). The implants are secured by suture to the surrounding soft-tissues and provide good and symmetrical contour correction (**987** and **988**).

Converse and Telsey (1971) described a tripartite mid-facial osteotomy which allows selective repositioning of the malar and lateral orbital walls in relation to the central facial pyramid

983   Malar osteotomy.

984 to 988   Malar augmentation with preformed Proplast 2 onlays (984 and **985,** patient before operation).

989   Tripartite osteotomy.

258

990 **991** **992** **993**

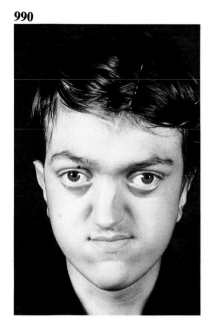
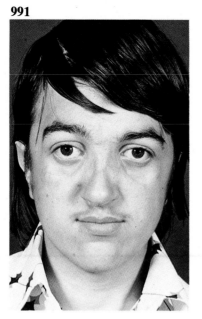
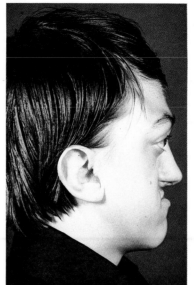
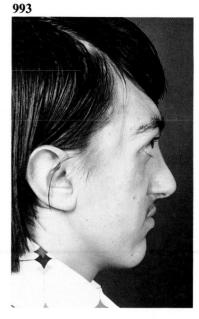

994

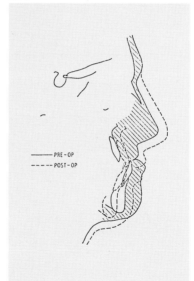

990 to 994   Full face and profile
changes following Le Fort 3
osteotomy.

(989). It may be considered as a Le Fort 2 with combination malar osteotomies, or as a divided Le Fort 3, and allows correction of the less severe types of total maxillary hypoplasia where the malar flattening is more pronounced laterally than anteroposteriorly. Great care that right/left symmetry is achieved is needed with this procedure.

Results in Le Fort 3 osteotomy. The indications for this kind of osteotomy are confined to the most severe panfacial deformities, and for practical purposes this means the craniostenotic syndromes. Some less severely deformed individuals will benefit from the procedure, but it should be emphasised that the complications are much greater than with lower level mid-third advancements, and the results are rarely fully satisfying to the surgeon, who understandably seeks to restore the face to complete normality.

The case illustrated (**990** and **992**) shows the result of a standard Le Fort 3 osteotomy (joint case with I.T. Jackson, Esq, FRCS) one year after operation (**991** and **993**). The changes are dramatic and can result in very considerable psychological reorientation for the patient, but the appearance of the full face view is never as pleasing as the profile improvement would lead one to expect. The patient should be warned that it will take at least a year for the tissues to settle down and that further minor operations may be necessary to finalise the result.

This patient was operated on before mandibular growth was complete, and a subsequent Le Fort 1 procedure has been carried out after growth ceased. The optimum time for surgery in the adolescent and young adult must be after the completion of facial growth, provided that no serious ocular problems dictate earlier interference.

Profile changes in Le Fort 3 advancement (**994**):
1. There is uniform advancement of the nose in a 1:1 ratio with the maxilla. Further bone grafting may well be necessary (there was only the minimum in this patient, at the bridge of the nose in the osteotomy gap), and this will modify the profile change accordingly.
2. The nasolabial angle is unaffected, but it may appear to be increased because the upper lip flattens and lengthens in profile.
3. Although controllable, there is a strong tendency for the maxilla to be inferiorly positioned, with slight increase in mid-facial height. If this does occur the mandible is auto-rotated posteriorly, setting back the chin, everting the lower lip and increasing labiomental curvature.

4. The stomion is advanced and lowered.
5. The upper lip shows more vermilion while the lower exhibits less. The overall balance of the lips is thus restored.

These changes are shown well in the tracing (**994**) of the case illustrated (**990** to **993**).

Variations of the Le Fort 3 osteotomy

The principal variations of the subcranial Le Fort 3 are as follows:
1. Inferior repositioning of the maxilla, using the vertical frontal spur.
2. The transverse frontal crescent.
3. Combined Le Fort 3 and Le Fort 1 osteotomies.

Beyond these variations of the basic pattern there lies the complex subject of transcranial Le Fort 3 osteotomies combined with cranial vault surgery, truly described as craniofacial surgery and beyond the scope of this book. Suggestions for further reading in this area are given in the Bibliography.

995

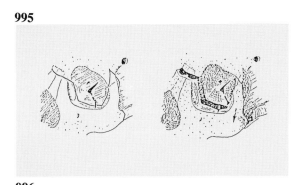

996

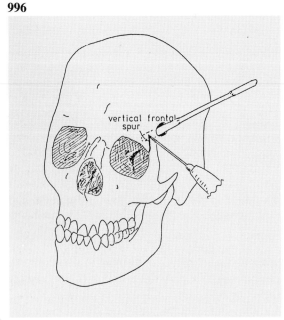

vertical frontal spur

Inferior repositioning of the total maxilla can be undertaken with the Le Fort 3, and in some circumstances will contribute to the correction of anterior open bite. This is especially true in Apert's syndrome, but it is usually necessary to combine the operation with a simultaneous or subsequent Le Fort 1 osteotomy to achieve a proper balance between anteroposterior movement and vertical correction at the different levels of the upper-face and the dentoalveolar region (see **1004** to **1006**).

That minor mid-facial lengthening is easily accommodated within the normal Le Fort 3 pattern already described has been demonstrated (**990** to **994**). However, if there is to be significant downward displacement of the maxilla, Tessier's *vertical frontal spur* (**995**), described in 1978, is self-retaining. The frontal bone above the lateral orbital rim is quite thick and a spur is cut as illustrated, carefully preserved during maxillary mobilisation, and fitted below the supraorbital ridge after maxillary advancement so that the vertical displacement is maintained. The spur may be cut up to 15mm in length according to Tessier. During sectioning of the frontal bone the thickness of the spur is measured to ensure that contact will be maintained after the planned forward movement of the maxillary bloc.

While sectioning the frontal bone in this procedure the semi-open-skull technique (also introduced by Tessier) is employed. A hole is made through the cranium above the spur area and lateral to the temporal crest, the dura is dissected with an elevator and protected with gauze. The frontal bone can then be cut without fear of dural damage (**996**).

The transverse frontal crescent (Tessier, 1978) is an important and useful modification of the basic Le Fort 3 patterns previously described. It is indicated in cases requiring simple forward movement of the mid-face, where the classic advancement would result in a sharp step at the superolateral orbital angle (**997** shows close-up of right lateral orbit after advancement following complete section of the lateral wall).

The osteotomy in this variation (**998**) is cut through the frontal bone along the crescent shaped lateral superior orbital rim, in continuity with the main section through the lateral orbital wall, instead of bringing the cut forwards in the frontozygomatic region. This preserves the contour of the upper and outer angle of the orbital rim.

The position of the cut is seen; a saw is used angled downwards and into the orbit, and after mobilisation of the mid-face the two 'crescents' are projected anteriorly as seen in **999**. The defects in the orbital wall are bone grafted with corticocancellous bone or split ribs, and the crescent is held forwards with split ribs placed across the two supraorbital crests behind the crescents (**1000**). The case shown (**1001**) is a

995 Le Fort 3: Tessier's vertical frontal spur.

996 Tessier's semi-open skull method (dural protection).

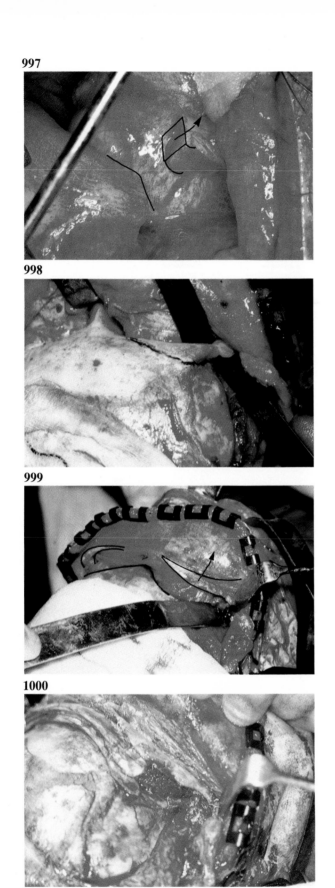

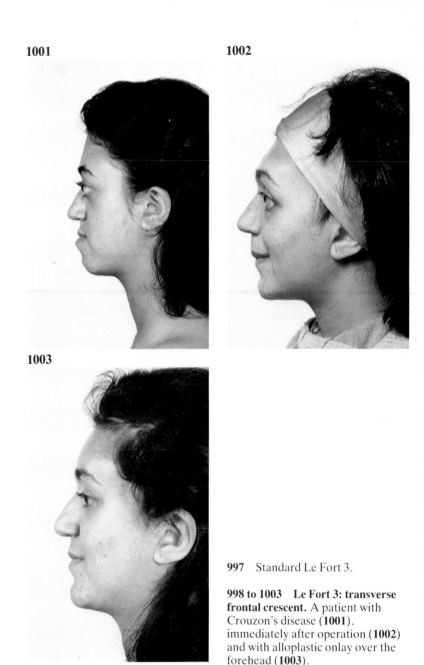

997 Standard Le Fort 3.

998 to 1003   Le Fort 3: transverse frontal crescent. A patient with Crouzon's disease (**1001**), immediately after operation (**1002**) and with alloplastic onlay over the forehead (**1003**).

typical Crouzon's disease for which frontal bone advancement was considered. With the technique described above, the supraorbital ridges appear too prominent immediately after operation (**1002**); however, with alloplastic onlay over the forehead (orthopaedic acrylic resin, methyl methacrylate, is recommended) a good cosmetic result is obtained (**1003**). This is most worthwhile and considerably reduces morbidity by comparison with transcranial Le Fort 3 and frontal bone advancement. The case shown was jointly undertaken with Derek Wilson Esq, FDSRCS (Eng).

As with the vertical frontal spur, this procedure is best undertaken with dural protection by the semi-open-skull method (**996**).

Combinations of Le Fort 3 and Le Fort 1 procedures are indicated in two ways.

Where the upper-facial retrusion is severe but the occlusion is normal the advancement of the Le Fort 3 block would create a severe postnormality in the occlusion. A simultaneous Le Fort 1 is undertaken, allowing the dentoalveolar segment to remain in its preoperative relationship with the mandible. More commonly, the degree of advancement required in the upper-face is greater than that at the occlusal level, but occlusal maxillary advancement is nevertheless indicated. In this event the upper-face can be advanced more than the lower.

The cuts (**1004**) shown were used to establish the differential advancement of the case shown preoperatively in **1005** and postoperatively in **1006** (Le Fort 3 minus Le Fort 1). This case was undertaken with I.T. Jackson Esq, FRCS, who also subsequently performed a revision rhinoplasty. The combination sometimes requires greater advancement at the Le Fort 1 level than in the upper-face. Great flexibility is possible (Obwegeser, 1969), including vertical repositioning at the lower level.

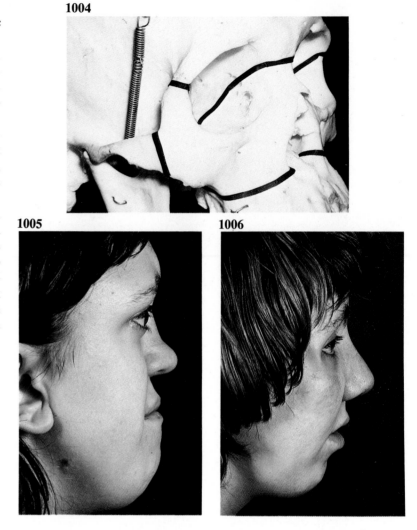

1004 to 1006   Combined Le Fort 3 and Le Fort 1 osteotomy.

Segmental alveolar maxillary osteotomies

These include (a) Anterior, (b) Posterior, and (c) Combined anterior and posterior procedures. These osteotomies are frequently undertaken in combination with other jaw surgery, especially in the anterior mandibular region or with forward sliding mandibular osteotomies (see, for example, **665, 666** and **667**) in the management of severe Class 2 malocclusions, or in bimaxillary alveolar protrusion (eg **801** to **807**). Other common examples occur with cases of anterior open bite confined to the anterior part of the jaws (as in **753** to **759**).

Anterior segmental osteotomies. This group includes (a) Corticotomy and inter-radicular osteotomy, and (b) Anterior maxillary osteotomy (premaxillary set-back with ostectomy, superior, inferior, or rotational repositioning, occasionally advancement with bone grafting). These procedures may be undertaken by any of three main approaches:
1. The Wassmund method
2. The Wunderer method
3. The Cupar method.

Corticotomy and inter-radicular osteotomy are rarely performed but have occasional uses, especially in the older patient with anterior spacing of the upper teeth where orthodontic correction is contra-indicated (usually for social reasons). The aim is to mobilise one or more teeth together with their immediate supporting structures.

This has been variously advocated by different authors since the International Dental Congress in Chicago in 1893 (Cunningham, 1894). At first it was done with immediate surgical repositioning of the segment and tooth or teeth at the time of operation, but later as a prelude to immediate postoperative orthodontic pressure. Merrill and Pedersen (1976) give an excellent review of the literature.

1007

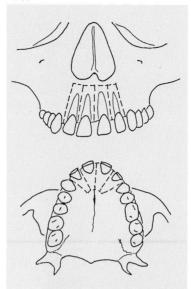

1007 to 1013   Corticotomy.

1008

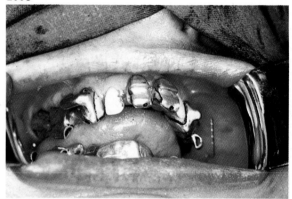

1009

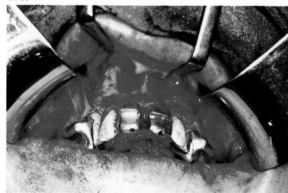

263

Köle's method is illustrated (**1007**) and consists of cortical cuts both labially and palatally (Köle, 1959). This method is easily adapted to the movement of one or two-tooth segments (Bell, 1973; Rayson *et al* 1975). The individual teeth to be moved are fitted with orthodontic bands or individual cap splints with open interdental areas incorporating some method of controlling postoperative elastics (**1008**). The labial (**1009**) and palatal (**1010**) cortices are exposed by reflection of appropriate mucosal flaps. The labial (**1011**) and palatal (**1012**) cuts are then made through the bony cortex only, the flaps are repositioned and heavy elastic traction applied immediately, directed in the manner appropriate to achieve rapid correction of the position and axial inclinations of the teeth concerned (**1013**, a case involving a forward sagittal split of the mandible). Barton (1973) combines this method with inter-radicular ostectomy, directing a bur between the teeth from the labial aspect but completing the supra-apical palatal and labial cuts through the cortical plates only from the palatal and labial aspects respectively. This leaves the teeth and their supporting bone dependent on the apical cancellous bone for nutrition, and it is about this bone that postoperative retraction is hinged.

The main problems to be overcome are those of blood supply and of damage to the teeth or their supporting tissues. Clinical experience indicates that *intact* apical cancellous bone is adequate for nutrition, and provided only cortical cuts are made supra-apically and distally the labial and palatal flaps may safely be raised for a one-stage procedure. Where a full-thickness bone cut is to be made from the labial to the palatal cortices, the palatal mucoperiosteum should be kept in place and the cuts made by 'feel' against a palpating finger. When transalveolar supra-apical cuts are made, maintenance of the palatal pedicle is mandatory; the alternative is a two-stage procedure with a 4 week interval between labial and palatal cuts. Damage to the periodontal tissues may be avoided by careful preoperative assessment of good quality intraoral radiographs and careful operative technique. Where there is little bone above the apices the cuts may be made into the pyriform fossa and the floor of the nose, but the nasal floor mucosa should be left in place rather than elevated. Fine fissure burs or small spear-point burs are used for the labial and palatal cuts until they approach the alveolar crest; then the cuts are completed with slim bibevel osteotomes. Mehnert (1973) uses a fret-saw, 0.25 mm wide, for this purpose.

Postoperative traction may be applied in many ways. The author uses separately cemented cap splints without inter-dental cover, grooved to receive elastic bands, which are stretched from hooks distal to the teeth to be moved on both sides (**1013**). Strong elastics are used and twisted to form one traction band per elastic. Usually two or three bands are used and they are sutured together to keep them within the channels on the splints. Movement usually occurs within a week, there being a common 'latent period' of 2 or 3 days before this

1010

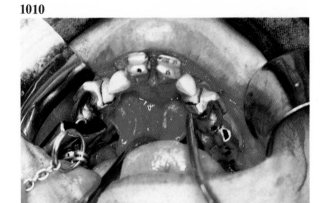

1011

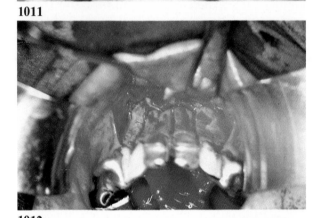

1012

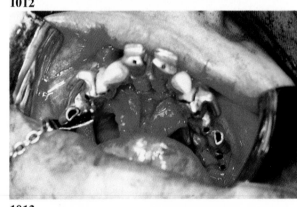

1013

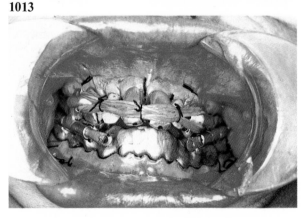

happens. The segments should be immobilised for 8 weeks, followed by the use of a retention appliance worn continuously for 6 months, and then at night for a further 3 months. This appliance is usually a simple acrylic plate with a labial bow attachment.

Indications for corticotomy. In younger patients with protrusion of the upper incisors and spacing, it is preferable to treat by orthodontic appliances alone. In older patients, or where orthodontic treatment is contra-indicated, corticotomy offers a quick and effective (but by no means reliable) method which can be tried. Great care is necessary to ensure a stable lip-to-tooth relationship postoperatively, or relapse will follow. The commonest indication is in Class 2 Division 1 cases with upper incisor spacing and skeletal postnormality, where corticotomy can be undertaken at the same time as mandibular advancement. Traction occurs during the early postoperative period and immobilisation concurrently with fixation for the main osteotomy. A typical case is illustrated (**1014** and **1015**).

Anterior maxillary osteotomy or ostectomy mobilises the anterior segment of the maxilla and allows repositioning in an upward, downward or rotational manner (by osteotomy alone) or in a posterior direction (if an ostectomy is performed). Rarely the segment may be advanced and the gap thus developed may be bone grafted. The simplest and commonest procedure is *anterior maxillary ostectomy*, illustrated in **1016**.

In this operation a premolar tooth is usually removed from each side of the maxilla and preplanned segments of bone are taken from the alveolar process at the sites of extraction. Where a space already exists in the premolar region the bone may be removed without the need for extraction of a tooth. Orthodontic treatment may be designed to transfer interdental spacing to the site of a proposed ostectomy. The two alveolar ostectomy sites are next connected across the palate with the removal again of the required amount of bone, as determined during preoperative model planning. Laterally, transverse cuts are made from the upper limits of the alveolar ostectomy sites, above the apices of the canine and incisor teeth, to the pyriform aperture of the nose. Finally the nasal septum is detached from the upper surface of the anterior palate with a grooved chisel. The anterior segment may now be set-back to the preplanned position, accurate localisation being secured with the appropriate method of fixation.

Where precise changes of axial inclination are involved, rotation into the required position is achieved partly by planning the shape of the alveolar (and perhaps also the supra-apical and nasal septal) ostectomies, and partly by the use of very precise splint localisation. For this purpose the East Grinstead pattern of localising plates is the most precise. Where the segment has to be repositioned superiorly bone must also be removed from the base of the nasal septum and from both transverse cuts to allow the necessary movement to occur. The midline of the alveolus may be split with an

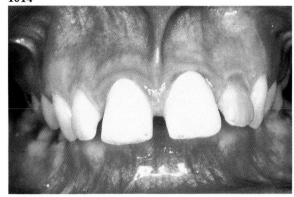

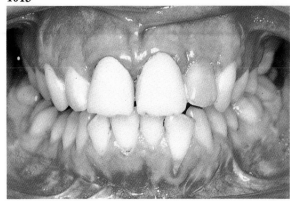

1014 and 1015 Protrusion of the upper incisors and spacing (**1014**) corrected by corticotomy and mandibular advancement.

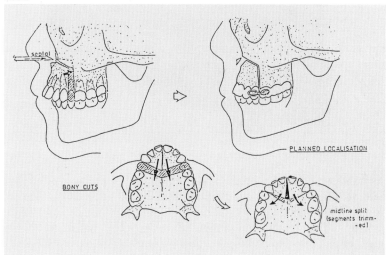

1016 Anterior maxillary ostectomy.

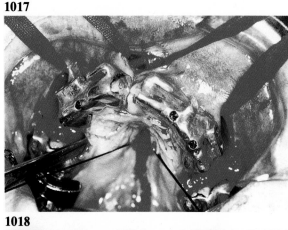

1018

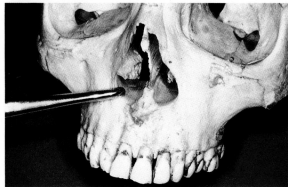

1019

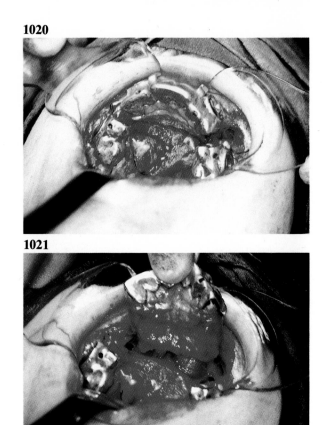

1017 to 1023 **Anterior maxillary osteotomy or ostectomy:** technique.

osteotome prior to final mobilisation in order to widen the intercanine distance and contour the upper arch to the lower. In this case separate splints must be made for each side and a system of central localisation built into the fixation, as for midline splitting in total maxillary osteotomy, see pp. 248, 249.

The technique of anterior maxillary osteotomy or ostectomy depends on the access chosen, and this has been discussed in detail (**559** to **564**). In the commonest method, the Wassmund technique (**562**), the bony cuts are mainly completed beneath mucoperiosteal tunnels, the soft-tissues being protected with an instrument. A Howarth's nasal raspatory is ideal under the palatal flaps (**1017**), and a pyriform rim retractor is passed

through the submucosal tunnel above the apices of the anterior teeth to hook around the angle of the pyriform aperture of the nose (**1018**). The alveolar ostectomy is performed, bilaterally, under direct vision. A preformed template can be used to construct the ostectomy, and if splints are being used this can be temporarily located onto the splints, while the site is marked out with a chisel in the same manner as for body ostectomy of the mandible (**1019**). The nasal septum is separated in the same manner as for Le Fort 1 osteotomy, but limiting the passage of the chisel to the anteroposterior depth of the premaxillary segment.

The Wassmund approach is recommended for all cases other than those requiring superior repositioning of the segment. Removal of the requisite amount of bone to allow upward movement is much easier with the Wunderer approach (**563**). Here the removal of the alveolar bone (or simple osteotomy cuts if no ostectomy is to be performed) and the transpalatal cut is performed under direct vision (**1020**). The transverse cuts are made as for the Wassmund technique and the nasal septum is dislocated with a curved chisel inserted through the palatal cut. A vertical midline incision on the labial aspect is contra-indicated; midline splitting during this technique is accomplished through an incision starting at the alveolar crest between the

1022

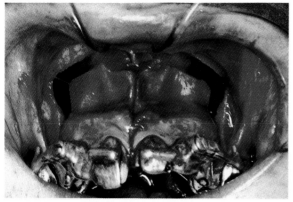

1023

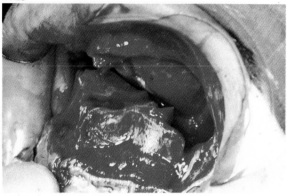

1024

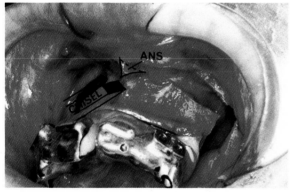

1024   **The anterior nasal spine.**

central incisors and passing back in the midline of the anterior palate until the transpalatal incision is reached. The osteotome is then inserted sagitally into the alveolus from the palatal aspect, protecting the labial pedicle with a guard finger during gentle malletting. The whole segment is then rotated forwards on its labial pedicle (**1021**) giving direct access to the nasal septum and nasal walls. This allows removal of the bone necessary to reposition the premaxillary segment superiorly.

The downfracture technique, originally described by Cupar (1954), is accomplished via a restricted horseshoe incision (**564**) and allows the transverse, septal and alveolar cuts to be made under direct vision (**1022**), the palatal cuts being completed through the ostectomy sites by 'feel', combined with some direct vision if the ostectomy site is large enough. After mobilisation and downfracture the superior aspect of the segment is available for trimming (**1023**). This technique is also useful for superior repositioning, and is ideal when a central ostectomy is required to eliminate a central diastema.

Anterior central ostectomy can also be performed by the Wassmund technique with an additional extension of the labial midline incision onto the palatal centreline from the labial aspect between the central incisor teeth. In these manoeuvres bone must be removed from the posteromedial aspects of the segments, to allow backward and medial rotation into their correct positions (Steinhauser, 1972). Fixation is similar to that used for lower labial segmental surgery. Intermaxillary fixation is unnecessary.

The anterior nasal spine (**1024**) should be detached during anterior maxillary osteotomy otherwise the effect of set-back on the nasolabial angle becomes too pronounced and there is a danger of distortion of the cartilaginous part of the nasal septum. The operation in any case has the effect of altering the nasolabial angle, usually by increasing it during set-back procedures. A chisel should be inserted below the anterior nasal spine (arrowed in the direction of chisel cut) and the spine detached from the maxilla with a sharp tap. The picture shows the spine still attached to the columellar base. It should be left there, although some operators prefer to remove it. Its position remains in its preoperative relationship to the columella and can be seen in postoperative radiographs. The result is a less pronounced widening of the nasolabial angle than otherwise occurs. This is true regardless of the basic technique used.

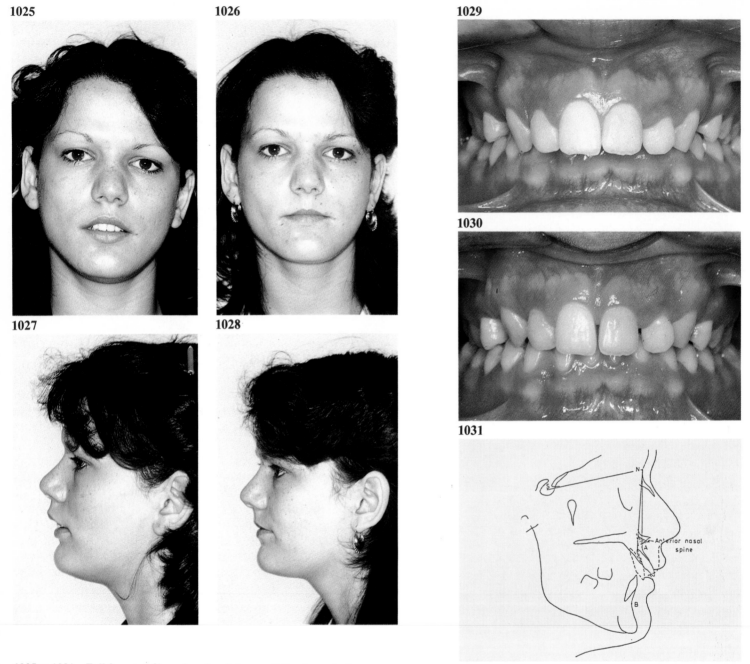

1025 **1026** **1029** **1030** **1031**

1025 to 1031   Full face, profile and occlusal changes following anterior maxillary ostectomy. (1025, 1027, 1029 preoperative.)

Results – anterior maxillary ostectomy. The results of this kind of surgery are localised in the anterior dentition and the associated soft-tissues – lips, paranasal region. The case shown in **1025** to **1031** is typical of simple premaxillary set-back with extraction of first maxillary premolars and a midline split to widen the anterior maxillary arch. Other more complex results can be seen elsewhere in this book.

Profile changes:

1. The nasal tip usually remains unaffected, especially if the anterior nasal spine is separated as described in **1024**. If not there may be marginal recession of the tip and the nasolabial angle becomes much more obtuse than necessary – the so-called Wassmund lip.

2. The nasolabial angle becomes more obtuse.

3. The vermilion border of the upper lip follows the upper incisor tip by about 60% of its movement, either forwards or backwards. The subnasale, however, moves only very slightly. There is a straightening, flattening and therefore

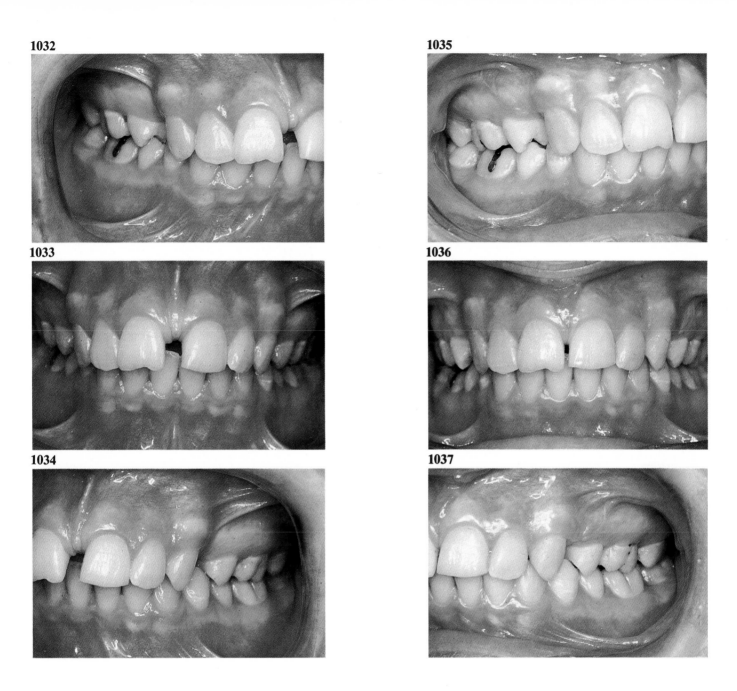

1032

1035

1033

1036

1034

1037

1032 to 1037 Occlusal changes following anterior central ostectomy (**1032** to **1034**, before operation).

(in profile) lengthening effect on the whole. This contrasts with the effect confined to the area overlying the incisor crowns which alone is set-back after orthodontic retroclination of proclined incisors.

4. The lower lip is removed from the lingual aspect of the upper incisors to the labial aspect, although the length of the lips and the incisors must be taken into account when assessing this. The labiomental curve is thus reduced, lip competence is restored, if not previously present, and lip balance is restored.

Anterior central ostectomy (**1032** to **1037**) as part of anterior segmental surgery is illustrated by this case and shows the rapidly obtainable correction possible. This case was done by the downfracture method and involves bilateral osteotomy at the site of previous premolar extractions.

1038

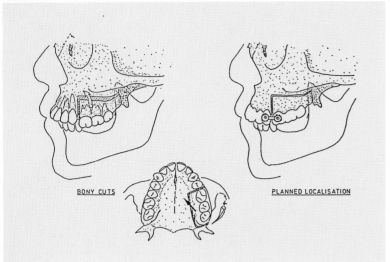

BONY CUTS   PLANNED LOCALISATION

1041

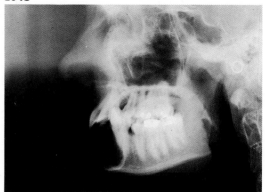

1042

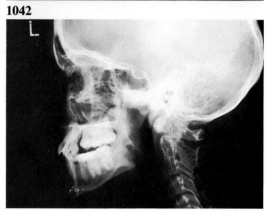

1038 to 1042 Posterior maxillary segmental osteotomy.

1039

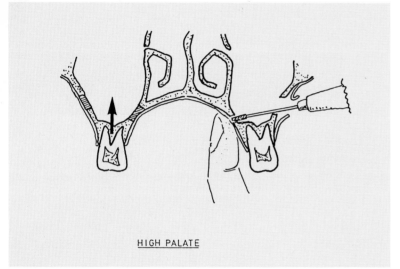

HIGH PALATE

1040

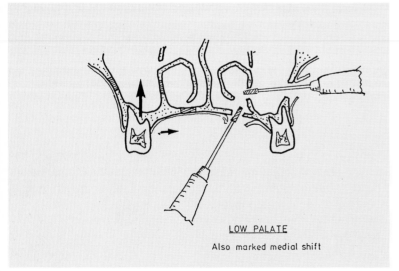

LOW PALATE

Also marked medial shift

270

Posterior maxillary segmental osteotomies were first described by Schuchardt (1959), but developed a bad reputation in Great Britain following reports of relapse. This was probably the result of poor case selection and poor technique; both case assessment and maxillary surgical technique were at a relatively primitive stage in the early 1960s. Posterior maxillary osteotomy is a useful technique and stable when applied to the correction of vertical maxillary alveolar excess, to the correction of transverse abnormalities in the posterior maxillary arch, or in combination with anterior maxillary osteotomy (see p. 272), and is reviewed by Hall and West (1976). Surgical access has been described (**565**).

Technique. The bony cuts are simple in design (**1038**) involving the removal of a planned segment of the lateral antral wall (or a simple bone cut if no upward displacement is planned), a corresponding palatal cut into the antrum, and vertical or transverse cuts connecting these anteriorly and posteriorly. For most cases the posterior cut is by simple pterygoid dysjunction as for total maxillary osteotomies, although occasions arise where a tooth or the tuberosity is left posteriorly. The anterior cut is most often in the premolar region. These cuts can usually be completed through the Küfner incision (**565***B*), or if a substantial alveolar ostectomy is to be performed in the premolar region a vertical limb can be carried from the anterior end of this incision to the neck of the tooth next but one to the ostectomy site. Transantral access to the palate, using a bur or osteotome is easy, provided that (a) the lateral ostectomy is wide enough to admit the instrument, and (b) that the palate is sufficiently vaulted to reach it directly (**1039**). Where the palate is very flat, or the lateral cut a simple osteotomy too narrow to admit an osteotome, then a palatal incision must be made (**1040**). The Perko incision (**565***C* or *D*) is recommended.

Schuchardt's original incisions were planned for a two-stage approach but this is never necessary, and indeed militates against adequate mobilisation – a possible cause of the early relapse problems associated with the method. Once down-fracture of the segment has been achieved the necessary obstructions to its movement can be easily reached through the lateral incision with bur or rongeurs, and a little careful elevation of the palatal mucoperiosteum medial to the mobilised segment is necessary to allow free movement into the planned position. Occasionally the greater palatine artery may be damaged; this does not prejudice the blood supply and bleeding can be stopped by careful pressure or electrocoagulation.

Fixation methods are as for other segmental procedures.

The case shown (**1041** and **1042**) illustrates one use of the method, where upward displacement of the posterior maxillary segments allowed a forward sagittal split of the mandible to be undertaken with rotation (and a genioplasty) (Case of J. Hovell Esq, FDS). Another example is shown in combination with posterior mandibular surgery (**809** to **811**); and yet another as part of combined anterior and posterior maxillary segmental surgery (**1046** and **1047**).

Indications. (a) Unilateral posterior crossbite, especially in older patients. Bilateral crossbite can be corrected in this way but either orthodontic expansion or total maxillary osteotomy with midline splitting is usually better.

(b) Excessive transverse width of the posterior maxilla.

(c) Over-eruption of a posterior maxillary segment, opposing an edentulous mandibular saddle. In such cases the denture should be fitted immediately fixation is removed.

(d) Vertical alveolar maxillary excess usually as a part of the so-called long face syndrome.

(e) To eliminate an unwanted edentulous space in the first molar/premolar region, where the occlusion will permit forward movement of the posterior maxillary segment.

(f) Rarely, in the closure of posterior open bite by inferior repositioning. This is the most likely type of case to relapse, especially in the movement of a lesser segment in secondary cleft cases. Where a moderate posterior open bite exists unilaterally the operation may be tried, but postoperative orthodontic retention is advised for at least 18 months.

Where the palatal shelf is low and flat, the osteotomies do not fully detach the segment from the maxillary residue, as the medial antral walls remain intact (**1040**). These are thin and can usually be broken by direct pressure; alternatively an osteotome may be needed. When segments are moved laterally to any extent it is important to consider the closure of the palate over the space(s) created; the latter should be bone grafted. If really wide movement is planned, the palatal cuts should be placed as far laterally as possible and the incision to the midline. If splints are used wiring is unnecessary, but a removable posterior palatal bar or plate is necessary to prevent rotational collapse of the tuberosity regions towards the midline.

1043

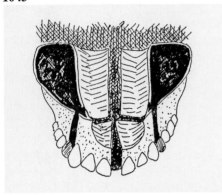

1044

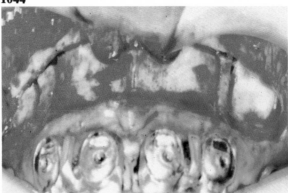

1048

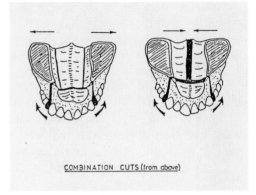

COMBINATION CUTS (from above)

1045

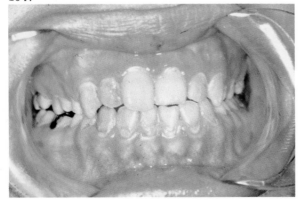

1046

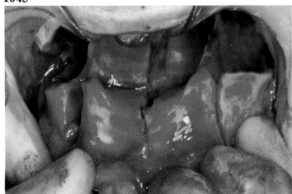

1047

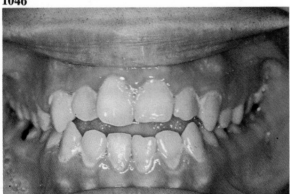

1043 to 1048   Combined anterior and posterior maxillary segmental surgery:
Technique (**1044** and **1045**); occlusal changes (**1046** and **1047**); types of
combined section (**1048**).

**Combined anterior and posterior maxillary segmental osteo-
tomy** is a most useful and logical extension of the principle of
downfracturing the maxilla at the Le Fort 1 level. The segmental movements discussed under anterior and posterior
segmental surgery may all be undertaken simultaneously while
the maxilla is in the downfractured position (**1043**), and at the
same time the maxilla as a whole may be repositioned as well
as the parts in relation to one another. Great care must be
taken not to detach the palatal mucoperiosteum from the
under surface of any of the segments, or sequestration will
ensue; but with moderate ease this is controlled by making all
cuts against a palpating finger in the palate and taking pre-
cautions against injudicious retraction of mobilised segments.

All buccal and labial cuts should be completed first (**1044**)
including removal of ostectomy segments from the alveolus or
lateral maxillary walls. Wide lateral posterior soft-tissue pedicles
should be maintained, as in **552** (arrowed). After downfracture
(**1045**) a variety of segments may be developed. The case
shown has been separated into four sections after extraction of
the two first premolars, anterior maxillary ostectomy with
midline split, and a further midline ostectomy between the two
posterior segments. Occlusal changes are illustrated (**1046** and
1047).

The commonest types of combined section are illustrated
diagramatically (**1048**), but much variation is possible. The
maxillary arch is commonly found to be deformed in anteroposterior and lateral combinations requiring retraction or
vertical displacement of the anterior segment combined with
expansion or contraction with vertical displacement of the
posterior segments. These are the cases suitable for combined
segmental surgery as an alternative to protracted orthodontic
treatment.

The whole subject of combined anterior and posterior segmental osteotomies is reviewed by West and Epker (1972) and
by Hall and West (1976).

SECTION 5

The management of special clinical groups exhibiting facial disharmony

Throughout this book the emphasis has been on clinical assessment, with descriptions of techniques applied to particular areas of facial skeletal abnormality. When the various surgical techniques are applied to particular cases there are certain groups of patients which require further consideration. In some there is a need to ensure that the full implications of the assessment process are taken into account when the surgical methods are applied to the individual case. An example of this is to be seen in the management of the vertical facial dysplasias. In others there are special technical difficulties, as in the secondary cleft palate group or in the correction of facial asymmetry. In yet others quite special techniques have to be described which differ from the standard operative procedures presented in Section 4. Again the asymmetries illustrate this difference.

In this section therefore the topics to be discussed are:

(a) The management of vertical facial dysharmony.

(b) The management of the secondary cleft lip and palate case.

(c) The management of facial asymmetry.

(d) Bimaxillary surgery.

The section is characterised by constant reference back to the preceding sections, where much of the case assessment and of the surgical 'bricks' has already been gathered.

The management of vertical facial disharmony

The different rotational growth patterns of the face, defined by Lavergne and Gasson (1978) have already been indicated in Section 1 together with the implications for anomalous growth. The two extremes most likely to present to the orthognathic surgeon are those of the short face syndrome (abnormal bimaxillary anterior rotational growth) and the long face syndrome (abnormal bimaxillary posterior rotational growth). The intermediate problems of high angulation anterior open bite on the one hand and low angle deep overbite on the other arise from anomalous divergent rotational growth of the two jaws or from anomalous convergent rotational growth respectively. All of these anomalies present as problems of vertical facial dysharmony, although there are also likely to be secondary sagittal and transverse disproportions.

The simplest observable feature of these cases may well be mandibular morphology (**122** to **125**) clinically, and divergence or convergence of cephalometrically determined antero-posterior planes (**126**) radiologically. Other clinical markers of vertical dysplasia are then sought in the full face examination (**221** and **250** to **255**) and a full cephalometric analysis of the vertical skeletal relationships is mandatory (**178** and **179**).

The clinical features of the commonest vertical dysplasias are to be found in Section 3, and include specifically:

1. Vertical mandibular excess (**303** to **307**)

2. Low angle mandibular deficiency (**332** to **338**)

3. High angle mandibular deficiency (**339** to **343**)

4. Vertical maxillary excess, including the majority of cases of the so-called long face syndrome (**365** to **368**)

5. Vertical maxillary deficiency, including the majority of cases of the so-called short face syndrome (**374** to **378**).

A special form of the low angle mandibular deficiency problem presents with the very deep overbite Class 2 malocclusion (**347** to **350**) which tends to present in later life when the lower incisors are traumatising the palate or the upper incisors the lower labial gingivae.

The surgical techniques which correct specific areas of vertical discrepancy are described in Section 4, some qualifying principles being stated in the relevant parts of Section 3. These techniques are:

1. *Mandibular advancement methods* (Section 4) especially sagittal splitting, the inverted-L osteotomy with bone grafting, and the C-osteotomy. These require to be considered with careful reference to the differences between high angle and low angle cases (**332** to **338** and **339** to **343**).

2. *Anterior mandibular augmentation and reduction* (**737** to **807**, **816** to **819**, **820** to **823**, and **832** to **838**) in both the subapical region of the chin and by repositioning the anterior dentoalveolar segments.

3. *Superior repositioning of the maxilla*, if necessary with differential vertical movement of the anterior and posterior components, either in one bloc or in several divided parts (**942** to **948** and **1043** to **1048**).

4. *Inferior repositioning of the maxilla* with interpositional bone grafting (**949** to **957**). This also can be undertaken with combined anterior and posterior differential movement.

It remains only to discuss and emphasise certain aspects of the detailed management of these cases.

The freeway space is of some importance in assessing vertical dysplasias. The mechanisms which determine the magnitude of the space between the occlusal surfaces of the teeth when the jaw is at rest are still not fully understood. For the orthognathic surgeon the significance of an excessive space is largely diagnostic, in order to detect both the presence of overclosure in occlusion (**1049**) and the effect on the profile that this overclosure produces by comparison with the profile when the jaw is at rest (**1050**).

In planning the profile an assessment needs to be made of the derotation which will result from, for example, inferior repositioning of the maxilla or raising the dentoalveolar component of the mandible relative to the ramus. This is best done by planning in these cases on photocephalograms prepared with the jaw in the rest position, or by deliberately derotating the mandible on the plan around the condylar axis (**1052**).

In most patients the effect of surgical impingement on the freeway space does not seem to matter; in some elderly people the altered vertical dimension may be difficult to accept. This can be tested in the following way. The patient shown in **1051** is clearly overclosed and prognathic; she seeks correction for functional reasons. The mandible is derotated on the photo-

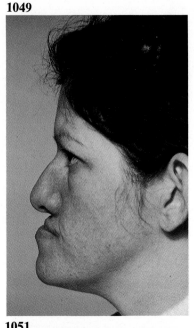

1049

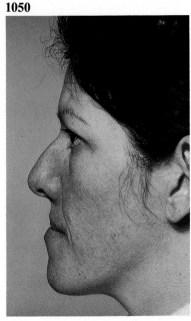

1050

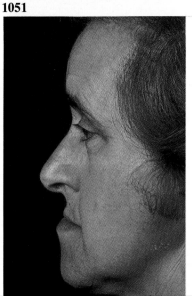

1051

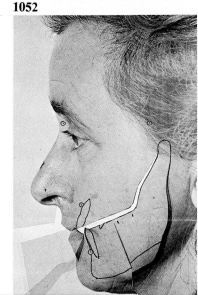

1052

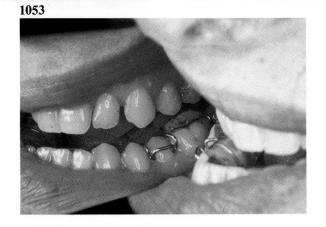

1053

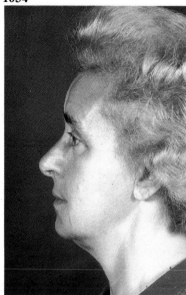
1054

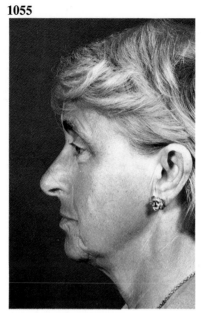
1055

In particular, elongation of the ramus against the ptery-gomasseteric investing tissues must be avoided (**127**). The relative contributions to the problem which result from the basic skeletal pattern and the soft-tissue morphology and behaviour patterns have been discussed in Section 2. In particular the possible influence of the tongue (**140** to **147, 169** and **170**) must be evaluated. The basic skeletal pattern may well indicate vertical dysharmony, which can be corrected surgically provided that full facial assessment is carried out and treatment planned accordingly.

Surgical options will range from simple anterior segmental surgery (maxilla or mandible, or both, see **752** to **759, 760** to **766** and **787** to **793**) to complex panfacial bimaxillary surgery (see **303** to **307** and **942** to **948**).

1049 **Effect on the profile of overclosure** in occlusion (**1049**) compared with when the jaw is at rest (**1050**).

1051 to 1055 **Correction of overclosure** by reducing the freeway space.

1056

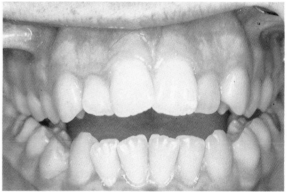

cephalogram, a correction made and a new freeway space estimated (**1052**). A bite-raising appliance is constructed to determine whether the patient can tolerate the reduced free-way space planned (**1053**), and in this case not only was the appliance tolerated but mastication was made more comfortable. Surgery was therefore undertaken by bilateral body ostectomy and a stable, comfortable and functional result obtained (**1054**). The same patient is seen 5 years after operation (**1055**). Some patients find this quite intolerable, and in these rare cases the excessive freeway space should be maintained. The trial bite appliance should be used in all such cases over 40 years of age.

Anterior open bite is not a diagnosis; it is a clinical sign which may be present in a number of different conditions and has many different causes. It must always be remembered that many cases of anterior open bite correct themselves during facial growth, without any interference from orthodontist or surgeon. The case shown here at 12 years of age (**1056** and **1057**) has spontaneously corrected itself by the age of 16 (**1058** and **1059**). This is clearly due to anterior rotational growth of the mandible, as comparison of the profiles shows. Stable results from the orthognathic surgical correction of anterior open bite depend on accurate diagnosis and the choice of appropriate techniques.

1057

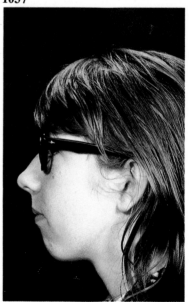

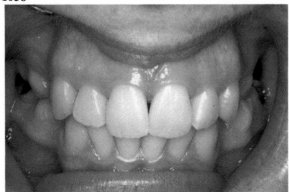

1058

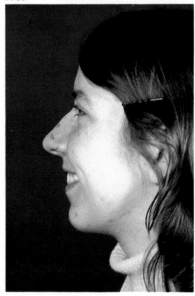

1059

 1056 to 1059 **Anterior open bite.** Spontaneous correction.

Complex bimaxillary correction of vertical dysharmony is often a matter for calculated compromises. There are certain limiting factors, of which the two most important are (1) The pterygomaxillary soft-tissue investment, already discussed in full, and (2) The upper lip to upper incisor relationship. The vertical positioning of the anterior maxilla must be related to the final lip/tooth position above all other considerations, and this frequently leads to compromise. The case shown in **1060** to **1070** illustrates both this and several other factors.

At initial presentation the most striking abnormality is the excessive display of upper incisor teeth with lip incompetence (**1060** and **1061**). The maxillary arch is contracted with anterior crowding (**1062**). One incisor is rotated and chipped. The SN:MP angle is high at 45°. Presurgical orthodontic treatment (carried out by N.S. Vasir Esq, BDS, MSc, FDS, D.Orth) achieves maxillary expansion and alignment of the upper anterior dentition (**1063**); the effects on the facial appearance are however minimal (**1064, 1065** and **1066**). Correction is by superior repositioning of the maxilla by Le Fort 1 combined anterior and posterior osteotomy, repositioning the anterior segment at a higher level than the posterior, to achieve good lip/tooth aesthetics (see tracing **1070**). This allows autorotation of the mandible, which is also split sagittally and advanced to achieve good intermaxillary occlusion. The chin thickness is augmented by a proplast onlay. The net result of these operations is a considerable improvement in both facial appearance and occlusion; the damaged incisor tooth can now be restored (**1067, 1068** and **1069**). However, study of the tracing raises several points of importance.

1060

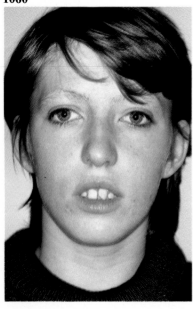

1061

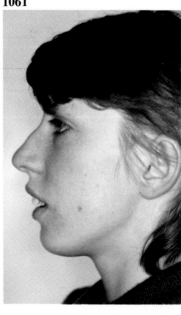

1062

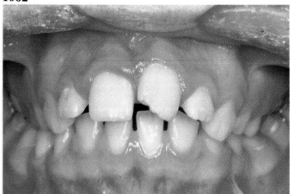

1060 to 1070 **Complex bimaxillary correction of vertical dysharmony.** Presurgical orthodontic treatment (**1063** to **1066**), **postoperative changes** (**1067** to **1070**).

1063

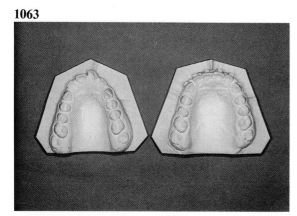

1064

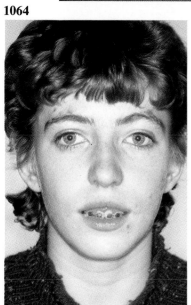

1065

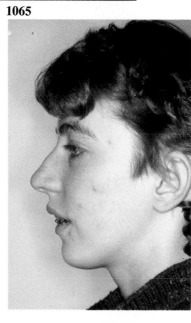

1066

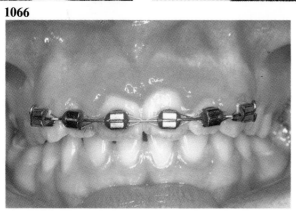

1067

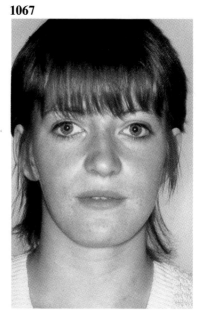

1068

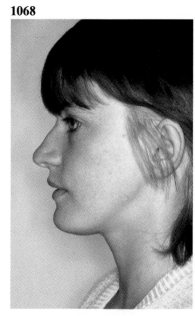

1069

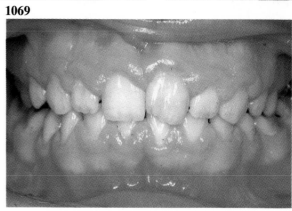

1070

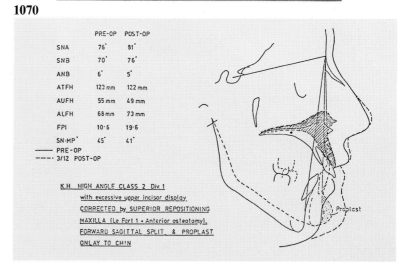

	PRE-OP	POST-OP
SNA	76°	81°
SNB	70°	76°
ANB	6°	5°
ATFH	123 mm	122 mm
AUFH	55 mm	49 mm
ALFH	68 mm	73 mm
FPI	10·6	19·6
SN·MP°	45°	41°

—— PRE-OP
----- 3/12 POST-OP

K.H. HIGH ANGLE CLASS 2 Div 1
with excessive upper incisor display
CORRECTED by SUPERIOR REPOSITIONING
MAXILLA (Le Fort 1 + Anterior osteotomy),
FORWARD SAGITTAL SPLIT, & PROPLAST
ONLAY TO CHIN

The preoperative FPI is normal at 10.6 while the postoperative balance is all wrong (FPI = 19.6). This has been brought about by elevation of the ANS during anterior maxillary shortening, thus reducing Anterior Upper Facial Height (AUFH) and increasing Anterior Lower Dental Height (ALDH). Skeletally the operation has decreased a relatively normal AUDH by 6mm and increased a relatively normal ALDH by the same amount. There remains an ANB difference after operation of 5° instead of 6° preoperatively. The total facial height has not been markedly altered relative to the cranial baseline, SN. The gonial angle has been increased.

Despite these observations the correction is successful. Partly this is due to the compromise introduced in respect of lip/tooth relationship; partly it reflects the unsatisfactory nature of estimating proportion by the use of the ANS when the latter point is moved during surgery, but not necessarily to the theoretically correct position in relation to the overall movement of the maxilla.

The correction of anterior open bite. The case (shown in **1071** to **1077**) serves to illustrate and should be contrasted with the case on p. 250 (**944** to **948**). The lip/tooth relationship here allows no scope for superior repositioning of the anterior maxilla, and indeed there was insufficient incisor display prior to operation. The posterior maxilla alone is therefore repositioned superiorly and the anterior maxilla inferiorly, thus allowing autorotation of the mandible. The latter is set-back by bilateral sagittal splitting, but the new occlusal plane, determined by the maxillary position, forces an actual increase in the slope of the mandibular plane.

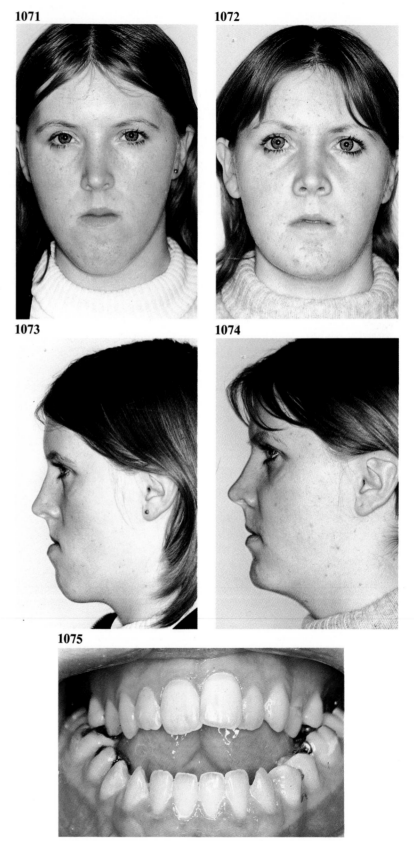

1071   1072

1073   1074

1075

1076

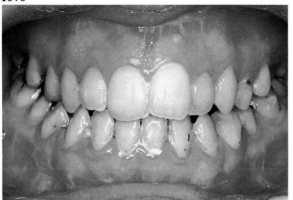

1077

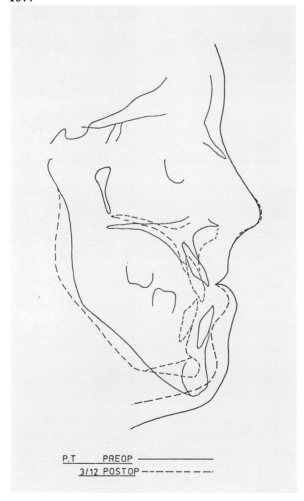

P.T   PREOP _____
3/12 POSTOP ----------

A forward sliding horizontal augmentation genioplasty improves the shape of the chin in both profile and full face views. The advancement of the maxilla fails to correct the effects of the short columella, and indeed the inferior repositioning anteriorly actually increases nasolabial angulation marginally. Stable correction of the anterior open bite is achieved (unchanged 4 years postoperatively).

Several cases of vertical correction scattered throughout this book illustrate the necessity for bimaxillary correction of most vertical dysplasias. This in itself probably helps to stabilise the results by distributing the tissue stresses widely. In the author's experience the stability of associated anteroposterior movements, especially maxillary advancement, is less than in advancement alone.

1071 to 1077   Correction of anterior open bite (1071, 1073, 1075 patient before operation).

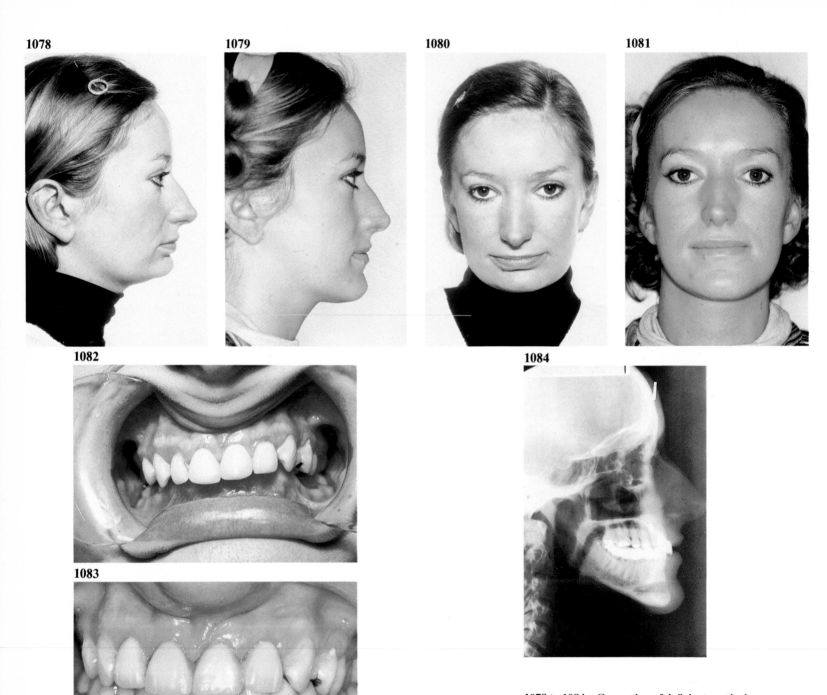

1078 to 1084 Correction of deficient vertical mandibular depth by mandibular advancement plus a subapical proplast implant (**1078, 1080, 1082**, patient before operation).

The Facial Proportion Index (FPI), described in Section 2 (**178** and **179**) is especially useful (apart from its diagnostic uses) in determining the amount of extra height which must be introduced subapically to restore deficient vertical mandibular depth (**832** to **838**).

The case shown here (**1078** to **1084**) should be compared with the almost identical case (**332** to **338**), both being low angle mandibular deficiency problems. Here the preoperative FPI is −2.8 (cf. −6.5 in **332** to **338**), while the postoperative FPI is 9.0 (cf. 0.0 in the comparative case). The difference is that in the former case correction by mandibular advancement alone achieved too little increase in lower-facial height, not recognising the contribution of the subapical deficiency of bone.

In the second case, shown here, mandibular advancement has been accompanied by a subapical proplast implant of 10 mm thickness (**1084**). The ATFH was 107 mm, AUDH 55 mm,

ALDH 52 mm. The FPI is therefore $\dfrac{52 \times 100}{107} - \dfrac{55 \times 100}{107} =$

48.6 − 51.4 = −2.8, or a difference of 12.8%. If the AUFH remains at 55 mm and should be 45% of the total then the ATFH should be 55 × 100 ÷ 45 = 122 mm. The ALFH should then = 122−55 = 67 mm. Photocephalometric planning will indicate the increased ALDH achieved by mandibular advancement alone (here = 4 mm, thus achieving an ALFH of 52 + 4 = 56 mm, while 67 mm is needed for vertical facial balance). Some 11 mm (67–56) still has to be found and thus a 10 mm thick Proplast 1 implant was chosen and inserted subapically (**1084**). In the radiograph shown an extra 2 mm of thickness due to temporary occlusal restorations (temporary bridge-work) has magnified the ALFH, and allowance has been made for this in calculating the actual postoperative figures, ATFH = 121 mm, AUFH = 55 mm, and ALFH = 66 mm, exactly the proportions aimed at.

The effects of vertical corrections on facial profile are to produce modifications of the basic qualitative patterns of change which characterise the osteotomies employed, these basic patterns having been described along with the surgical techniques in Section 4.

The tracings shown here illustrate the modifications of simple mandibular set-back introduced by vertical displacement of the anterior mandible at the same time. In (**1085**A) the mandible is set-back in the standard way for comparison. Note that this is a case with a preoperative flattening of the labio-mental curve of such magnitude that the supramentale is raised to the level of the lower incisor crowns; the considerable set-back required has some effect in lowering it. The effect of less set-back, but some elevation of the anterior dentition (**1085**B) is to reduce or eliminate the downward and lingual displacement of stomion, and may actually advance the upper lip fractionally at the F point.

1085

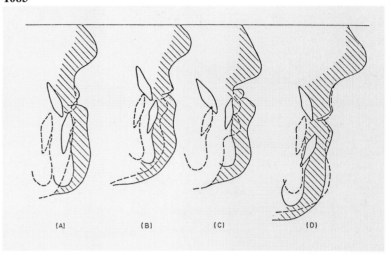

1085 Modifications of mandibular set-back introduced by simultaneous vertical displacement of the anterior mandible.

These effects are greater the greater the elevation and the less the set-back. Correction of overclosure (**1085**C) leads to real unrolling of the upper lip, with drop-back of the upper vermilion and great increase in the amount exposed, an increased drop in the stomion, and exaggeration of the labio-mental curvature. In (**1085**D) we see the effect of real closure of open bite with rotation of the pogonion forwards. Apart from reduction of the lower-facial height there is a tendency to advance the upper lip.

1086

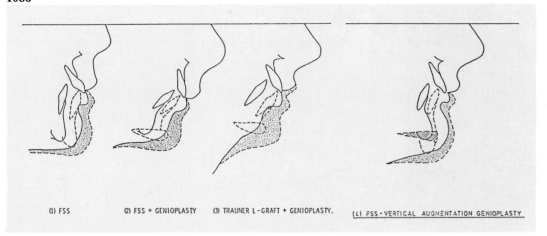

(1) FSS   (2) FSS + GENIOPLASTY   (3) TRAUNER L-GRAFT + GENIOPLASTY.   (4) FSS • VERTICAL AUGMENTATION GENIOPLASTY

1087

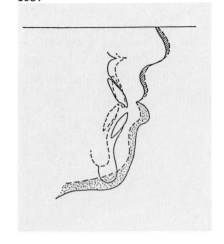

1086 **Effects on facial profile of vertical corrections** in combination with mandibular advancement.

1087 **Reduction in vertical mandibular height** (with mandibular set-back and maxillary surgery).

1088

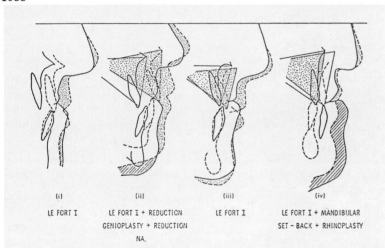

(i)   (ii)   (iii)   (iv)

LE FORT I   LE FORT I + REDUCTION   LE FORT I   LE FORT I + MANDIBULAR
    GENIOPLASTY + REDUCTION   SET-BACK + RHINOPLASTY
    NA.

1088 **Effect of vertical maxillary movement.**

In mandibular advancement cases, with or without separate reduction or augmentation of the anterior mandibular height, there is usually some increase in lower facial height, excluding the high angle cases. Lowering the whole anterior segment has its main effect on the depth of the labiomental curve, flattening it out to a greater extent as the degree of inferior repositioning increases, **1086** (1). This recontouring is greater still if a horizontal augmentation genioplasty is added, **1086** (2), but a significant 'tilting' effect which throws the lower incisor crowns further forwards than the pogonion, **1086** (3), will counteract this effect. Where significant vertical augmentation occurs, **1086** (4) the labiomental curve is again straightened but now the menton is lowered, and the contour of the chin improved.

Reduction in vertical mandibular height is usually associated (see **1087**) with pan-facial surgery in the correction of long faces. The labiomental curve starts too flat and reduction

improves it while raising the chin and neck line. The changes shown in **1087** are typical.

The effect of vertical maxillary movement (**1088**) is to modify the basic qualitative changes of profile described (see p. 246). In (i) the basic pattern is shown for comparison, the changes of simple Le Fort 1 advancement. Superior repositioning is shown in (ii) with slight rotation. The nasal tip is seen to be more acutely tilted forwards and upwards, although the 3 to 1 relationship with the A·point is maintained. The greater projection of the upper incisor tips is reflected in the lip profile, and the effect of mandibular autorotation is shown. The reverse effects are seen in inferior repositioning (iii), with the nose less projected and a slight drop in the columellar profile. The everting effect on the lower lip is accentuated, despite the very moderate change effected in the case traced. The effect of bimaxillary correction in a cleft case is shown in (iv).

The management of secondary cleft lip and palate cases

It is not intended to present in this book any account of the overall management of the cleft palate problem; the reader is referred to the many standard texts covering both the primary and secondary stages. It is intended to discuss the management from the standpoint of the orthognathic surgeon, and this is almost entirely confined to the secondary case, starting in early adolescence. The cleft palate child presents at three stages, and it is well to think of management in terms of these periods.

(1) *In infancy*. After the initial surgical closure of the palate, or lip and palate, the parents main concern during this stage is for *speech*. Nasal escape and poor articulation compel interference in order to fit the child into its social environment, and particularly to allow proper integration into the school for educational purposes. There is a strong argument for minimal surgical interference in order to prevent inhibition of maxillary growth (see Section 1).

Therefore some surgeons advocate the early closure of the lip and posterior palate, but argue that the anterior palate should be left until the child is much older. It is likely then, that for many years to come, there will be great variation in the degree of surgical interference; but the pressures are strong for at least pharyngoplasty, lip closure and posterior palatal closure, and some children will be subjected to additional operations on the anterior palate and nose (especially the alar base and columellar regions). The orthognathic surgeon has no useful role apart from advising surgical moderation to minimise growth inhibition.

(2) *During the period of mixed dentition*. The main concern during this period is to begin a total assessment of the individual child. There is relatively little that the orthodontist can do until the permanent teeth have erupted. Surgically, a *poor lip scar* may be revised, taking care to restore the circumoral musculature if this has not been done. If it is apparent that maxillary growth is sufficient to preclude the likelihood of a later maxillary osteotomy, then a *patent anterior oronasal fistula* may be closed and bone grafted (see pp. 288 to 297). If there is doubt then closure may be delayed. The matter of sequence is discussed later in this section.

However if the case seems likely to involve orthognathic surgery, then the whole problem should be carefully assessed and the timing of surgery planned, together with the appropriate timing of presurgical orthodontics if that is necessary. If the maxilla is to be advanced there should be no interference with the retromaxillary soft-tissues (pharyngoplasty) until after the osteotomy. Otherwise both the pharyngoplasty and the osteotomy are likely to be compromised later. Rhinoplasty should be deferred until after closure of a still patent oronasal fistula for reasons which will be discussed later.

(3) *During the period of permanent dentition*. At this time, and as early in the period as possible, orthodontic expansion of collapsed segments and alignment of the arches should be undertaken, followed by closure of the anterior fistula. If maxillary surgery is to be undertaken this is timed according to the priorities discussed on pp. 298 to 302. The object of surgery should be total and radical reconstruction of the deformity.

The anatomy of the problem is fully described in textbooks on cleft palate surgery. The orthognathic surgeon is concerned with the following anatomical problems:

1. A patent anterior oronasal fistula and adjacent under-development of the nasal sill with alar distortion.

2. Poor lip scarring and function.

3. Maxillary arch collapse.

4. Maxillary hypoplasia.

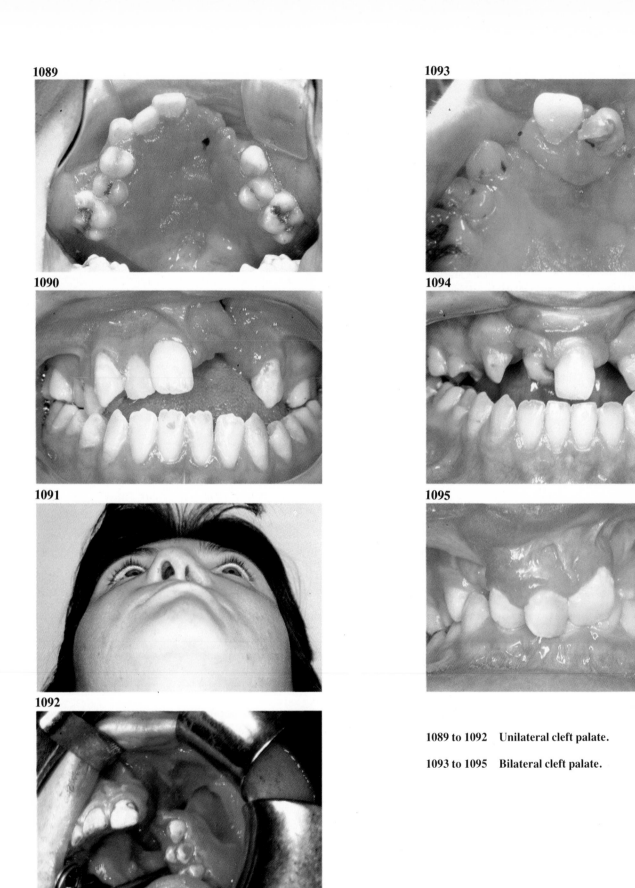

1089

1090

1091

1092

1093

1094

1095

1089 to 1092   Unilateral cleft palate.

1093 to 1095   Bilateral cleft palate.

A patent oronasal fistula is usually present, despite attempts at closure in infancy. Even when effective closure has been obtained there is nearly always a deficiency of underlying bone, and usually the closure has been undertaken in the presence of transverse maxillary collapse, thus acting against effective expansion. A typical unilateral cleft is illustrated (**1089** and **1090**). Because there is an underlying bony cleft, always much larger than the soft-tissue gap might indicate, there is secondary soft-tissue distortion. The anterior nasal spine is absent or rudimentary and there is hypoplasia of the bone at the lateral margin of the lower pyriform aperture on the affected side. The premaxilla is rotated towards the normal side, carrying the base of the columella with it, and the alar cartilages on the cleft side lie low and posteriorly placed on the hypoplastic maxillary base beneath.

Thus the typical nasal base deformity (**1091**), with deviation of the columella and alar base distortion. The defect can be displayed in its entirety at operation (**1092**), showing the absence of the nasal spine and nasal sill, the unsupported nasal floor and the displacement of the nasal septum to the intact side, leaving a pronounced vomerine spur from front to back of the cleft. The inferior turbinate often hypertrophies into the cleft area. In bilateral cases the fistula forms a Y-shaped defect and the premaxillary segment (the prolabium) is isolated between the arms of the Y. It is usually retroclined with real loss of alveolar bone at the site of the cleft on each side (**1093** and **1094**). The premaxillary segment may be grossly rotated (**1095**).

A poor lip scar following primary or subsequent surgery may be a cosmetic problem at rest (**1096**), and if the orbicularis has not been repaired the divided muscle will cause lateral bunching during function. If a patient with this defect is asked to whistle, this bunching can be seen, **1097** and **1098** (arrowed in **1098**). In the bilateral case the typical 'whistling deformity' is fully developed (**1099**). This functional defect is sufficient indication for lip revision with muscle repair.

1096

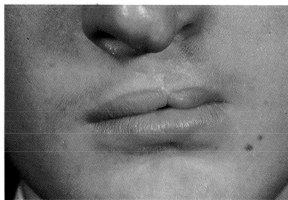

1098

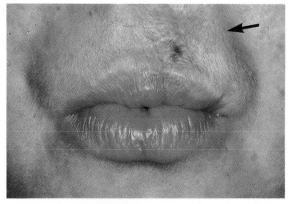

1097

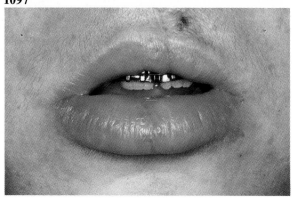

1099

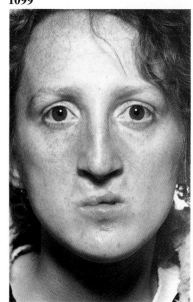

1096 **Lip scar** following surgery.

1097 and 1098 **Lateral bunching** during function. **1097**, lips at rest; **1098**, whistling.

1099 **Typical 'whistling deformity'** in a bilateral case.

1100

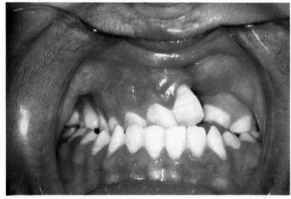

1101

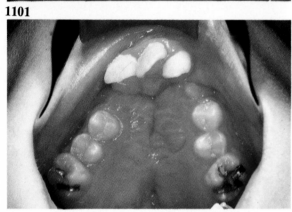

1102

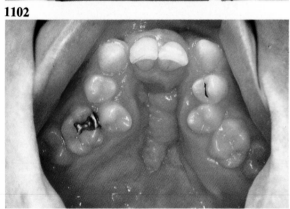

1100 to 1102 **Maxillary collapse** in unilateral cleft (**1100**) and in bilateral cleft (**1101** and **1102**).

1103

1104

1105

1106

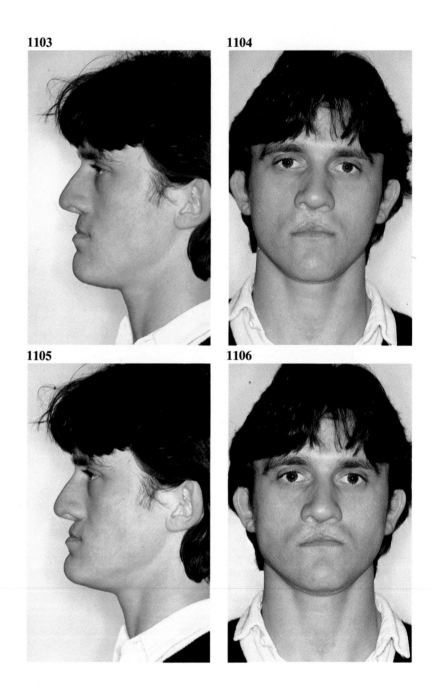

1107

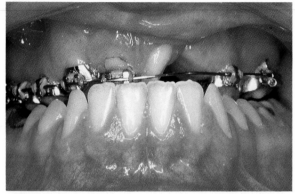

1108

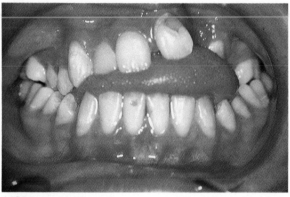

1109

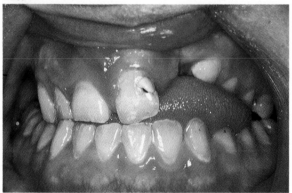

1103 to 1107   Supra-apical maxillary hypoplasia.

1108 and 1109   Differential vertical hypoplasia.

Maxillary collapse is almost always present to some degree. In unilateral cases there is most often rotational collapse of the lesser segment with a smaller degree of medial displacement of the greater segment (**1100**). In bilateral cases the posterior segments collapse medially and the anterior segment usually collapses posteriorly, as in **1101**. Sometimes gross collapse of the dentition occurs (**1102**).

Maxillary hypoplasia may occur at the low level equivalent to supra-apical hypoplasia (**1103** and **1104**). There is frequently a failure of vertical development, which can be seen when the patient brings the teeth into occlusion (**1105** and **1106**). This is a bilateral case with marked maxillary retrusion at the occlusal level (**1107**), but the overclosure is exaggerating the degree of retrusion. This always requires careful assessment in cleft cases. Sometimes there is differential vertical hypoplasia, with deficiency anteriorly, or in the region of the lesser segment (**1108** and **1109**). Lesser segment failure often leads to a curved open bite with the canine (if present) and the first premolar at a higher level than the rest of the segment.

This kind of vertical problem is difficult to correct for two reasons. First, the curve of the occlusal line of the segment makes it impossible to bring all the teeth into occlusion with the lower dentition; either an anterior or a posterior open bite is inevitable; and orthodontic repositioning of the individual teeth seems difficult to achieve and unstable if achieved. This brings the second problem into focus, which is the inherent tendency to vertical relapse after surgical or orthodontic repositioning.

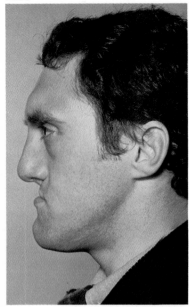

1110

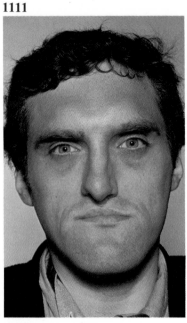

1111

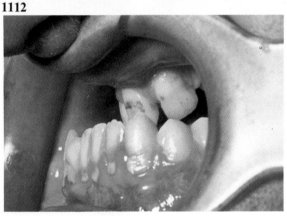

1112

Hypoplasia is sometimes more widespread, extending to involve the nasomaxillary area of the mid-face, correctable by Le Fort 2 osteotomy. Again vertical failure of maxillary growth is usually associated and overclosure in occlusion may suggest gross mandibular protrusion (**1110** to **1112**). This case shows some underdevelopment of the malar regions also.

Real mandibular prognathism occurs in some cleft palate patients, compounding the deformity (**1113**).

Closure of Oronasal Fistulae

The steps in closing fistulae are as follows:

Preliminary

Reconstruct the primary defect. The maxillary arches must be expanded to produce correct arch form and alignment. This inevitably enlarges the size of the fistula, demonstrating the actual bony deficiency. This preliminary step (which may be orthodontic or surgical) is absolutely essential if good facial contour is to be restored. Collapsed arches mean that the overlying soft-tissues are collapsed inwards; this is especially true of the alar base(s). Alignment is not always possible, as in the case illustrated for closure.

Stage 1   Excise the fistula

Stage 2   Close the nasal floor

Stage 3   Bone graft the defect

Stage 4   Close the oral layer over the bone graft.

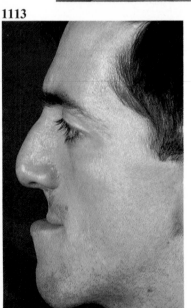

1113

1110 to 1112   Extensive hypoplasia involving the nasomaxillary area of the mid-face.

1113   Mandibular prognathism complicating maxillary hypoplasia, in a cleft palate case.

These four stages are demonstrated in the case shown in **1089** to **1090** and here after surgical expansion (**1114** and **1115**). The patient refused orthodontic treatment and arch alignment has therefore not been undertaken, with resulting occlusal compromise. Comparison of **1089** with **1115** shows that bilateral Le Fort 1 osteotomies have been used to expand the maxilla, both greater and lesser segments being moved outwards.

1114

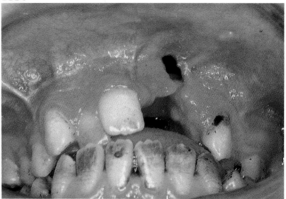

1115

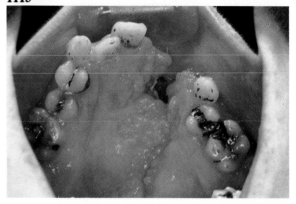

1114 and 1115   Surgical expansion of maxillary arches. (Compare with **1089** and **1090**.)

1116

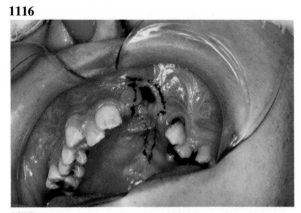

1117

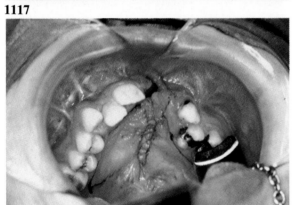

1118

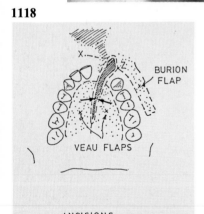

1116 to 1123   Excision of the fistula.

1119

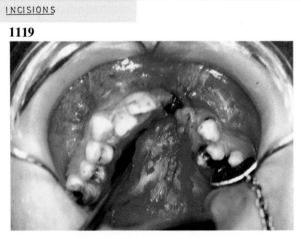

1120

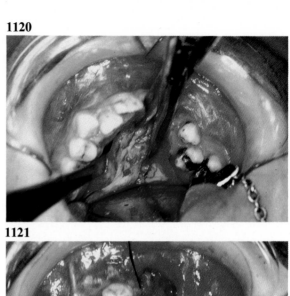

1121

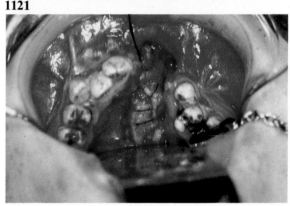

1122

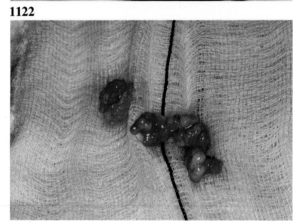

1123

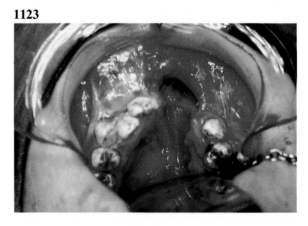

Stage 1

Excision of the fistula. The fistula is marked out (**1116**) and Veau flaps drawn on the palate (**1117** and **1118**). The lateral edge of the Veau flap on the side of the greater segment is incised and the flap raised from the lateral aspect until the lateral edge of the bony fistula can be felt with the periosteal elevator (**1119**). A Howarth's nasal raspatory is ideal for periosteal elevation. McIndoe's scissors are next inserted so that one blade lies under the Veau flap as far medially as it is possible to get while still beneath good mucoperiosteum (**1120**). The medial edge of the Veau flap is now cut with the scissors, including as much good mucoperiosteum as possible, but not encroaching on friable or hyperplastic tissue in the fistula.

The same is repeated for the Veau flap on the lesser segment. Both flaps are reflected and held below a tongue retractor, leaving the fistula in the midline (**1121**) (sutured over for demonstration purposes). The vestibular extension of the fistula is circumferentially incised and dissected from the underlying tissue, taking care not to 'button-hole' through into the nasal floor apart from the fistula itself (**1121**). All tissue in the fistula (ie where there should be bone) is excised and discarded (**1122**), leaving a clean defect with the nasal mucosa cut cleanly (**1123**).

Stage 2

Closure of the nasal floor. The nasal mucosa is carefully elevated from the nasal septum medially and the lateral wall of the nose laterally. The dissection is carried forwards subperiosteally to define the whole of the bony defect and the pyriform rim on both sides (**1124**). This facilitates final development of septal and lateral nasal wall flaps for closure of the nasal floor (**1125**) (taken from a different case with the lip split). At this stage the hypertrophied turbinate may be trimmed back and the vomerine spur chiselled from the nasal septum, in order to improve the airway. It should be possible to pass an endotracheal anaesthetic tube along the nasal cavity after this has been done, without obstruction. The nasal floor is next sutured from the back forwards, using 3/0 chromic catgut on small ¾ Round Denis Brown needles, or similar. If difficulty is encountered posteriorly, a Reverdin needle is useful. Closure should be complete (**1126**).

Where the cleft is too narrow in the palate for access, or 'bridges' of old bone graft are present, the cleft should be gently widened with a chisel, taking away the bony bridges or the edges of a narrow cleft. This greatly simplifies nasal floor closure, and the subsequent bone grafting quickly restores the lost tissue.

1124

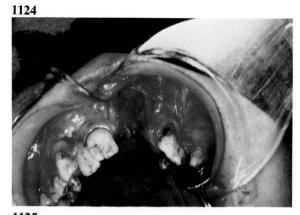

1125

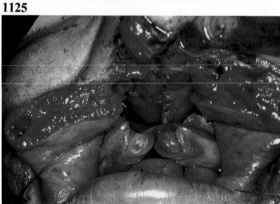

1126

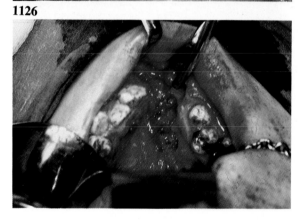

1124 to 1126   Closure of the nasal floor.

1127

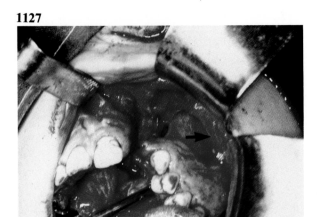

1128

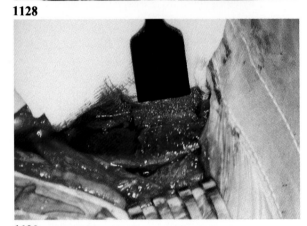

1129

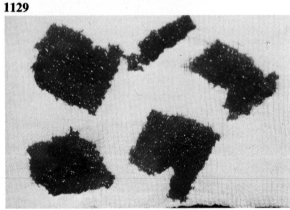

1130

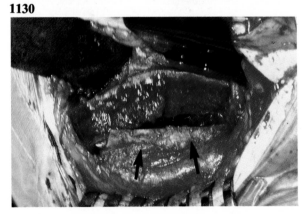

1131

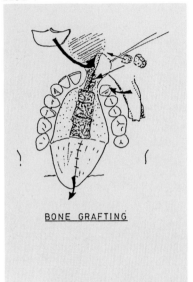

BONE GRAFTING

1127 to 1132   Bone grafting the defect.

1132

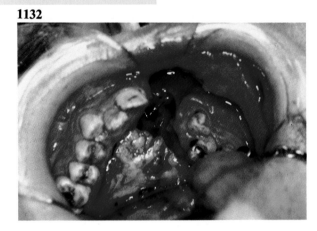

Stage 3

Bone grafting the defect. Wherever there is hypoplastic bone, as in the area below the alar base, the overlying periosteum is incised to allow a pocket to accommodate bone grafts. The whole area is displayed and the amount of bone required can be assessed (**1127**).

The lateral incision in the sulcus is the inferior limb of the flap to be used in closure of the anterior soft-tissue defect (see **1133** to **1135**) and it helps to gain good access all round if this incision is made at this stage (arrowed). The illium is opened and the crest reflected with attached periosteum in order to gain access to the cancellous bone beneath. Fillets of thin bone can be cut from the intact hip (**1128** and **1129**), leaving a clear working base in the ilium before replacement of the crest, arrowed in **1130**. This bone is then packed into the cleft area as indicated (**1131**). Fillets are laid over the palatal defect and are rolled up to build up the alveolar defect.

Similarly the alar base area is built up, and finally a piece of thin cortical bone is contoured to finalise reconstruction of the nasal sill. It is helpful to suture the two Veau flaps together in the midline before packing bone along the palatal cleft (**1132**).

Stage 4

Closure of the oral layer has already been started by joining the Veau flaps prior to packing the palate with bone (**1131**). The secondary defects remaining laterally after medial rotation of the Veau flaps are left to epithelialise, with just one or two sutures placed anteriorly to hold them in place (**1133**). The anterior defect may be closed by rotating a long cheek flap taken from the mucosa of the cheek on the cleft side, and based on the lip (**1118**, **1131** and **1133**). This is ascribed to Burion, and will be termed a 'Burion Flap'. A small horizontal incision ('x' in **1118**) is cut to be opened out into a V and receive the leading point ('z' in **1118** and **1133**) of the flap as it is swung round (arrowed in **1134**). The flap is carefully sutured into the defect to complete closure (**1135**). The whole procedure may be undertaken at the same time as lip revision, which considerably simplifies access and clear visualisation.

Alternative flaps for closure of the oral layer are shown (**1216**) and the indications for their use are discussed. Sliding gingival flaps are particularly indicated in smaller fistulae where the palatal extension is small; the great advantage of these flaps is that 'wear and tear' oral mucoperiosteum is transferred to the crest of the alveolar ridge, and this certainly improves the chances of underlying teeth erupting satisfactorily into functional occlusion.

1133

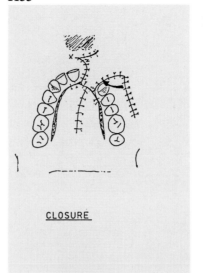

CLOSURE

1133 to 1135 Closure of the oral layer.

1134

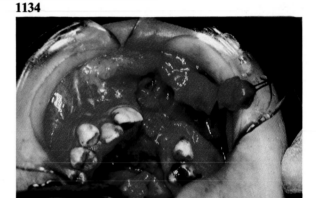

1135

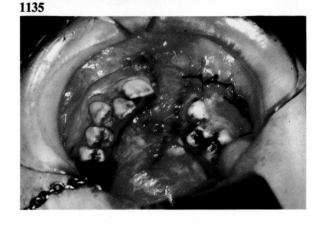

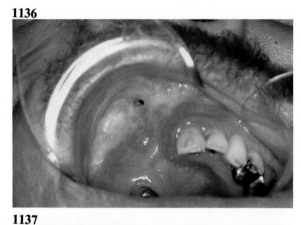

1136

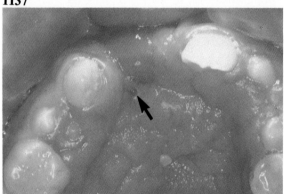

1137

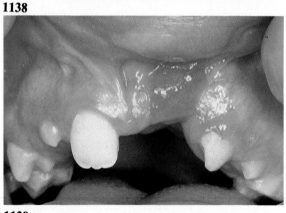

1138

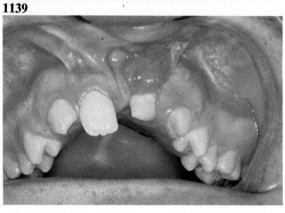

1139

Bone grafting is important because (1) It helps to maintain the expanded maxilla, (2) It converts the cleft maxilla into a solid one piece upper jaw, which can then be dealt with as a single unit if osteotomy is necessary (but see also pp. 304 to 309), (3) It is difficult to obtain complete closure without the three separate layers, nasal floor, bone, oral mucosa, (4) It is essential in order to reconstruct the nasal sill and build up the alar base so that subsequent rhinoplasty can be undertaken with the two alar bases more or less on symmetrical bony supports. The latter is important if cosmetic correction is to be achieved. (5) Finally, after the bone has settled down the alveolus is a better shape for subsequent dental bridging or prosthetic appliances. Without bone, old repairs sometimes break down many years later (**1136**).

A repaired fistula and cleft is shown in **1137** and **1138**. A little area of sequestration is common at the site shown (arrowed), and provided small chips of bone have been used in this area (where the three flaps join together), the small sequestrum separates or is lifted away and epithelialisation is the rule. It is helpful to cover these areas with a small dental plate for a few weeks (many cases are still in orthodontic retention anyway, and a new retention plate must be constructed immediately postoperatively). Teeth often erupt through the bone grafted area (**1139** shows the previous case 2½ years postoperatively) and sometimes these are useful for abutments. Where this occurs through a Burion flap, however, the gingival attachment is poor. Sliding gingival flaps yield better results where tooth eruption through (or orthodontic movement into) bone grafted areas is anticipated.

Sulcus depth is always reduced in the area of a buccal advancement flap, and the use of Burion flaps is no exception (**1140** and **1141**). The situation can always be saved by a local vestibuloplasty, if necessary using a skin graft (**1142**).

Very large fistulae can sometimes be closed using modifications of the same technique, as here in a postsurgical case (**1143**). There is always sufficient tissue for nasal floor closure (**1144** and **1145**). The sutures are left long and carried through the oral layer to eliminate dead space and haematoma formation. After bone grafting (**1146**), buccal advancement flaps are used for oral closure (**1147**). If such large cavities can be made to heal (**1148**), the same principle is readily applied to large clefts. Alternatively tongue flaps can be raised and sutured into large palatal defects with considerable success (**1149** to **1152**).

1136 Breakdown of repaired fistula many years later (bone grafting had not been used).

1137 to 1139 Repaired fistula and cleft. 1139 Tooth erupting through bone grafted area.

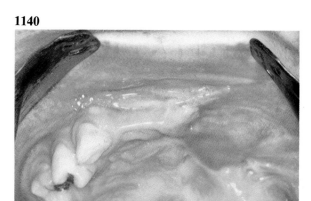

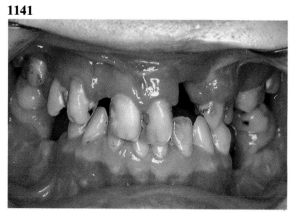

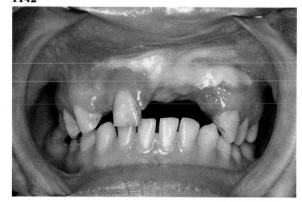

1140 and 1141   **Buccal flaps:** reduction in sulcus depth.

1142   **Local vestibuloplasty.**

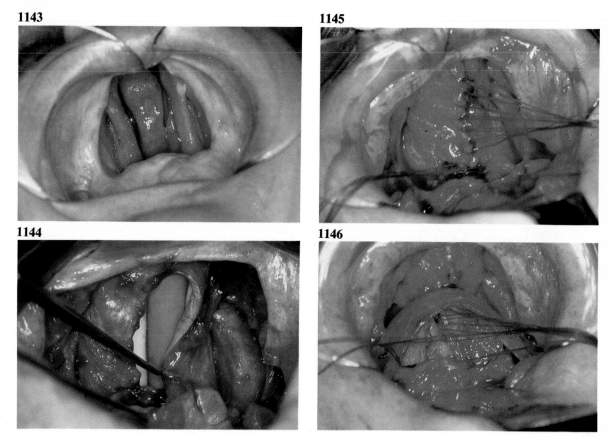

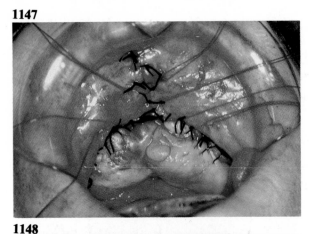

1147

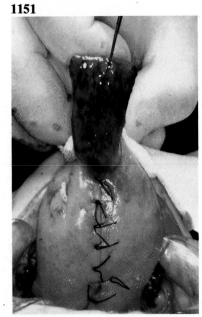

1151

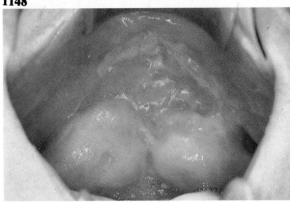

1148

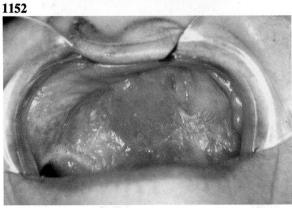

1152

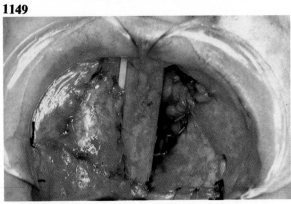

1149

1143 to 1152 **Closure of very large fistulae.** Use of tongue flaps (**1149** to **1152**).

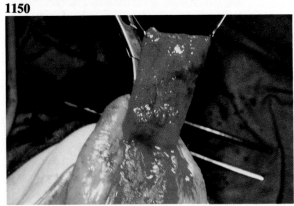

1150

Bilateral clefts are closed by a similar technique with one important modification. The prolabial segment is attached only to the anterior septum; this is divided with a chisel after excision of the fistulae, and fractured forwards in the manner of the Wunderer procedure, being sustained on its labial pedicle. This simplifies access to the nasal floor for development of flaps, and allows the segment to be repositioned in a more forward location, which is invariably necessary. The sequence shows a typical case prior to orthodontic expansion (**1153** and **1154**), after orthodontic treatment (**1155** and **1156**), and after closure of the fistulae as described, including advancement of the premaxillary segment (**1157** and **1158**). The small tooth rudiment seen in **1153** and **1155** has been removed prior to closure.

1153

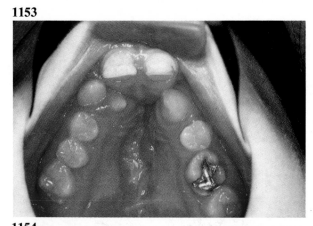

1157

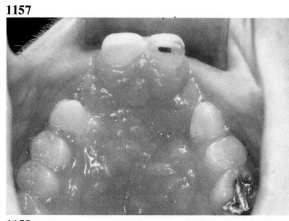

1154

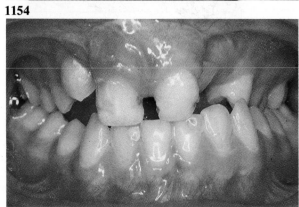

1158

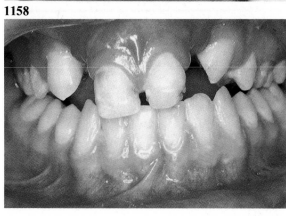

1155

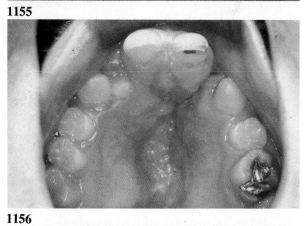

1153 to 1158   Closure of fistulae in bilateral cleft.

1156

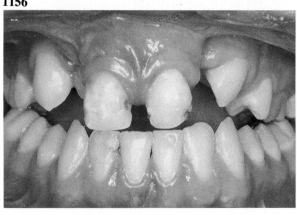

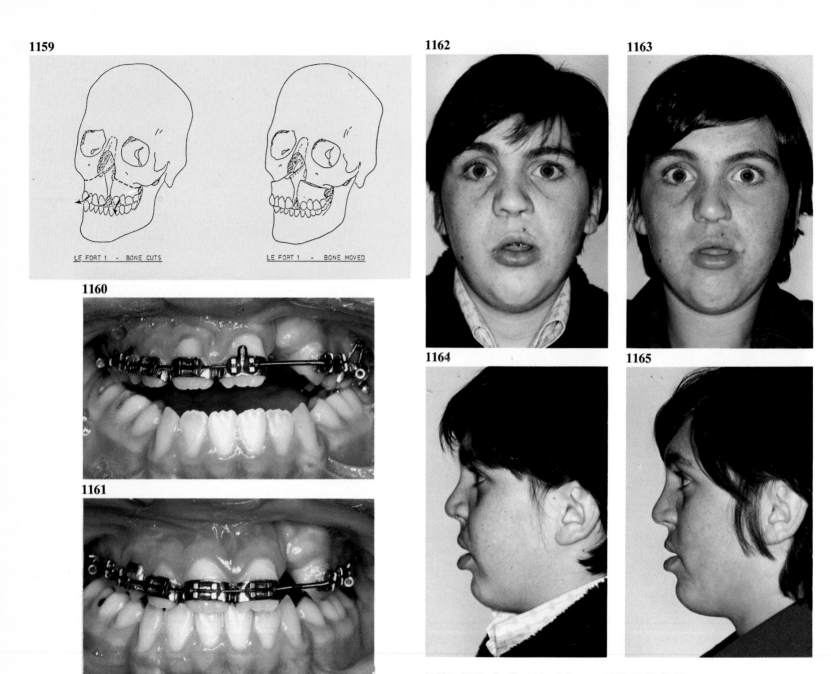

1159 to 1165   Le Fort 1 in cleft cases 1160, 1162, 1164 patient before operation.

Management priorities

Two major considerations arise in the management of the secondary cleft case:

1. *The type of maxillary osteotomy.* At what level should surgery be undertaken, Le Fort 1, 2 or 3? Should surgery be unilateral or bilateral?

2. *The timing of osteotomy* in relation to fistula closure.

In considering these two matters opportunity will be taken to discuss technical difficulties peculiar to the cleft palate case when undertaking maxillary osteotomies.

The choice of osteotomy lies between the Le Fort 1 and its variants, and osteotomies at a higher level than the Le Fort 1.

1166

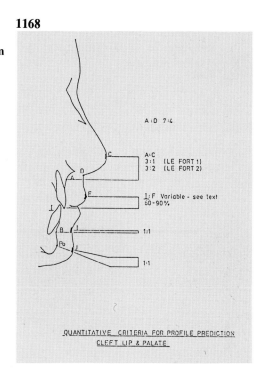

1167

**1166 and 1167
Rotational correction
– Le Fort 1.**

1168

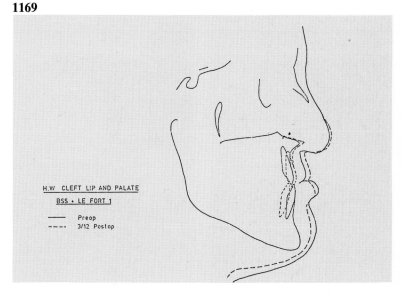

QUANTITATIVE CRITERIA FOR PROFILE PREDICTION
CLEFT LIP & PALATE

1169

H.W CLEFT LIP AND PALATE

BSS + LE FORT 1

—— Preop
---- 3/12 Postop

Type of osteotomy

The Le Fort 1 in cleft cases (**1159**) has the following indications:

(a) It applies to the *commonest level* of maxillary hypoplasia in cleft palate patients, and it allows simultaneous correction of vertical maxillary deficiency (see **1103** to **1106**). A typical correction is shown (**1160** to **1165**).

(b) It offers the *greatest flexibility* in movement of the alveolar segments. In particular vertical and rotational repositioning can be achieved by the Le Fort 1, and only by the Le Fort 1. Typical rotational movement is shown in **1166** and **1167**. The high canine on the left has been removed, and the vertical differential (discussed in **1108** to **1109**) is seen to be a problem with the lesser segment. This flexibility is very important. Transverse expansion, differential anteroposterior repositioning, and possible left/right variation are easily accomplished. The segments can be moved in two or three parts. None of this is possible in Le Fort 2 or 3 osteotomies alone.

(c) Specific profile changes occur in cleft cases (**1168**). Nasal tip advancement is reliably one third of maxillary advancement at the Le Fort 1 level. The A point is really nonexistent but the most anterior part of the maxillary alveolar outline can be located. This nasal tip movement is more reliable than in non-cleft cases (Freihofer, 1977).

There is an improved columellar slope. Subnasale moves about four sevenths of the maxillary advancement. (Freihofer, 1976). The skin/vermilion junction moves with the upper incisor tip in relation to its thickness and 'stretchability'. This means that a heavily scarred lip may move 80% to 90% of the tooth movement, while a good muscle repair will result in a lip that moves more like the non-cleft lip, approximating 60% of the movement. However, this is the least predictable and most unreliable of all profile predictions. The lip lengthens, flattens and the stomion moves down and forwards in general, but great variation occurs. A typical change is seen in **1169**.

Indications for the Le Fort 1 are therefore:

1. Lower nasolabial profile disproportionately retruded in relation to the upper mid-face.

2. Differential right/left movement of the alveolar segments needed.

3. Vertical maxillary insufficiency.

The Le Fort 1 will not correct infraorbital recession, nor recession of the nasomaxillary base. Examples of three very different types of case are shown in **1170** to **1179**.

The Le Fort 2 osteotomy (**1180** and **1181**) is increasingly used in those cases where the demands of profile are for advancement of the nasal tip, dorsum and bridge by bringing forwards the base of the nasal skeleton, and full face requirement is for infraorbital advance. It is incompatible with simultaneous Le Fort 1, as this creates too many fragments for control. If combined with mandibular surgery it allows full tilting of the maxilla about the nasal bridge, with alteration of the occlusal plane (**1182**).

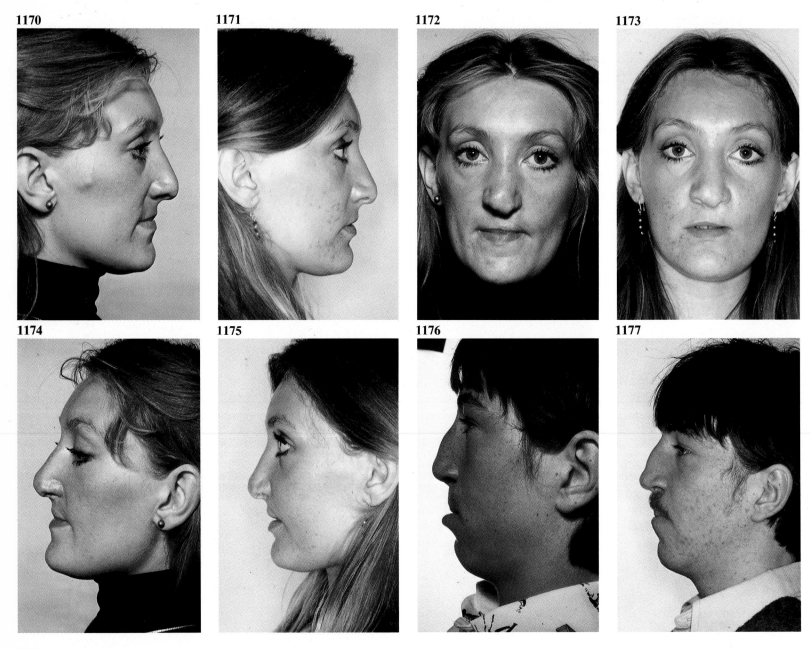

1170 1171 1172 1173

1174 1175 1176 1177

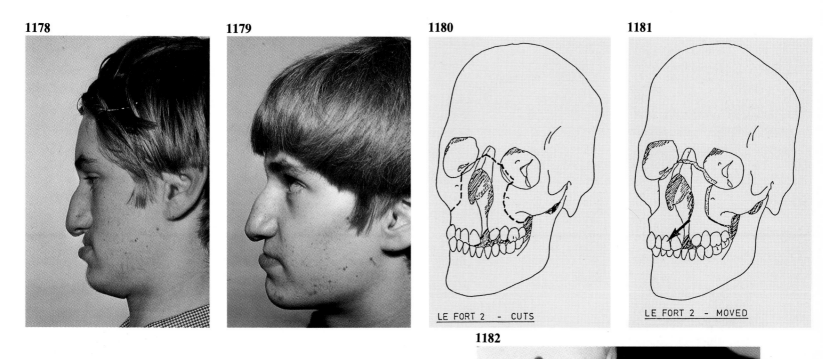

1178

1179

1180

LE FORT 2 - CUTS

1181

LE FORT 2 - MOVED

1170 to 1179   Three cleft cases treated by Le Fort 1.

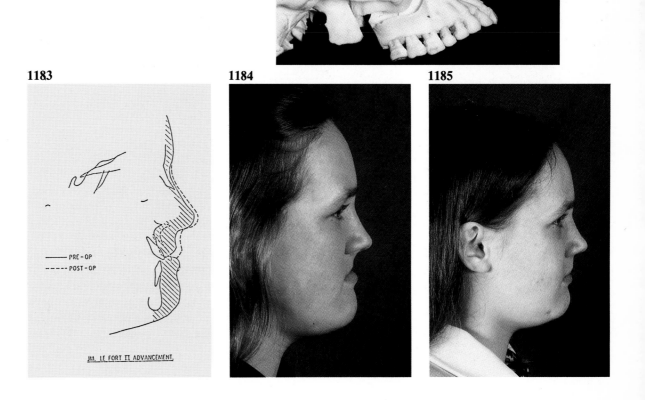

1182

1183

—— PRE-OP
---- POST-OP

JM. LE FORT II ADVANCEMENT.

1184

1185

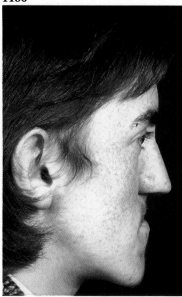
1186

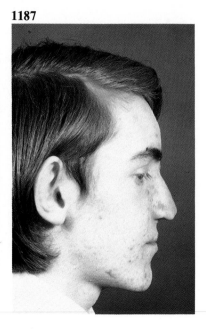
1187

1184 to 1187   Le Fort 2 in cleft cases. (Joint cases with I.T. Jackson, FRCS).

1. The infraorbital rim is advanced, and this can be extended laterally as for the non-cleft patient.

2. It advances the nasomaxillary base allowing greater movement of the tip than the Le Fort 1 for the same advancement of the maxilla, but without the same differential effect between the upper nasal profile and the lower (see **1183**, a typical cleft profile change, seen clinically **1184** to **1185**).

3. It is easier to combine with rhinoplasty, especially in the area of the nasal bridge.

4. It allows increase in vertical height of the maxilla, but not decrease (rarely indicated in cleft cases).

5. It allows pure expansion from a nasal bridge fulcrum, but this tends to produce buccal inclination of the lateral maxillary segments.

6. There is greater security of blood supply to the alveolar segments. This is useful where the blood supply has been seriously reduced by previous palatal surgery or by a very large fistula (wide posteriorly). This is also useful for simultaneous closure of clefts with maxillary advancement (**1215**).

The Le Fort 2 is not suitable for bilateral cleft cases unless there has been previous, and completely successful, closure of the fistulae, with conversion of the three part maxilla to one solid bony bloc. Otherwise great difficulty will be experienced in mobilising the anterior maxillary alveolar region.

Where the Le Fort 2 is used to inferiorly reposition the maxilla, the cut should be made anterior to the lacrimal apparatus, and the medial canthal attachment retained at the higher level on the cranial residue. Tissue can be brought down from the glabella to lengthen the nose.

The Le Fort 3 osteotomy is very rarely indicated in cleft palate cases unless these are associated with craniostenotic syndromes, when the indications are as for the latter. No particular technical difficulties arise over and above the problems of lower level osteotomies in cleft cases. A typical case is shown (**416** to **423**). Occasionally gross malar and orbital hypoplasia may suggest Le Fort 3 correction but reference should be made to p. 117 (**404** to **409**). Probably the most common indication is when the case requires differential movement of upper and lower mid-face (the lower movement may be lateral or rotational) and a Le Fort 3 is combined with a Le Fort 1 to achieve this (remembering that the Le Fort 2 and Le Fort 1 cannot be combined simultaneously).

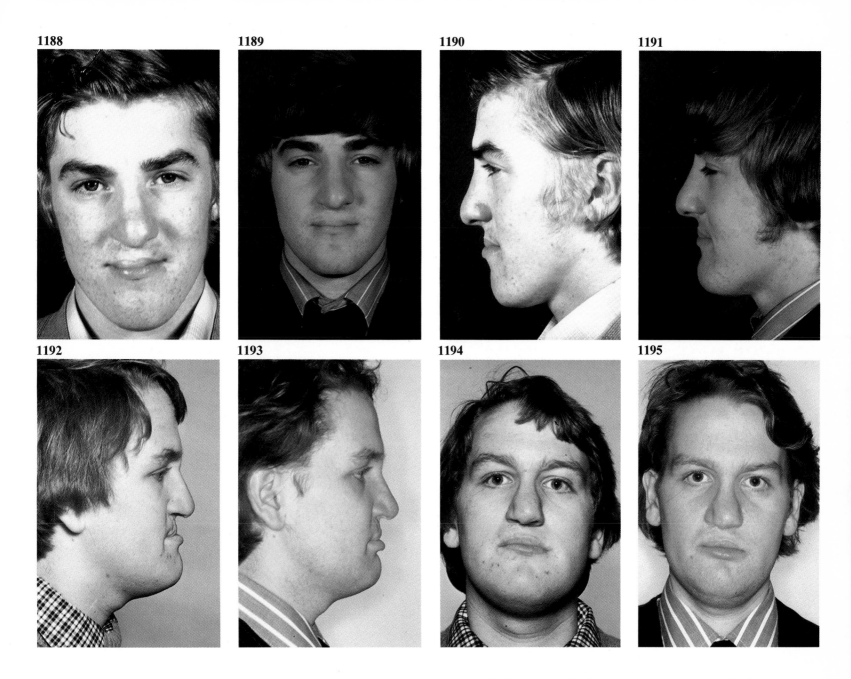

1188 to 1191 Mandibular symphyseal ostectomy.

1192 to 1199 Bilateral sagittal split combined with Le Fort 1 maxillary advancement.

Mandibular set-back plays an important part in the management of secondary cleft palate cases. The operator should be more ready to compromise on profile ideals in view of the acknowledged difficulty in fully mobilising some cleft maxillae and advancing them far. It is better to accept a little compromise and balance the correction with the mandible, even if the problem is entirely maxillary. Judgment is necessary in these cases. Secondly, bimaxillary corrections increase perioral suppleness; so also does mandibular symphyseal ostectomy (already discussed (**771** to **774**)). A further case is shown here (**1188** to **1191**).

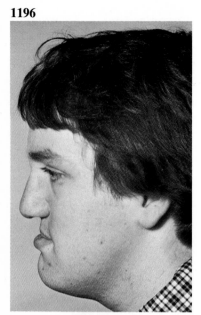

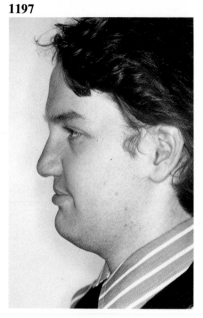

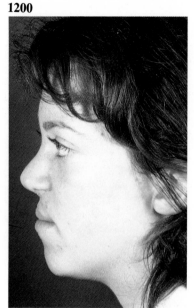

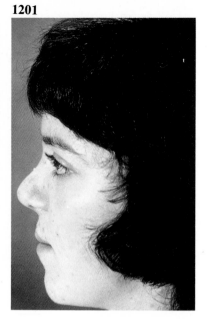

1198

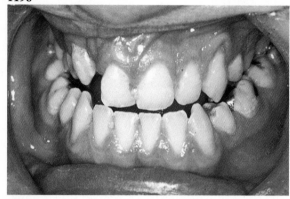

1200 and 1201   Lower labial segmental set-back.

1199

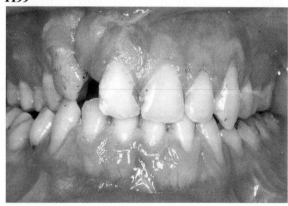

A typical 'compromise' case is shown (prior to lip or nasal surgery) in **1192** to **1199**, with tracing shown on p. 299 (**1169**). A bilateral sagittal split was combined with Le Fort 1 maxillary advancement, and the fistula will be closed at a later date. Simple lower labial segmental set-back (**1200** and **1201**) can be quite useful, again especially because of the loosening effect around the perioral tissues.

Sequence and Timing

When it is anticipated that a maxillary osteotomy is necessary and that closure of an anterior fistula must be undertaken, the question of timing is important.

Ideally, before any osteotomy is performed both maxillary and mandibular growth should be *complete*. The case shown (**1202** and **1203**), was operated on (Le Fort 1) before mandibular growth was complete, and initially a nice result was obtained (**1204** and **1205**). However, 18 months later (**1206** and **1207**), apparent relapse has occurred. In fact mandibular growth has re-established a Class 3 malocclusion. Once occlusal lock has been lost, relapse is certain in cleft cases.

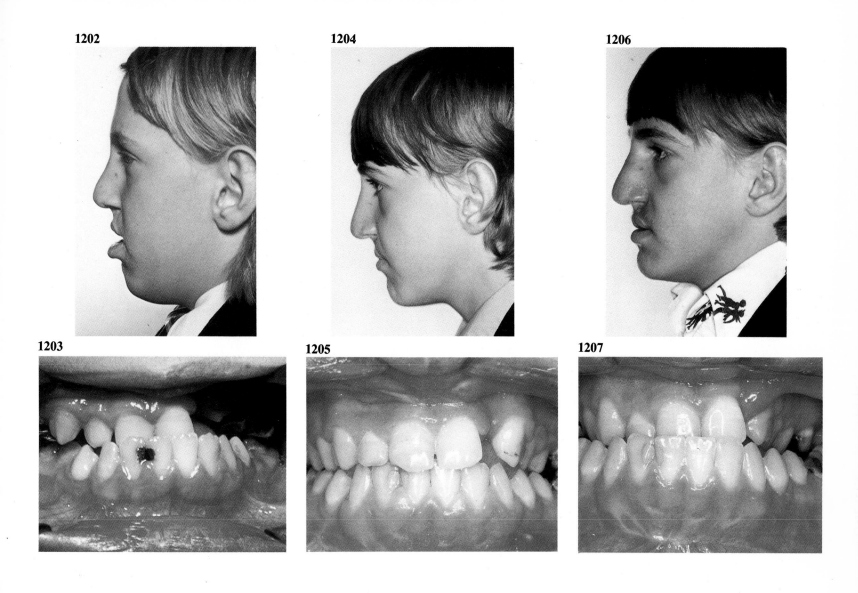

1202 to 1207   Relapse in a cleft case operated on (Le Fort 1) before
mandibular growth was complete.

The Choice for sequence is:

(a) Fistula first, maxilla later. The fistula can be closed before completion of growth.

(b) Maxilla first, fistula later. Here both must await completion of growth.

(c) Simultaneous closure of fistula and advancement of the maxilla, again after growth is finished (Henderson and Jackson, 1975).

The latter option is rarely undertaken, but the principles and problems will be discussed next.

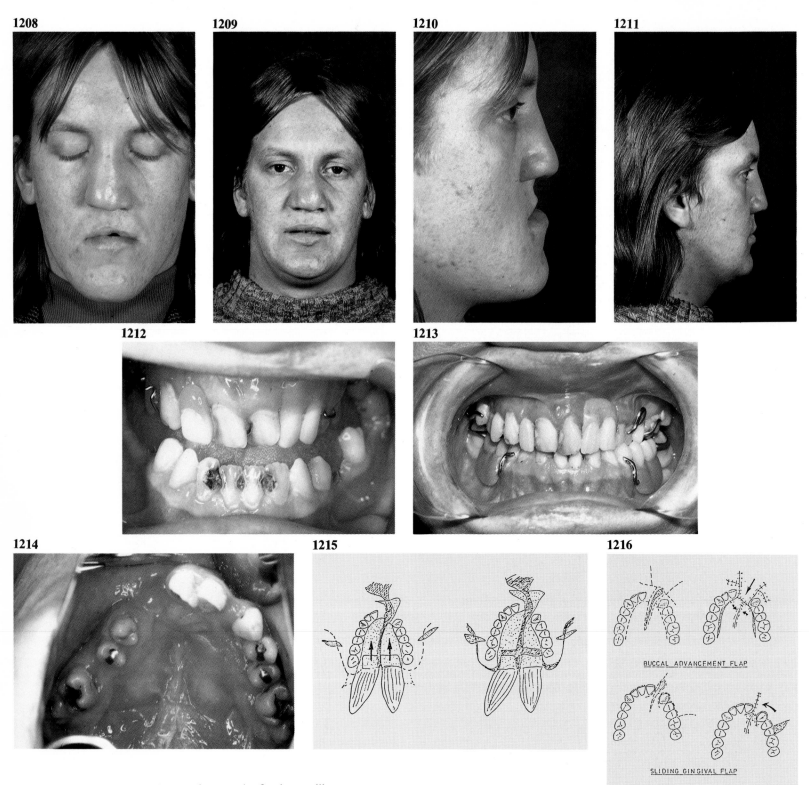

1208 to 1214 **Simultaneous closure** of an anterior fistula, maxillary advancement, mandibular set-back, lip revision and first stage rhinoplasty.

BUCCAL ADVANCEMENT FLAP

SLIDING GINGIVAL FLAP

306

Simultaneous closure of an anterior fistula, maxillary advancement, mandibular set-back, lip revision and first stage rhinoplasty were undertaken in this patient (**1208** to **1214**) (joint case
with I.T. Jackson Esq, FRCS).

1. If the level is Le Fort 1 simultaneous fistula closure is not
   compatible with a horseshoe incision (because Veau flaps
   would then devitalise the alveolar fragments). Therefore
   the downfracture method cannot be used and the osteotomy
   has to be completed under vestibular tunnels (see **555**).
   This is a serious disadvantage. The method of retromolar
   maxillary osteotomy described by Converse and Shapiro
   (1952) and applied to the cleft case by Wake (1976) theoretically overcomes the problem (**1234** to **1236**). The difficulties are discussed when the technique is described.
   Minor closures, where very small bony clefts are present,
   are possible if a Veau flap is raised from one side (usually
   the lesser segment) and the Burion flap from the other, thus
   maintaining the blood supply to the one side from the
   vestibule and to the other from the palate. Great care is
   needed, and palatal flaps should not be raised until all
   osteotomy cuts in the buccal walls have been completed
   without compromising the vestibular pedicles. Burion flaps
   should not be raised from a segment to which the palatal
   blood supply is to be interrupted. On the whole simultaneous closure is best avoided when the osteotomy is to be
   at the Le Fort 1 level.

2. If the level is Le Fort 2 simultaneous closure is quite
   possible, and at the alveolar level the method to be followed
   is that of the modified Converse/Wake technique (**1215**).
   This works well, the tunnelling is less and therefore easier.
   The Burion flap is kept high in the cheek and the blood
   supply seems to be quite adequate.

3. If the lesser segment, or the premaxillary segment, of a
   bilateral case only are to be rotated, it is easier to maintain a
   good vestibular blood supply, and simultaneous closure
   may be possible. This will depend on the size of Burion flaps
   required. Simple buccal advancement flaps can be used in
   some of these cases (**1216**). Where the fistula is very large a
   buccal advancement flap is also useful. Where small unilateral
   or bilateral fistulae exist sliding gingival flaps (**1216**) are
   indicated. These transfer 'wear and tear' oral mucoperiosteum
   to the alveolar crest. If teeth are likely to erupt into the
   bone grafted area, then these sliding flaps are especially
   useful; a much greater likelihood of eruption and a greatly
   improved gingival attachment result.

The logical sequence is to close the fistula first, after orthodontic maxillary expansion and before growth is complete.
This helps with speech and function, and after the bone
grafted maxilla has fully united the maxillary downfracture is
relatively simple, although separation of the nasal floor from
the upper aspect of the palate is sometimes tedious. It is

1217

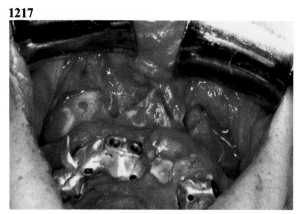

1218

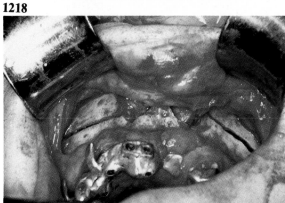

1219

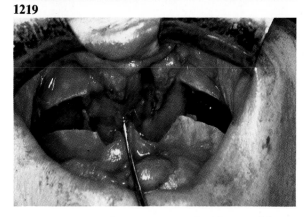

1217 to 1219   Maxillary osteotomy after closure of the
fistula.

interesting to observe how effective bone grafting has been
(**1217**), and the osteotomy cuts are made in the normal way
(**1218**), followed by routine downfracture (**1219**).

This case is a unilateral cleft and the ideal sequence is
therefore:

1. Orthodontic expansion and alignment after tooth eruption,
   say aged 11 to 13, followed by

2. Closure of the fistula, followed by (after completion of
   growth)

3. Maxillary osteotomy, followed by

4. Final orthodontic alignment with retention for at least 1 year, followed by

5. Anterior bridgework to replace missing teeth and provide further retentive support.

But this plan robs the maxillary osteotomy of any scope for segmental or directional flexibility, and the palate may reopen during mobilisation if union has been less complete than anticipated. The sequence is most suitable for those cases presenting early, with good orthodontic control and acceptance and relatively simple sagittal advancement without left/right variation, at either Le Fort 1 or 2 levels.

Other surgery is best fitted into this pattern. Closure of the fistula must precede rhinoplasty, and Le Fort 2 must always precede rhinoplasty (or there is a real and disturbing tendency for the two sides to separate at the nasal bridge during mobilisation). Lip revision can be undertaken at the same time as fistula closure, and pharyngoplasty (secondary) should be deferred until after maxillary osteotomy. It is preferable if bridgework is done last.

More often *alveolar flexibility is indicated* with two- or three-part differential movement at the Le Fort 1 level. Here the sequence must be changed to:

Preliminary orthodontics as indicated, but

1. Allow maxillary growth and mandibular growth to be completed, followed by

2. Maxillary advancement and other segmental movements at the Le Fort 1 level in 2 or 3 segments, followed by

3. Retention for 6 months, using a transpalatal plate as part of the retention device, followed by

4. Closure of the fistula, followed by

5. Further retention for at least 1 year, followed by

6. Final bridgework

The case illustrated (**1220** to **1223**), first had a Le Fort 2 osteotomy (**1224** to **1226**), then fistula closure (**1227** to **1230**), and finally bridgework (**1231** and **1232**). There is a slight occlusal compromise in the selection of Le Fort 2 (for cosmetic reasons) and losing the flexibility of Le Fort 1, in the absence of orthodontic perseverance; but the result is satisfactory.

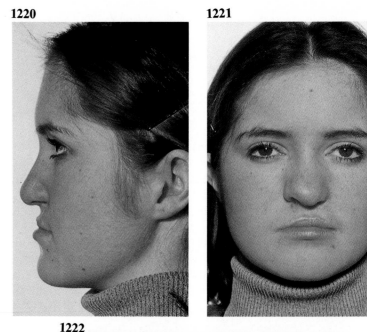

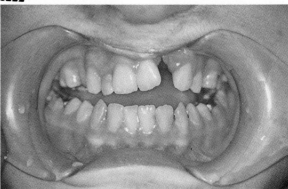

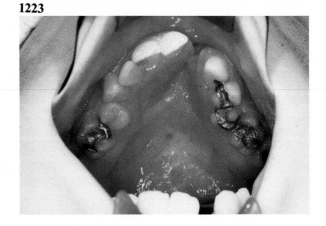

1220 to 1232   **Le Fort 2 osteotomy (1224 to 1226) before** fistula closure (**1227** to **1230**) and bridgework (**1231** and **1232**). (Bridgework by G. Kantorowicz Esq.)

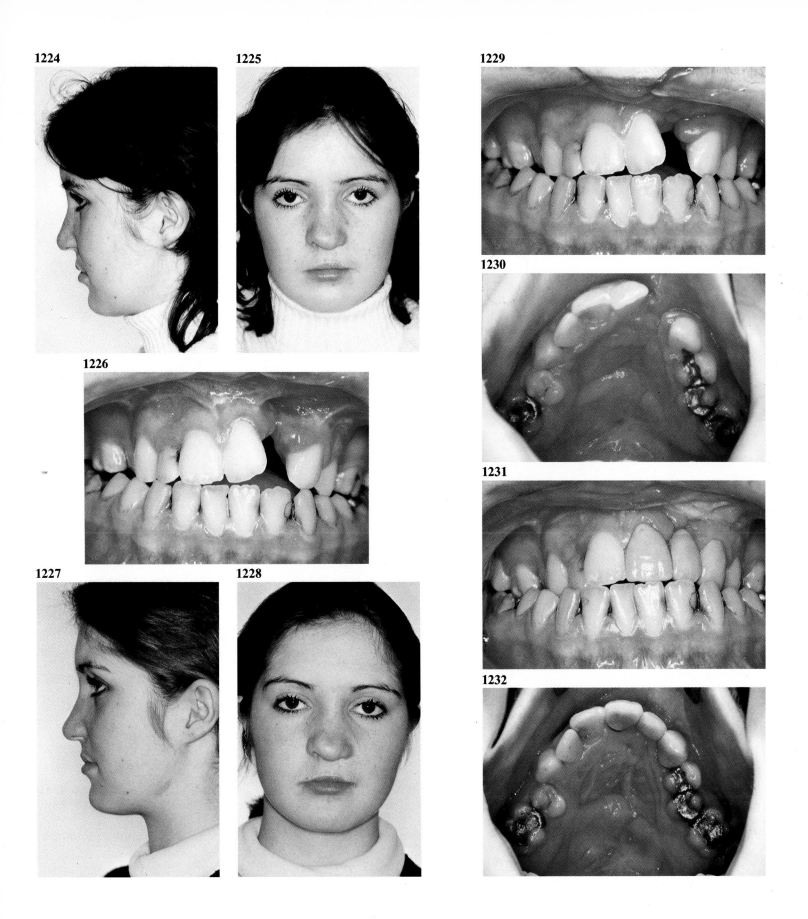

Technical difficulties and modifications

The approach to Le Fort 1 and 2 osteotomies in cleft cases should not be dissimilar to the routine non-cleft patient. There is always greater difficulty in mobilising the maxilla because of the effect of scarring from previous surgery and the shortage of soft-tissues; for the same reasons the tendency to postoperative relapse is greater. Great care (and sometimes effort) is required to make sure that *adequate mobilisation* is achieved at operation.

If there is resistance the tissues behind the maxilla should be separated from the posterior edge of the hard palate, which is much easier if the downfracture method is being employed. The finger should be passed round the posterior maxilla to determine the sites of tethering, and scars incised. If a pharyngo-

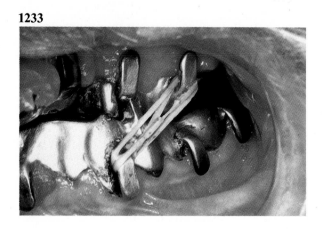

1233   Postoperative elastic traction.

plasty is holding things up it should be divided, regardless of the inevitable need for it to be repeated later. Bone grafting is essential. The maxilla may be overcorrected and fixation should be long (2½ to 3 months). Postoperative elastic traction should be employed; initially the splints may be left on for this (**1233**).

The modified technique of Converse and Shapiro (1952) and Wake (1976) is applicable to both Le Fort 1 and Le Fort 2 osteotomies. The buccal cuts are completed under muco-periosteal tunnels, and provided the vestibular pedicles are intact at this stage, the Veau flaps are fully reflected. The palate is cut transversely as shown (**1234**), and the maxilla is separated from the pterygoid plates from the palatal side under direct vision. The posterior hard palate is thus left in its original position and so the restraining soft-tissues attached posteriorly to the palate are not stretched, making mobilisation easier and with less danger of speech compromise (**1235**). Bone grafting is completed (A in **1236**) and the cleft (B in **1236**) can be closed.

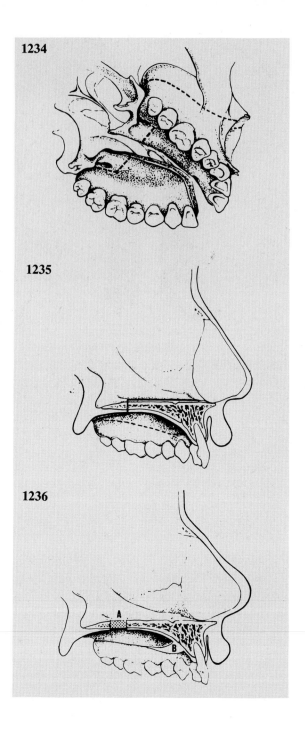

1234 to 1236   Modified technique of Converse and Shapiro (1952) and Wake (1976). (Reproduced by kind permission of Michael Wake Esq, FDS.)

There is a danger of a small oronasal fistula remaining anteriorly with this method, and it is time consuming. If the contour of the maxilla is very irregular, cutting the lateral osteotomies under tunnels can also be difficult. The patient should be prepared for maxillary advancement only, if technical problems are encountered at operation, the fistula then being closed at a separate operation later. This method combined with Le Fort 2 osteotomy where applicable is the best method of simultaneous closure and osteotomy (see **1215**).

The management of facial asymmetry

The treatment of facial asymmetry presents many special problems.

Complex three-dimensional distortions of the facial skeleton are very difficult to restore to symmetry, and the interaction of associated soft-tissue anomalies together with the effects of continuing growth during childhood and adolescence all combine to complicate both the assessment and treatment of superficially similar cases. Reference should be made to preceding sections for necessary preliminary material to this discussion:

Section 1, pp. 16 to 22 – aetiology and pathogenesis.

Section 2, pp. 71 to 75 – assessment of facial symmetry.

Section 3, pp. 121 to 138 – clinical presentation.

To some extent treatment of the congenital asymmetries will depend on the surgeon's views of the aetiology, still controversial for a number of conditions.

Basic considerations

1. *Control of growth processes.* In individual cases, especially those presenting during the growing period, there is sometimes a possibility of affecting the growth to allow more balanced facial development. This may be done by:

(a) Inhibition of potentially excessive growth. An example of this is seen in slowing down condylar growth by high condylectomy or condylar shave as a treatment of unilateral condylar hyperplasia (see Section 1, **36** to **39**; also **1244** to **1248**).

(b) Stimulation of potentially deficient growth. This may be seen in the early and active mobilisation of an ankylosed temporomandibular articulation in order to stimulate mandibular growth in response to restored function.

It may be argued that these two treatment methods are incompatible with the same view of condylar growth and function; that the condyle is a primary growth centre for the mandible, or that it maintains compensatory temporomandibular spacing in response to mandibular growth by functional demand. The two clinical situations described represent ab-normal growth responses, and there can be no certainty in our present state of understanding about the factors operating. On the one hand it is necessary to take a somewhat pragmatic view of these debates, and on the other to avoid unjustified rationalisation of the techniques used.

2. *Correction of spatial asymmetry.* With proper case assessment the site and nature of spatial abnormality, both hard and soft-tissue, should be ascertained. To correct these asymmetries may prove to be technically very difficult indeed, partly because of the infinitely varied gradations of anatomical change from one part of the face to another in all three dimensions; partly because of the pressures of deficient soft-tissues or the unbalanced effects of soft-tissue functions.

Fortunately, most facial asymmetries are simple abnormalities of mandibular morphology, easily corrected by intelligent application of standard osteotomy techniques applied unequally on the two sides of the face. Examples are shown (**958** to **964** and **1249** to **1263**).

Stages of Assessment

1. Determine the influence of deviant mandibular closure patterns (see Section 2, **229** to **236**).

2. Determine (by clinical and radiographic examination) the exact site(s) of abnormality, both primary and secondary, and attempt to relate the case to one of the recognised clinical conditions (described in Section 3, **424** to **512**). Assess the likelihood of an acquired or congenital aetiology. Full use will need to be made of full face analysis, PA and orthopantomographic radiology, and model study. Specifically, the condylar head (presence or absence, size and shape), condylar necks, mandibular rami and bodies should be compared for right/left morphological differences. The muscular processes should be assessed as indicators of muscle activity, and the soft-tissues examined at rest and in function.

The transverse planes of the face, especially the occlusal plane, should be assessed for transverse tilting. The occlusion should be examined to determine the presence of crossbites or lateral open bites. Where the occlusal plane is tilted transversely, a decision should be made as to whether this is due to vertical maxillary excess on one side or deficiency on the other, as this has an important bearing on treatment. Any other maxillary compensations should be noted, and asymmetry of the orbits, malar, temporal or frontal bones evaluated.

A logical correction can then be planned. All primary defects or deficiencies should be reconstructed prior to spatial reconstruction, and all secondary anomalies corrected, although there are exceptions to this (*vide infra*).

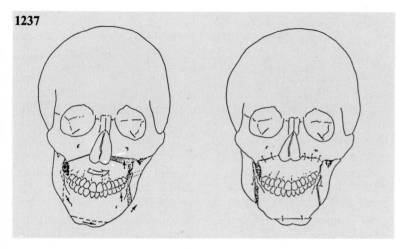

1237　Unilateral maxillary shortening.

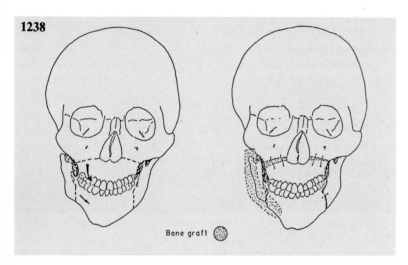

1238　Unilateral maxillary lengthening: Obwegeser method.

Bone graft ⊙

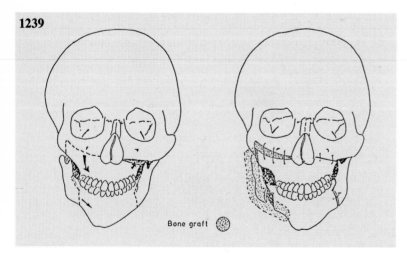

Bone graft ⊙

1239 to 1243　Unilateral maxillary lengthening (after Brami *et al*).

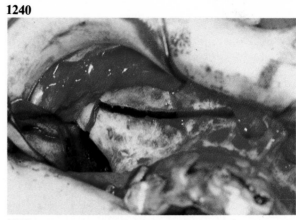

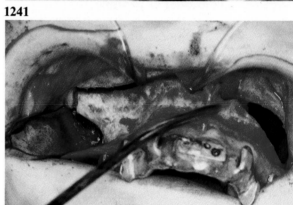

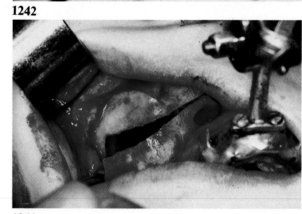

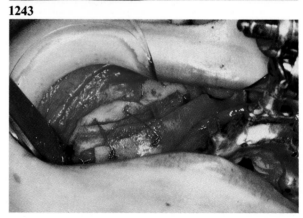

The place of maxillary osteotomy in the correction of asymmetry usually involves either lengthening one side of the maxilla or shortening the other with simultaneous adjustment of the mandible. The maxillary distortions are usually secondary to primary asymmetry in the mandible, but if they are to be corrected then maxillary correction must take place before the mandible can be brought into position, albeit at the same operation.

There are two basic approaches: (a) Unilateral maxillary shortening, or superior repositioning, is a simple extension of total maxillary shortening, a planned section being taken out of the elongated side and the maxilla rotated up into position (**1237**). Midline correction can be undertaken by left/right rotation at the same time. (b) Unilateral maxillary lengthening, or inferior repositioning, is more complex. The method of Obwegeser (1971) (**1238**), is by simple downward rotation following standard Le Fort 1 cuts, with interpositional bone grafting on the elongated side. This is, in the author's experience, likely to relapse.

The method of Brami *et al* (1974) is followed (**1239**), with the cut on the short side being made into the zygomatic buttress, and carried below the infraorbital nerve into the pyriform aperture of the nose (**1240**). If the problem of occlusal slope is severe, regardless of the site of abnormality, correction should be distributed between the long and short sides (**1241**), thus stabilising the result after rotation (**1242**) by filling the gap on the lengthened side with an interpositional bone graft (**1243**). This works well and remains stable.

In summary therefore maxillary surgery is indicated:

(1) To correct transverse tilting of the maxillary occlusal plane.

(2) To centralise the maxillary midline.

(3) To correct unilateral maxillary collapse, in any plane.

Where the occlusal plane is tilted down secondary to unilateral mandibular or condylar hyperplasia, maxillary correction is not strictly necessary. Simple condylectomy will be followed in due course by spontaneous correction of the occlusal plane under the influence of the muscles of mastication. Correction may be undertaken to hasten the final result or to make easier a pan-facial correction. Sometimes simple posterior maxillary ostectomy will suffice to correct simple compensatory maxillary alveolar hyperplasia on one side. Provided the mandible is corrected at the same time, the result is stable. An acrylic wafer may be made as an intermediate guide during surgery.

Unilateral condylar hyperplasia presents in the mid-teens and the recommended treatment is to arrest or retard condylar growth on the affected side when it is estimated that the mandible has attained adult size on that side. Inevitably this is a somewhat subjective and uncertain estimation. Hovell (1963)

1244

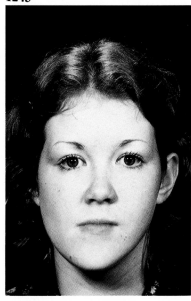

1245

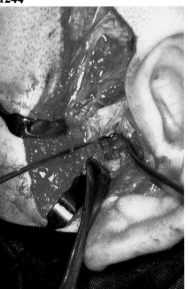

1246

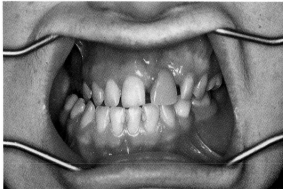

1247

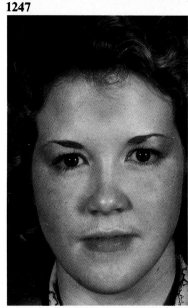

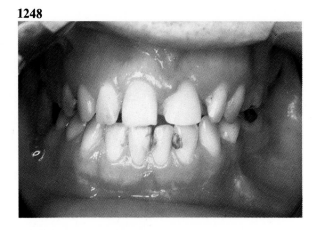

1248

1244 to 1248 Correction of unilateral condylar hyperplasia (1245 and 1246) by high condylar shave (1247 and 1248, 2 years after operation).

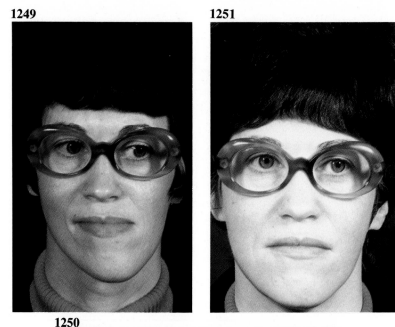

1249 **1251**

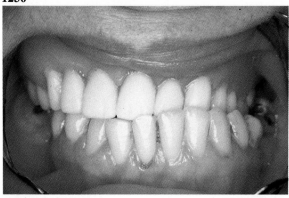

1250

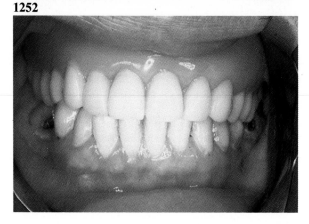

1252

1249 to 1252 Correction of fully developed unilateral condylar hyperplasia by unilateral body ostectomy and a new upper denture.

recommended condylectomy, but the high condylar shave (Henny and Baldridge, 1957) is the treatment of choice. In this procedure the condyle is exposed, usually around 15 years of age, by the method outlined in Section 4 (**569** to **576**). At the stage shown in **575** the articular surface of the condyle is cut away with a bur to a depth of about 2 mm. This is shown in **1244,** with the mandible distracted downwards, thus exaggerating the appearance of the excision, but bringing the cut condylar surface into view.

The case shown in **1245** and **1246** at 14 years of age is seen again in **1247** and **1248** 2 years later. The compensatory effect of inhibiting the abnormal condylar growth on the left side by high condylar shave is clearly seen.

In the fully developed condition (unilateral condylar hyperplasia) spatial correction is required. In the simpler type of case, where maxillary occlusal sloping is not important, an ostectomy of the mandibular body on one side may suffice, as in the case shown in **1249** and **1250** where the upper dentition is replaced by a prosthesis. After unilateral body ostectomy on the right side, and a new denture, the symmetry of the face is restored (**1251** and **1252**).

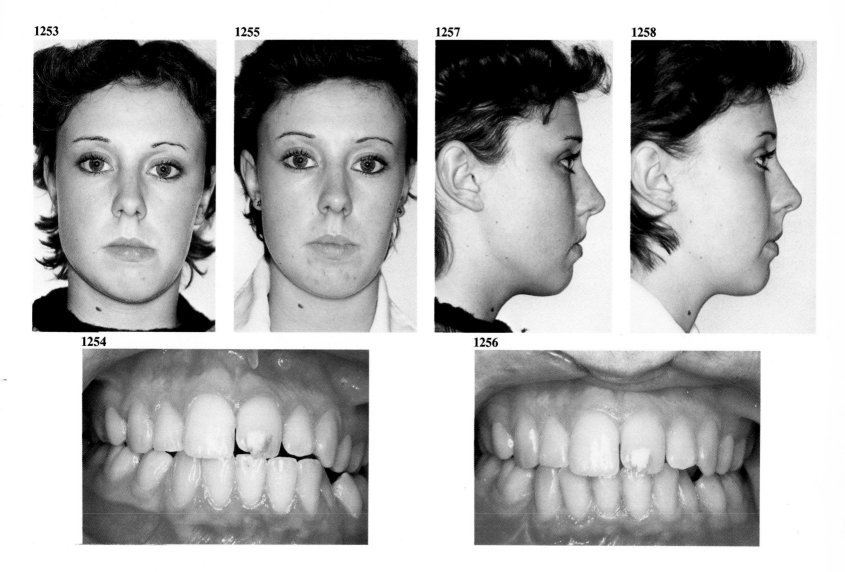

1253

1255

1257

1258

1254

1256

In the fully dentate case (**1253** and **1254**) it is also sometimes possible to achieve full correction by this method, here by extraction of 4| and body ostectomy (**1255** and **1256**). The effect on profile is minimal (**1257** and **1258**). However, it is often necessary in these cases to undertake a relieving osteotomy (usually a sagittal split) on the contralateral side to enable the occlusion to be corrected. Note, however, a common problem in the postoperative result of both these cases (**1251** and **1255**).

There is a flattening of the contralateral aspect of the lower-face in the canine/premolar region which is not corrected by centralisation of the jaw. This can be corrected at the time of surgery by a proplast implant (**1259**) applied to the flat area via an intraoral incision. The result of correction by right sided sagittal split plus left sided proplast onlay with a relieving left sided osteotomy is seen in the case shown in **1260** and **1261** (preoperatively) and **1262** and **1263**, 3 months after correction.

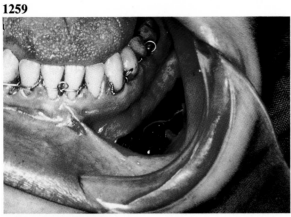

1259

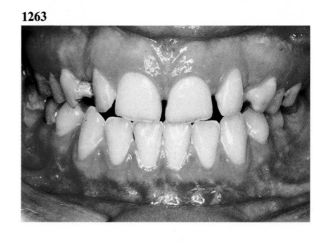

1263

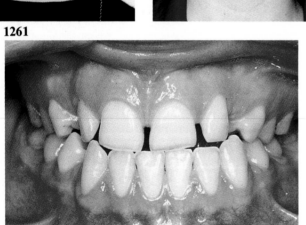

1260

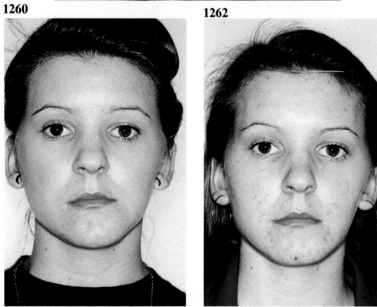

1262

1253 to 1258 Correction of unilateral condylar hyperplasia by body ostectomy and extraction of 4 .

1259 to 1263 Correction of unilateral condylar hyperplasia by right sided sagittal split plus left sided proplast onlay with a relieving left sided osteotomy (**1262** and **1263**, patient 3 months after correction).

1261

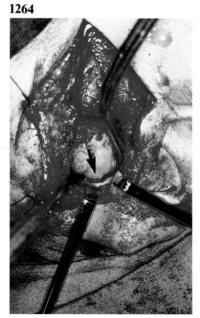

1264

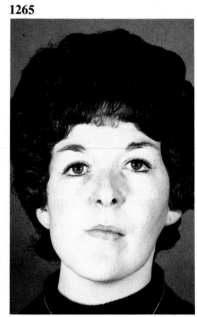

1265

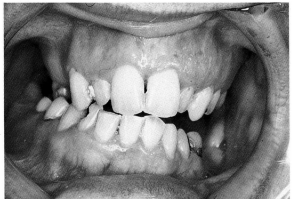

1266

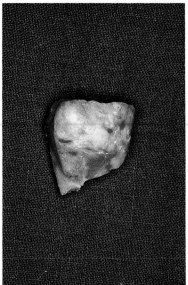

1267

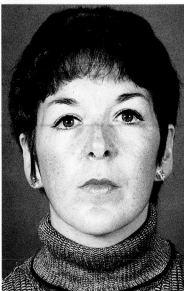

1268

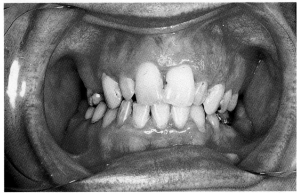

1269

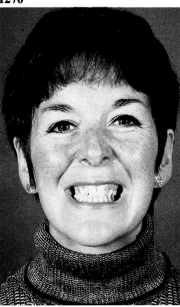

1270

1264 Condylectomy: exposure of the condyle.

1265 to 1270 Osteochondroma (**1265** and **1266**) treated by condylectomy.

Condylectomy is indicated in osteochondroma of the condylar head and in enlargement of the condyle in hemihypertrophy of the mandible. It is also necessary in the correction of bony ankylosis, but in this condition large areas of bone below and medial to the condyle usually require excision and the problem is of a different kind. The condyle is exposed as previously described, and the pathology demonstrated (**1264**). (The case of osteochondroma previously illustrated in **463** to **465** and reproduced here in **1265** and **1266**. The cut across the condylar neck has already been made in **1264** (arrowed), and the enlarged condyle is excised (**1267**). Postoperatively in this type of case a dramatic improvement occurs (**1268** and **1269**) because at the later age of presentation there is little or no secondary maxillary tilting. If the technique of approach is followed as described, no facial nerve weakness should be encountered postoperatively (**1270**).

In **hemihypertrophy of the mandible** condylectomy may be performed, as the condyle is usually enlarged (**437** to **443**). This must usually be combined with reduction of the lower border, but as the inferior alveolar neurovascular bundle is usually displaced to the lower border itself, the nerve must be delivered from the mandible after the buccal plate has been removed and before the lingual plate is reduced (**1271**).

The case shown here (**1272** to **1276**) has had these two procedures alone, refusing sagittal correction which was indicated by profile examination (**1277** and **1278**). Nevertheless, reasonable symmetry has been restored. The occlusion remained unaltered, there being posterior molar contact prior to operation (**1274**). Other procedures which may be indicated are contralateral ramus division, and ipsilateral posterior maxillary ostectomy or asymmetrical superior repositioning of the whole maxilla (**1271**).

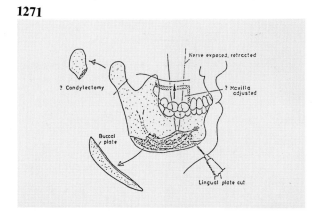

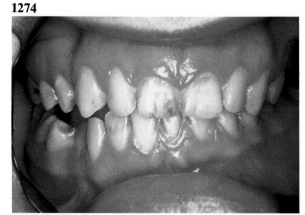

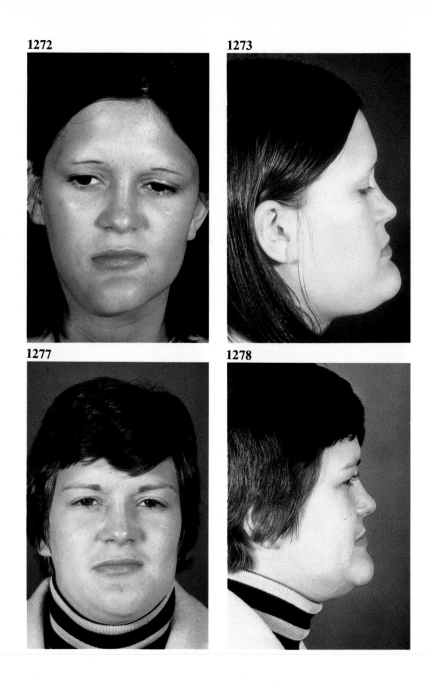

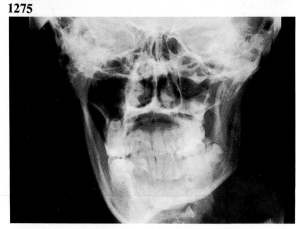

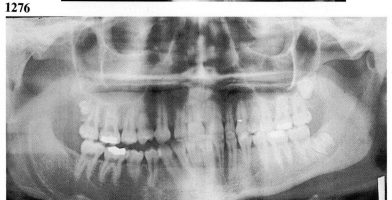

1271 to 1278   Reduction of mandibular hemihypertrophy.

A compensatory genioplasty with a slide to the flatter side is often necessary when a condition has been present for a long time and secondary genial compensation has occurred. In this case (**1279**) an osteochondroma of the left condyle in an older patient has been treated by condylectomy and a centralising sliding genioplasty (**1280**).

Full correction therefore often requires bimaxillary surgery which in turn requires careful three-dimensional planning on full skeletal models (**1281** and **1282**). This case, shown clinically (**1283**, **1285** and **1287**) required maxillary advancement with left/right correction, and asymmetrical mandibular setback, the relative amount on the two sides being determined

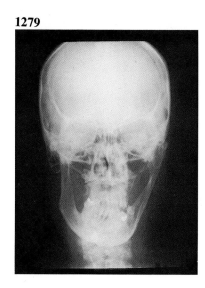

1279

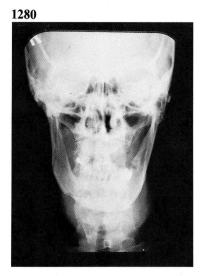

1280

1279 and 1280 **Osteochondroma of the left condyle** in an older patient (**1279**) treated by condylectomy and a centralising sliding genioplasty (**1280**).

on the models. The results are shown (**1284, 1286** and **1288**). In profile, as the tracing shows (**1289**), there is much less change than in anteroposterior deformity cases.

1281 and 1282 **Skeletal models** for three-dimensional planning of bimaxillary surgery.

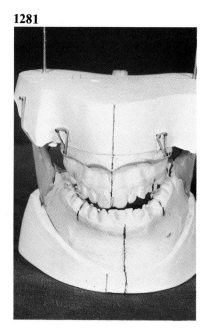

1281

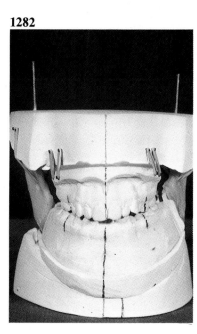

1282

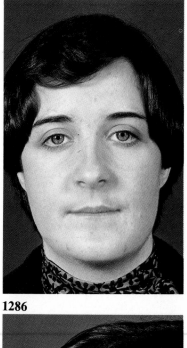

1283

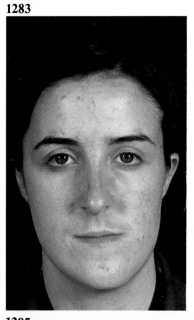

1284

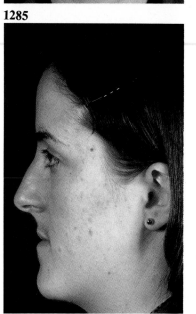

1285

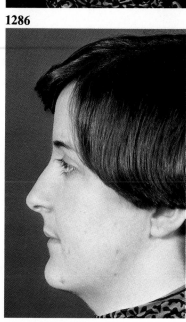

1286

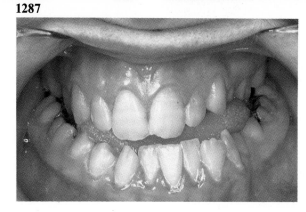

1287

319

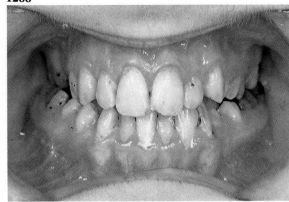

1288

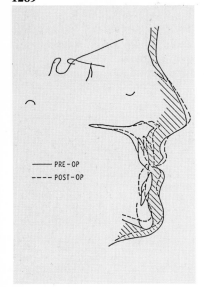

1289

— PRE-OP
---- POST-OP

1283 to 1289   Correction of facial asymmetry by maxillary advancement with left/right correction, and asymmetrical mandibular set-back.

Congenital unilateral mandibular hypoplasia

This, in all its forms, presents the most difficult group of asymmetries for treatment. There are those who maintain that all treatment of the hemifacial microsomic patient should be deferred until growth is complete, the argument being that the shortage of investing soft-tissues will inevitably cause relapse during the growing stages. Others have maintained that enlargement of the deficient mandibular ramus during growth (usually by serial bone grafting across the ramus) will help to stimulate whatever soft-tissue potential for growth is present.

In the former camp are Hovell (1962) and Obwegeser (1974). Longacre *et al* (1961), and Stark and Saunders (1962) argue for earlier intervention. Towers (1976) takes the balanced view that the result of such earlier interference will depend on the degree of abnormality present in the individual (see Section 2, p. 46). He considers that where there are positive indicators of activity in the masticatory muscles on the affected side, this favours early intervention; and that their absence argues for non-interference until growth is complete. Such indicators are 'the presence of a condyle, however rudimentary,

a reasonably sized coronoid process, a masseteric process at the angle of the mandible and a degree of antegonial notching, however slight . . .' (Towers, 1976).

The author agrees with this view, but finds that the majority of cases coming under surveillence do not have these favourable prognostic signs thus balancing the decision in favour of conservative early management and late radical correction. The principles governing the management of hemifacial microsomia apply also to other unilateral mandibular hypoplasias of congenital origin, but the prognostic signs are usually much more favourable. According to Hovell (1960) this suggests localised disturbance at one or both condylar growth centres, an assumption which can probably be justified no longer. Nevertheless the practical deduction is demonstrably true, and early surgical interference by ramus augmentation is of permanent benefit.

A further factor has entered the picture during the last decade. With the development of microvascular surgery has come the possibility of introducing soft-tissue flaps by vascular anastomosis, thus increasing soft-tissue volume in deficient areas, if not actually introducing functional elements. It is still too early to assess the effect of free flap augmentation during the growing period, although throughout the world many cases are now under observation following this kind of intervention. The preliminary reports appear promising.

Ramus augmentation during the growing period is usually undertaken by serial bone grafting or by sagittal splitting (**1290**). The ages of 8, 12, and 16 where the condition is severe, or 10 and 15 if less severe are recommended. Hovell (1960) indicates the advantages of this timing which allows for sufficient bone at the donor sites (rib or hip). The size of the graft is determined on a mandibular model, and an acrylic overlay is made for the upper teeth to maintain the lateral open bite developed by the elongation of the ramus at operation. This is maintained during fixation. After the splints are removed an additional bite-raising appliance is made and fitted.

The approach is via a submandibular incision extended posteriorly and all muscular attachments are fully separated from the distal segments of bone. Horizontal ramisection above the lingula (or by removal of the outer plate and displacement of the neurovascular bundle) is carried out, the acrylic overlay is fitted to the teeth, and bone inserted in the gap which is developed in the ramus. In the very young a rib is used, but in the adolescent hip is better. IMF is advisable and maintained for 10 weeks (Hovell). After removal of fixation the acrylic bite-raising appliance is fitted immediately, and over the ensuing 3 months all occlusal contact is relieved from the splint over the most distal maxillary tooth, thus controlling its eruption into occlusion with the mandibular molar.

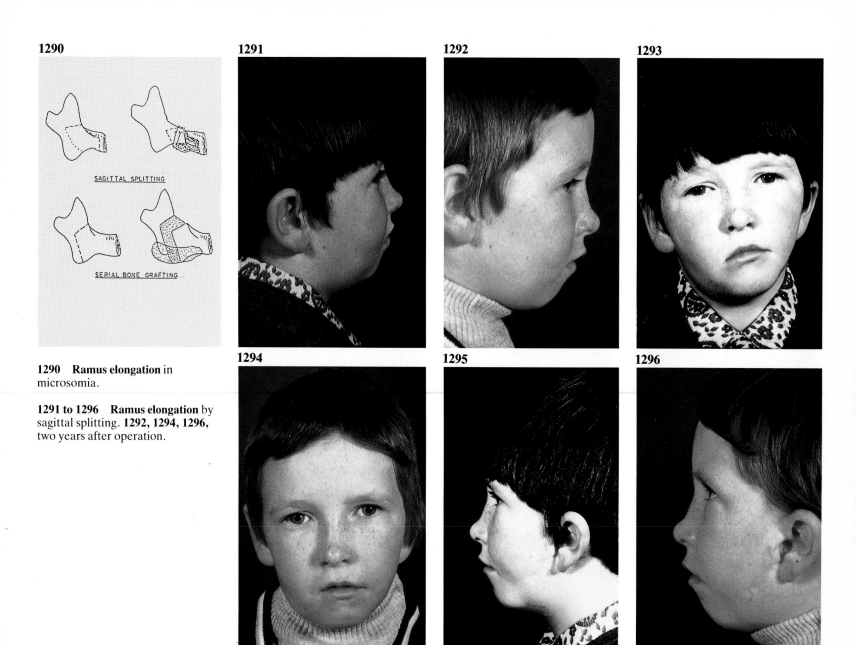

1290 Ramus elongation in microsomia.

1291 to 1296 Ramus elongation by sagittal splitting. **1292, 1294, 1296,** two years after operation.

The case shown (**1291** to **1296**) was treated by the alternative method, attributed to Rowe and mentioned by Caldwell and Gerhardt (1974) of sagittal splitting. Postoperative control is the same as for serial bone grafting, and the split tends to result in end-to-end approximation of the distal and proximal segments rather than the usual overlap associated with the technique. Provided intraoral access is adequate to carry out the procedure it seems to work well. In the case shown there is a 2 year interval between the immediately preoperative pictures (**1291, 1293** and **1295**) and the postoperative comparisons.

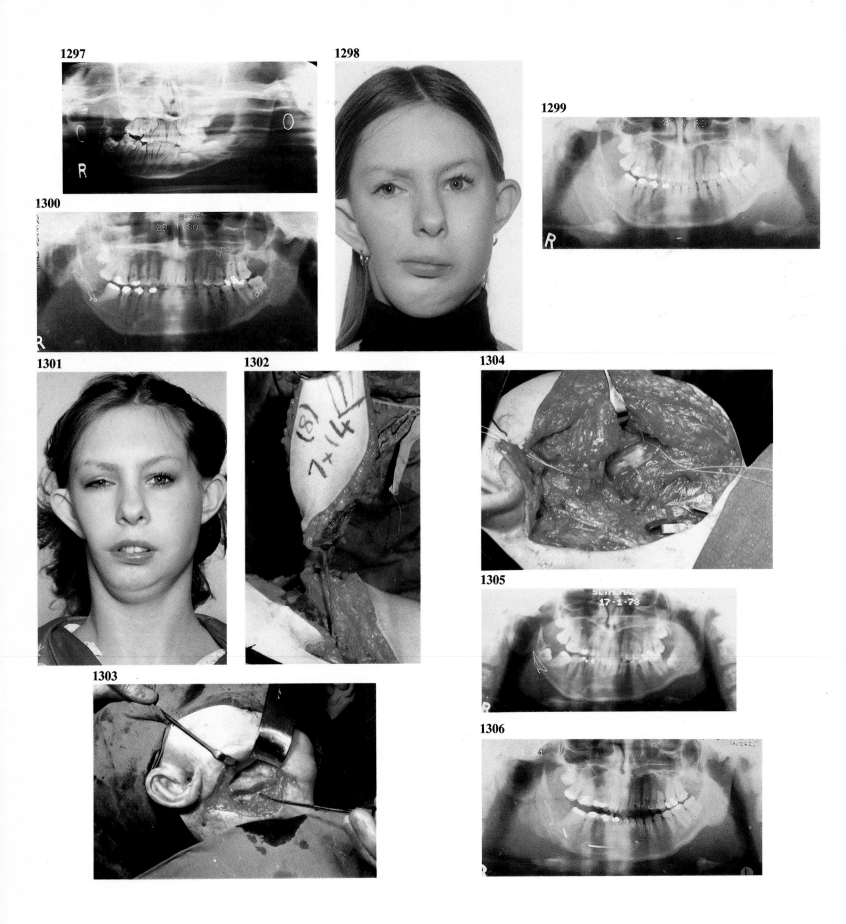

322

1307

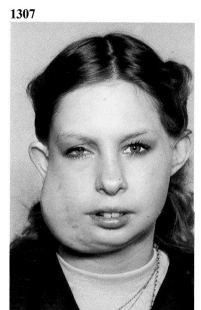

1308

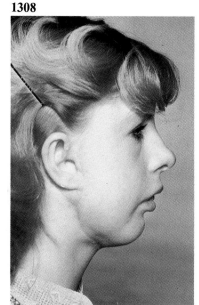

1309

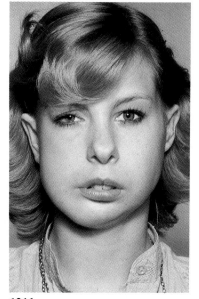

1310

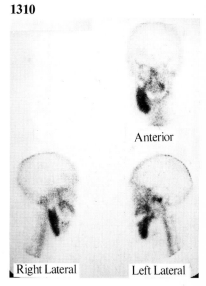

Anterior

Right Lateral   Left Lateral

An illustrative case of facial microsomia (also shown **483** to **489**) is shown in **1297** to **1312**. At the age of 6 years and 9 months a rib graft was inserted in the right mandibular ramus, but such shortage of soft-tissue was found that only a reduced amount of bone could be inserted, and the patient is shown after this at the age of 10 (**1297**) and at 14 years (**1298** and **1299**).

At the age of 16, growth being nearly complete, the maxilla was levelled by the method shown (**1239**) and an L-shaped osteotomy with iliac crest bone grafting was carried out on the right ramus, with a relieving osteotomy on the left side (**1300** and **1301**). This shows levelling of the oral commissure and some improvement in overall symmetry, but still very gross shortage of tissue bulk on the right side, inhibiting full bony correction and maintaining severe residual deformity.

At the age of 17 therefore, a free flap was transferred from the left hip (**1302**) including part of the iliac crest and overlying groin flap to augment the right side of the face (**1303** and **1304**). (Microvascular free flap surgery by Brian Mayou Esq, FRCS). This was deliberately overdone (**1305** and **1306**) and subsequently reduced until most of the skin could be eliminated, leaving substantial augmentation of the subdermal hard and soft-tissues (**1307, 1308** and **1309**). A bone scan shows the vitality of the transferred bone 2 weeks after transfer (**1310**). Finally, at 19 years of age, a premaxillary ostectomy and proplast augmentation of the left mandible was undertaken (**1311** and **1312**).

1311

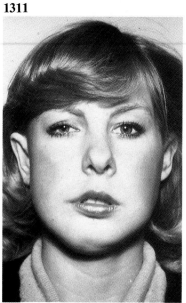

1312

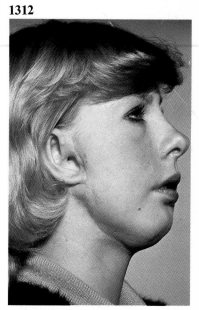

1297 to 1312   Patient with facial microsomia treated over a number of years.

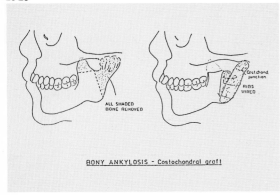

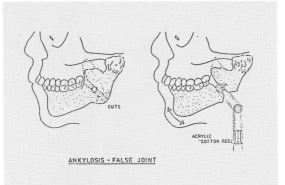

BONY ANKYLOSIS - Costochondral graft

ANKYLOSIS - FALSE JOINT

1313 and 1314   Management of temporomandibular joint ankylosis.

The management of **temporomandibular joint ankylosis** is regarded as outside the field of orthognathic surgery and a separate subject in its own right. It is not dealt with in this volume beyond indicating the place of radical excision of the bony mass in the region of the affected condyle, usually by a combination of submandibular and preauricular access incisions; and the insertion of a costochondral graft to restore the joint function (**1313**). Energetic postoperative exercise is necessary, including forcible opening under general anaesthesia at intervals over the first postoperative year.

If re-ankylosis occurs (as it frequently does) an angle operation to produce a false joint below the area of adventitious bone formation is recommended; the author uses an acrylic 'cotton-reel' wired to the proximal segment and allowing rotational and translational movement of the distal segment; this technique was originally described by McComb of Perth, Western Australia, and further experience recorded by Sethi, *et al* (**1314**).

Bimaxillary surgery

Scattered throughout this book are many examples of the need, both the planning need and the treatment need, for jaw corrections to involve both jaws frequently by bimaxillary total osteotomy. Facial dysharmony has been shown to be due either to combinations of primary abnormalities arising in different parts of the facial skeleton and its soft-tissue investment, or to primary abnormalities in one area causing secondary deformations in another. Harmonious aesthetics and satisfactory function with stability is only likely to be achieved when each contributory anatomical abnormality is corrected; otherwise compromise must result.

1315 to 1318   Bimaxillary sagittal abnormality corrected by Le Fort 2 maxillary advancement and bilateral sagittal splitting of the mandible with set-back.

1319 to 1324   Long face syndrome corrected by maxillary repositioning, mandibular set-back and genioplasty.

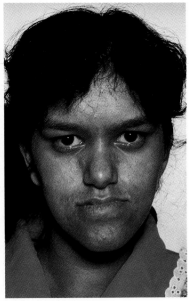
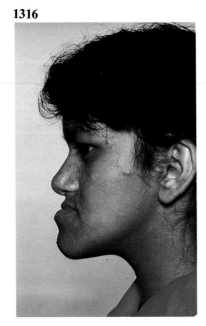
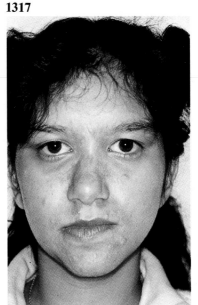
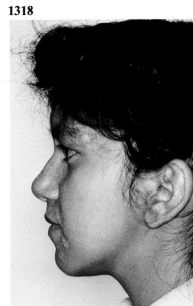

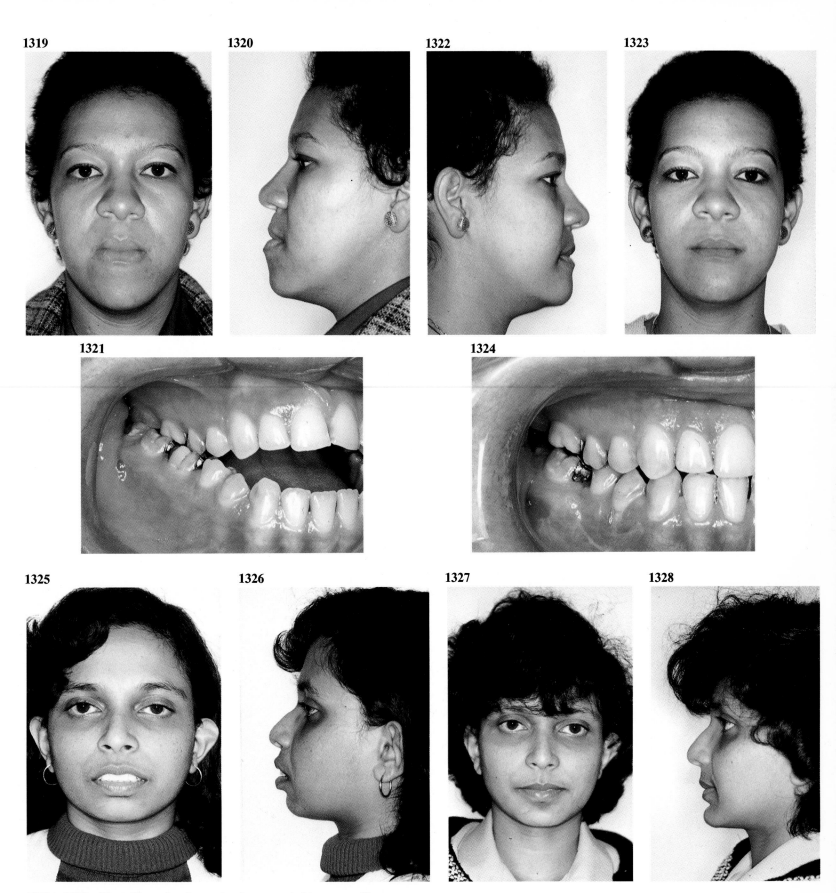

1319

1320

1322

1323

1321

1324

1325

1326

1327

1328

1325 to 1328 **Bimaxillary alveolar protrusion** corrected by premaxillary ostectomy and anterior mandibuloplasty.

325

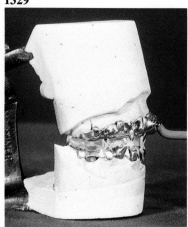
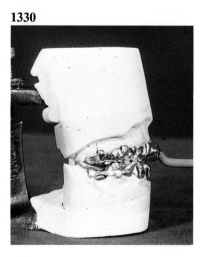

1329 to 1330 Models showing technique of bimaxillary surgery.

It is desirable to achieve as much as possible at one main operation. The advantages of simultaneous bimaxillary surgery are evident:

(a) The patient undergoes one major procedure with one period of intermaxillary fixation, of hospitalisation, and of anaesthesia with all the attendant discomfort and potential hazards.

(b) An awkward intermediate malocclusion is avoided.

(c) The danger of the patient refusing further surgery in an unacceptable stage of occlusal compromise is avoided.

(d) When the jaws are moved in opposite directions at the same time the balancing effect on the soft-tissues is maximised. Thus restriction of the oropharyngeal airway by backward displacement of the mandible is counteracted by enlargement of the tongue space by maxillary advancement; and postoperative soft-tissue tensions are balanced to some extent, improving postoperative stability. The only real disadvantage is the increased operating time at one sitting, although with modern anaesthetic techniques this is mainly a physical problem for the surgeon. Most procedures can be completed in 4 to 5 hours, many in much less.

Indications

In summary, bimaxillary surgery is indicated in

1. Bimaxillary sagittal abnormalities, as the case shown (**1315** and **1316**), corrected by Le Fort 2 maxillary advancement and bilateral sagittal splitting of the mandible with set-back (**1317** and **1318**).

2. Many facial asymmetries, as described earlier in this section.

3. Bimaxillary vertical growth abnormalities, often associated with anterior open bite; the illustrations **1319, 1320** and **1321** are of a typical long face syndrome corrected by maxillary repositioning, mandibular set-back, and genioplasty (**1322, 1323** and **1324**).

4. Bimaxillary alveolar protrusion (**1325** and **1326**), corrected by bimaxillary anterior jaw surgery, here by premaxillary ostectomy and anterior mandibuloplasty (**1327** and **1328**), involving the loss of 4 first premolars.

5. Cases requiring primary correction in one jaw with alteration of the occlusal plane.

The technique involves the use of an intermediate overlay or wafer representing the occlusal relationship when one jaw has been repositioned to the planned degree (**1329**). It matters little whether the mandible or the maxilla is operated on first; whichever it is can be repositioned into the wafer and fixed (by interosseous wiring or craniomaxillary fixation). The other jaw is then sectioned, the wafer removed and the jaws secured in the position of planned occlusion (**1330**). Internal suspension methods of fixation are best avoided if the planned position of each jaw is to be retained relative to the other jaw. All orthognathic surgery demands that great care be taken to actually perform the jaw movements in the operating room which were planned in the clinic, and there is great scope for individual variation in the detailed methods by which this is achieved. Upon this, and upon rational planning and meticulous surgical technique, will depend the longterm stability of the results obtained.

BIBLIOGRAPHY

Section 1: Variations and Anomalies in the Growth and Development of the Facial Tissues

Craven, A.H. (1958). A radiographic cephalometric study of Central Australian aborigines. *Angle Orthodont.*, **28**, 12–35.

David, D.J., Poswillo, D. and Simpson, D. The Craniosynostoses; Natural History, Diagnosis and Management. Springer, New York, 1982.

Davoody, P.R. and Sassouni, V. (1978). Dentofacial pattern differences between Iranians and American caucasians. *Am. J. Orthodont.*, **73**, 667–75.

Festing, M.F.W. and Wolff, G.L. (1979). Quantitative characters of potential value in studying mutagenesis. *Genetics*, **52**, s173–s179.

Fraumeni, J.F. *et al.* (1967). Wilms tumour and congenital hemihypertrophy. *Pediatrics*, **40**, 886–899.

Gasson, N. and Lavergne, J. (1977). The maxillary rotation; its relation to the cranial base and the mandibular corpus. An implant study. *Acta Odontol. Scand.*, **35**, 89–94.

Moss, M.L. and Crikelair, G.F. (1960). Progressive facial hemiatrophy following cervical sympathectomy in the rat. *Arch. Oral Biol.*, **1**, 254–258.

Moss, M.L. (1968). The primacy of functional matrices in orofacial growth. *Dent. practit. dent. Rec.*, **19**, 65–73.

Poswillo, D. (1966). Fetal posture and causal mechanisms of deformity of the palate, jaws and limbs. *J. Dent. Res.*, **45**, 584–596.

Poswillo, D. (1973). The pathogenesis of the first and second branchial arch syndrome. *Oral Surg.*, **35**, 302–328.

Poswillo, D. (1974). The pathogenesis of submucous cleft palate. *Scand. J. Plast. Reconstr. Surg.*, **8**, 34–41.

Poswillo, D. (1974). Otomandibular deformity: pathogenesis as a guide to reconstruction. *J. max-fac. Surg.*, **2**, 64–72.

Poswillo, D. (1975). The pathogenesis of the Treacher Collins syndrome (mandibulofacial dysostosis). *Brit. J. Oral Surg.*, **12**, 1–26.

Safra, M.J. and Oakley, G.P. (1975). Association between cleft lip with or without cleft palate and prenatal exposure to diazepam. *Lancet*, **ii**, 478–480.

Slone, D., Shapiro, S., Heinonen, O.P. *et al.* (1976). Maternal drug exposure and birth defects. pp. 265–277 *in*: Kelly, S. *et al.* (Ed.). *Birth Defects, Risks and Consequences.* New York, Academic Press.

Sulik, K.K., Johnson, M.C. and Ambrose, L.J. (1979). Phenytoin (dilantin) induced cleft lip and palate in A/J mice: a scanning and transmission electron microscopic study. *Anat. Rec.*, **195**, 243–255.

Warbrick, J.G. (1960). The early development of the nasal cavity and upper lip in the human embryo. *J. Anat.*, **94**, 351–362.

Section 2: Assessment and Treatment Planning of Facial Disproportion

Bell, W.H. and Dann, J.J. (1973). Correction of dentofacial deformities by surgery in the anterior part of the jaws. *Amer. J. Orthod.*, **64**, 162.

Bell, W.H., Proffit, W.R. and White, R.P. (1980). *Surgical Correction of Dentofacial Deformities.* W.B. Saunders Co., Philadelphia.

Berkovitz, B.K.B., Holland, G.R. and Moxham, B.J. (1978). *Colour Atlas and Textbook of Oral Anatomy.* Wolfe Medical, London.

Broadbent, B.H. Sr., Broadbent, B.H. Jr. and Golden, W.H. (1975). *Bolton Standards of Dentofacial Developmental Growth.* C.V. Mosby, Co., St. Louis.

Dann, J.J., Fonseca, R.J. and Bell, W.H. (1976). Soft-tissue changes associated with total maxillary advancement: a preliminary study. *J. Oral Surg.*, **34**, 19.

Downs, W.B. (1948). Variations in facial relationships: their significance in treatment and prognosis. *Amer. J.Orthod.*, **34**, 812.

Freihofer, H.P.M. Jr. (1976). The lip profile after correction of retromaxillism in cleft and non-cleft patients. *J. Max-fac. Surg.*, **4**, 136.

Freihofer, H.P.M. Jr. (1977). Changes in nasal profile after maxillary advancement in cleft and non-cleft patients. *J. Max-fac. Surg.*, **5**, 20.

Henderson, D. (1974). The assessment and management of bony deformities of the middle and lower-face. *Brit. J. Plast. Surg.*, **27**, 287.

Henderson, D. (1976). Photocephalometric prediction and its influence on the surgery of symmetrical facial deformity. *Hunterian Lecture.* R.C.S. England, London.

Hershey, H.G. and Smith, L.H. (1974). Soft-tissue profile change associated with surgical correction of the prognathic mandible. *Amer. J. Orthod.*, **65**, 483.

Holdaway, R.A. (1976). *The 'V.T.O.'.* University of Texas Press, Houston.

Hovell, J.H. (1961). Orthodontic considerations in the surgical correction of mandibular prognathism. *Transactions Europ. Orthodontic Soc. 1961.* pp. 205 *et seq.*

Hovell, J.H. (1965). Variations in mandibular form. *Annals RCS (Eng).*, **37**, 1.

Krogman, W.M. and Sassouni, V. (1957). *Syllabus in Roentgenographic Cephalometry.* Centre of Research in Child Growth, Philadelphia.

Lavergne, J. and Gasson, N. (1978). Influence of jaw rotation on the morphogenesis of malocclusion. *Amer. J. Orthod.*, **73**, 658.

Lines, P.A. and Steinhauser, E.W. (1974). Soft-tissue changes in relationship to movements of hard structures in orthognathic surgery – a preliminary report. *J. Oral Surg.*, **32**, 891.

Lockwood, H. (1974). A planning technique for segmental osteotomies. *Brit. J. Oral Surg.*, **12**, 102.

McEwen, J.D. and Martin, J. (1967). The rapid assessment of cephalometric radiographs. *Dent. Pract.*, **17**, 195.

McIntosh, R.B. (1970). Orthodontic surgery: comments on diagnostic modalities. *J. Oral Surg.*, **28**, 249.

Merrifield, L.L. (1966). The profile line as an aid in critically evaluating facial aesthetics. *Amer. J. Orthod.*, **52**, 804.

Moss, M.L. (1968). The primacy of functional matrices in orofacial growth. *Dent. Pract. Dent. Rec.*, **19**, 65.

Opdebeeck, H. and Bell, W.H. (1978). The short face syndrome. *Amer. J. Orthod.*, **73**, 499.

Petraitis, B.J. (1951). A cephalometric study of excellent occlusion and Class 1 malocclusion of children and adults. *MSD Thesis.* Univ. of Washington.

Plint, D.A. and Ellisdon, P.S. (1974). Facial asymmetries and mandibular displacements. *Brit. J. Orthod.*, **1**, 227.

Poswillo, D.E. (1974). Otomandibular deformity: pathogenesis as a guide to reconstruction. *J. Max-fac. Surg.*, **2**, 64.

Powell, S.J. and Rayson, R.K. (1976). The profile in facial aesthetics. *Brit. J. Orthod.*, **3**, 207.

Rakosi, T. (1981). *An Atlas and Manual of Cephalometric Radiography.* Wolfe Medical, London.

Reidel, R.A. (1957). An analysis of dentofacial relationships. *Amer. J. Orthod.*, **43**, 103.

Ricketts, R.M. (1957). Planning treatment on the basis of the facial pattern and the estimate of its growth. *Angle Orthod.*, **27**, 14.

Ricketts, R.M. (1972). The value of cephalometrics and computerised technology. *Angle Ortho.*, **42**, 179.

Robinson, S.W., Speidel, T.M., Isaacson, R.J. and Worms, F.W. (1972). Soft-tissue profile change produced by reduction of mandibular prognathism. *Angle Orthod.*, **42**, 227.

Sassouni, V. (1964). *The Face in Five Dimensions,* 2nd edition. Morgantown, W. Va. West Virginia University Press.

Steiner, C.C. (1953). Cephalometrics for you and me. *Amer. J. Orthod.*, **39**, 729.

Steinhauser, E.W. (1973). Advancement of the mandible by sagittal ramus split and suprahyoid myotomy. *J. Oral Surg.*, **31**, 516.

Tweed, C.H. (1954). The Frankfort-mandibular incisor angle (FMIA) in orthodontic diagnosis. *Angle Orthod.*, **24**, 121.

Waite, D.E. and Worms, F.W. (1974). Orthodontic and surgical evaluation and treatment of maxillomandibular deformities. Chapter in *Current Advances in Oral Surgery.* W.B. Irby (Ed.). C.V. Mosby Co., St. Louis.

Section 3: Clinical Presentation of Facial Disproportion

Beckers, H.L. (1977). Masseteric muscle hypertrophy and its intraoral surgical correction. *Jour. Max-Fac. Surg.*, **5**, 28.

Bell, W.H. (1977). Correction of the short face syndrome – vertical maxillary deficiency: a preliminary report. *J. Oral Surg.*, **35**, 110.

Bell, W.H., Creekmore, T.D. and Alexander, R.G. (1977). Surgical correction of the long face syndrome. *Amer. J. Orthod.*, **71**, 40.

Bell, W.H. and McBride, K.L. (1977). Correction of the long face syndrome by Le Fort 1 osteotomy. *Oral Surg. Oral Path. and Oral Med.*, **44**, 493.

Binder, K.M. (1962). Dysostosis maxillonasalis, ein arhinencephaler Missbilungskomplex. *Dtsch. zahnarzil. Z.*, **17**, 438.

Converse, J.M., Horowitz, S.L., Valauri, A.J. and Montandon, D. (1970). The treatment of nasomaxillary hypoplasia. A new pyramidal naso-orbital maxillary osteotomy. *Plast. and Reconstr. Surg.*, **45**, 527.

Gonzales-Ulloa, M. and Stevens, E. (1968). The role of chin correction in profileplasty. *Plast. and Reconstr. Surg.*, **41**, 477.

Goodman, R.M. and Gorlin, R.J. (1977). *Atlas of the face in genetic disorders,* 2nd edition. C.V. Mosby Co., St Louis.

327

Gorlin, R.J. and Pindborg, J.J. (1964). *Syndromes of the head and neck*. McGraw-Hill Book Co., New York.

Hall, H.D. and West, R.A. (1976). Combined anterior and posterior maxillary osteotomy. *J. Oral Surg.*, **34**, 126.

Heard, G.M.C. (1962). Nerve sheath tumours and Von Recklinghausen's disease of the nervous system. *Annls. RCS.*, **31**, 229.

Henderson, D. and Jackson, I.T. (1973). Nasomaxillary hypoplasia – the Le Fort 2 osteotomy. *Brit. J. Oral Surg.*, **11**, 77.

Henderson, D. (1980). Nasomaxillary hypoplasia. Chapter in '*Surgical correction of dentofacial deformities*'. Bell, W.H., Proffit, W.R. and White, R.P. (Eds.). W.B. Saunders Co., Philadelphia.

Küfner, J. (1971). Four year experience with major maxillary osteotomy for retrusion. *J. Oral Surg.*, **29**, 549.

Müller, H. and Slootweg, P.J. (1981). Maxillofacial deformities in neurofibromatosis. *J. Max-fac. Surg.*, **9**, 89.

Opdebeeck, H. and Bell, W.H. (1978). The short face syndrome. *Amer. J. Orthod.*, **73**, 499.

Pindborg, J.J. and Hjørting-Hansen, E. (1974). *Atlas of diseases of the jaws*. Munksgaard, Copenhagen.

Poswillo, D.E. (1973). The pathogenesis of the first and second mandibular arch syndrome. *Oral Surg. Oral Path. and Oral Med.*, **35**, 302.

Schendel, S.A., Eisenfeld, J., Bell, W.H., Epker, B.N. and Mishelevich, D.J. (1976). The long face syndrome: vertical maxillary excess. *Amer. J. Orthod.*, **70**, 398.

Tessier, P. (1979). Facial Clefts. Chapter in '*Plastic surgery in infancy and childhood*'. J.C. Mustardé (Ed.). Churchill Livingston, London.

Towers, J.F.T. (1975). The management of congenital and acquired deformity of the mandibular condyle in children. *Cartwright Prize Essay, Royal College of Surgeons England, 1970–75*.

West, R.A. and Epker, B.N. (1972). Posterior maxillary surgery: its place in the treatment of dentofacial deformities. *J. Oral Surg.*, **30**, 562.

Wolford, L.M., Walker, G., Schendel, S.A., Fish, L.C. and Epker, B.N. (1978). Mandibular deficiency syndrome. 1. Clinical delineation and therapeutic significance. *Oral Surg. Oral Path. and Oral Med.*, **45**, 329.

Section 4 – Part 1: Surgical Access to the Facial Skeleton

Al-Kayat, A. and Bramley, P. (1979). A modified preauricular approach to the temporomandibular joint and malar arch. *Brit. J. Oral Surg.*, **17**, 91.

Axhausen, G. (1931). De operative freilegung des Keefergelenks. *Chirurg.*, **3**, 713.

Bell, W.H. (1969). Revascularisation and bone healing after anterior maxillary osteotomy; a study using adult rhesus monkeys. *J. Oral Surg.*, **27**, 249.

Bell, W.H. (1973). Biologic basis for maxillary osteotomies. *Amer. J. Phys. Anthrop.*, **38**, 279.

Bell, W.H. (1975). Total maxillary osteotomy. In *Oral Surgery: a Step by Step Atlas of Operative techniques*. W.H. Archer (Ed.). W.B. Saunders Co., Philadelphia.

Bell, W.H., Fonseca, R.J., Kennedy, J.W. and Levy, B.M. (1975). Bone healing and revascularisation after total maxillary osteotomy. *J. Oral Surg.*, **33**, 253.

Borges, A.F. and Alexander, J.E. (1962). Relaxed skin tension lines, Z-plasties on scars, and fusiform excision of lesions. *Brit. J. Plast. Surg.*, **15**, 242.

Converse, J.M., Horowitz, S.L., Valauri, A.J. and Montandon, D. (1970). The treatment of nasomaxillary hypoplasia: a new pyramidal naso-orbital maxillary osteotomy. *Plast. Reconstruct. Surg.*, **45**, 527.

Cupar, I. (1954, 1955). Die chirurgische Behandlung der Form; und Stellungsveranderungen des Oberkiefers. *Osterr. Z. Stomatol.*, **51**, 565 (1954). *Bull. Soc. Cons. Acad. R.P.F. Jougos.*, **2**, 60 (1955).

Davidson, A.J. (1956). Endaural condylectomy. *Brit. J. Plast. Surg.*, **8**, 64.

Epker, B.N. (1969). A modified anterior maxillary osteotomy. *J. Max-fac. Surg.*, **27**, 939.

Gibson, T.G. and Kenedi, R.M. (1967). Biomechanical properties of skin. *Surg. Clin. N. Amer.*, **47**, 279.

Gibson, T. (1978). Translation of 'On the anatomy and physiology of the skin'. Professor K. Langer (Ed.), 1861. *Brit. J. Plast. Surg.*, **31**, 3.

Küfner, J. (1970). Experience with a modified procedure for correction of openbite. In *Transactions of the IIIrd International Conference of Oral Surgery*. R.V. Walker (Ed.). E & S Livingston, London.

Langer, K. (1861). See translation by Gibson, T. (1978) (above).

McGregor, I.A. (1975). *Fundamental techniques of plastic surgery, and their surgical applications*. 6th edition. Churchill Livingston, London.

Nelson, R.L., Path, M.G., Ogle, R.G., Jensen, G.D., Olsen, D.V., Sokoloski, P.M. and Meyer, M.W. (1978). Quantitation of blood flow after anterior maxillary osteotomy: investigation of three surgical approaches. *J. Oral Surg.*, **36**, 106.

Perko, M. (1972). Maxillary sinus and surgical movement of the maxilla. *Intern. J. Oral Surg.*, **1**, 177.

Risdon, F. (1934). Ankylosis of the temporomandibular joint. *J. Amer. Dent. Ass.*, **21**, 1933.

Rowe, N.L. (1972). Surgery of the temporomandibular joint. *Proc. Roy. Soc. Med.*, **65**, 383.

Schuchardt, K. (1959). Experiences with the surgical treatment of deformities of the jaws: prognathia, micrognathia, and openbite. In *Proc. 2nd Congress of Internat. Soc. Plast. Surgeons*. A.G. Wallace (Ed.). E & S Livingston, London.

Tessier, P. (1973). The conjunctival approach to the orbital floor in congenital malformation and trauma. *J. Max-fac. Surg.*, **1**, 3.

Wassmund, M. (1927). *Fracturen und Luxationen des Gesichtsschadels*. Berlin, 1927.

Wunderer, S. (1963). Erfahrungen mit der operativen Behandlung hochgradiger Prognathien. *Dtsch. Zahn-Mund-Kieferheilk.*, **39**, 451.

Section 4 – Part 2: The Techniques of Facial Bone Osteotomy

Banks, P. (1977). Pulp changes after anterior mandibular subapical osteotomy in a primate model. *J. Max-fac. Surg.*, **5**, 39.

Barton, P. and Rayne, J. (1969). The role of alveolar surgery in the treatment of malocclusion. *Brit. Dent. J.*, **126**, 11.

Barton, P. (1973). Segmental surgery, section in Symposium on the treatment of Class 2 Facial Deformity. *Brit. J. Oral Surg.*, **10**, 265.

Bell, W.H. and Condit, C.L. (1970). Surgical-orthodontic correction of alveolar bimaxillary protrusion. *J. Oral Surg.*, **28**, 578.

Bell, W.H. and Levy, B.M. (1970). Revascularisation and bone healing after anterior mandibular osteotomy. *J. Oral Surg.*, **28**, 196.

Bell, W.H. (1973). Immediate surgical repositioning of one- and two-tooth dento-osseous segments. *Intern. J. Oral Surg.*, **2**, 265.

Bell, W.H. and Kennedy, J.W. (1976). Biological basis for vertical ramus osteotomies – a study of bone healing and revascularisation in adult rhesus monkeys. *J. Oral Surg.*, **34**, 215.

Bell, W.H., Creekmore, T.D. and Alexander, R.G. (1977). Surgical correction of the long face syndrome. *Amer. J. Orthod.*, **71**, 40.

Binder, K.M. (1962). Dysostosismaxillo-nasalis, ein arhinencephaler Miß bildungskomplex. *Dtsch. zahnarzte. Z.*, **17**, 438.

Blair, V.P. (1907). Operations on the jaw bone and face. *Surg. Gynae. and Obst.*, **4**, 67.

Booth, D.F., Dietz, V. and Gianelly, A.A. (1976). Correction of Class 2 malocclusion by combined sagittal ramus and subapical body osteotomy. *J. Oral Surg.*, **34**, 630.

Bradley, P.F. and Kincaid, L.C. (1974). The use of the rhesus monkey in research into alveolar surgery. *Brit. J. Oral Surg.*, **12**, 70.

Caldwell, J.B., Hayward, J.R. and Lister, R.L. (1968). Correction of mandibular retrognathia by vertical L-osteotomy: a new technique. *J. Oral Surg.*, **26**, 259.

Converse, J.M. and Shapiro, H.H. (1952). Treatment of developmental malformations of the jaws. *Plast. Reconstr. Surg.*, **10**, 473.

Converse, J.M. and Telsey, D. (1971). Tripartite osteotomy of the mid-face for orbital expansion and correction of the deformity in craniostenosis. *Brit. J. Plast. Surg.*, **24**, 365.

Cunningham, G. (1894). Methode sofortiger Regulierung von anomalen Zahn-Stellungen. *Oester-Ung Vjschr. Zahnheilk.*, **10**, 455.

Cupar, I. (1954). Die chirurgische Behandlung der Form-und Stellurgsveranderungen des Oberkeifers. *Ost. Z. Stomat.*, **51**, 565.

Dal Pont, G. (1961). Retromolar osteotomy for the correction of prognathism. *J. Oral Surg., anaesth., and Hosp. Dent. Serv.*, **19**, 42.

Dingman, R.O. (1944). Osteotomy for correction of mandibular malrelation of developmental origin. *J. Oral Surg.*, **2**, 239.

Epker, B.N. (1977). Modifications in the sagittal osteotomy of the mandible. *J. Oral Surg.*, **35**, 157.

Ernst, F. (1927). Progenie, *in* Kirschner, M. and Nordmann, O. *Die Chirurgie*, Vol. 4, Part 1 page 802. Berlin. Urban and Schwarzenberg.

Fitzpatrick, B.N. (1974). Alveolar osteotomy – splint design. *Brit. J. Oral Surg.*, **11**, 266.

Fitzpatrick, B.N. (1977). Total osteotomy of the mandibular alveolus in reconstruction of the occlusion. *Oral Surg.*, **44**, 336.

Flint, M. (1964). Chip bone grafting of the mandible. *Brit. J. Plast. Surg.*, **17**, 184.

Foster, M.E. and Henderson, D. (1981). Anterior mandibuloplasty. *Brit. J. Oral Surg.*, **19**, 258.

Ginestet, G. (1939). Traitement chirurgical du mordex apertuf du prognathisme. *Rev. Stomatol (Paris).*, **41**, 4.

Gray, J.C. and Elves, M.W. (1979). Early osteogenesis in compact bone isografts: a quantitative study of the contribution of the different graft cells. *Calcified Tissue Intern.*, **29**, 225.

Gray, J.C. and Elves, M.W. (1981). Osteogenesis in bone grafts after short-term storage and topical antibiotic treatment: an experimental study in rats. *J. Bone & Joint Surg.*, **63**, 441.

Hall, H.D. and West, R.A. (1976). Combined anterior and posterior maxillary osteotomy. *J. Oral Surg.*, **34**, 126.

Henderson, D. and Jackson, I.T. (1973). Nasomaxillary hypoplasia – the Le Fort 2 osteotomy. *Brit. J. Oral Surg.*, **11**, 77.

Henderson, D. (1980). Nasomaxillary hypoplasia, *in* Bell, W.H., Proffit, W.R. and White, R.P. *Surgical Correction of Dentofacial Deformities*. Philadelphia. W.B. Saunders Co.

Hicks, K.A. and Bradley, J. (1974). A method of fixation following the vertical midline split during the anterior maxillary osteotomy. *Brit. J. Oral Surg.*, **11**, 265.

Hunsuck, E.E. (1968). A modified intraoral sagittal splitting technique for correction of mandibular prognathism. *J. Oral Surg.*, **26**, 249.

Kent, J.N., Homsey, C.A.and Hinds, E.C. (1975). Proplast in dental facial reconstruction. *Oral Surg. Oral Medicine. Oral Path.*, **39**, 347.

Köle, H. (1959). Surgical operations on the alveolar ridge to correct occlusal abnormalities. *Oral Surg.*, **12**, 277, 413, 515.

Kostechka, F. (1931). Analyse critique de la therapeutique chirurgicale des anomalies d'occlusion. *8th Congress Dentaire Internat. Sect XII*, **235**, 241.

Küfner, J. (1971). Four year experience with major maxillary osteotomy for retrusion. *J. Oral Surg.*, **29**, 549.

Le Fort, Réné (1900). Fractures de la machoire superieure. *Cong. Intern. Med. (Paris) Sect. Chir. Gen.*, **275**.

Lockwood, H. (1974). A planning technique for segmental osteotomies. *Brit. J. Oral Surg.*, **12**, 102.

Marx, R.E., Kline, S.N., Johnson, P., Malinin, T.I., Mathews, J.G. and Gambill, V. (1981). The use of freeze dried allogenic bone in oral and maxillofacial surgery. *J. Max-fac. Surg.*, **39**, 264.

McIntosh, R.B. and Carlotti, A.E. (1975). Total mandibular alveolar osteotomy in the management of skeletal (infantile) apertognathia. *J. Oral Surg.*, **33**, 921.

Mehnert, H. (1973). Die interalveolare Osteotomie im Oberkiefer. *Dtsch. Zahn Mund Kieferheilkd.*, **61**, 289.

Merrill, R.G. and Pedersen, F.W. (1976). Interdental osteotomy for immediate repositioning of dental-osseous elements. *J. Oral Surg.*, **34**, 118.

Obwegeser, H.L. (1964). Indications for surgical correction of mandibular deformity by sagittal splitting technique. *Brit. J. Oral Surg.*, **1**, 157.

Obwegeser, H.L. (1969). Surgical correction of small or retrodisplaced maxillae. The 'dish-face' deformity. *Plast. and Reconstr. Surg.*, **43**, 351.

Obwegeser, H.L. (1971). Deformities of the jaws, *in* Mustarde, J.C. *Plastic Surgery in Infancy and Childhood*. Edin. and Lond., E & S Livingstone.

Peterson, L.J. (1978). Posterior mandibular segmental alveolar osteotomy. *J. Oral Surg.*, **36**, 454.

Poswillo, D.E. (1972). Early pulp changes following reduction of anterior openbite by segmental surgery. *Intern. J. Oral Surgery.*, **1**, 87.

Rayson, R.K., Houston, W.J.B. and Howe, G.L. (1975). A surgical approach to the treatment of permanent incisor teeth in infraocclusion: two case reports. *Brit. J. Orthod.*, **1**, 237.

Robinson, P.P. (1980). Reinnervation of teeth following segmental osteotomy in the cat. *J. Dent. Res. Special issue DI*, 1341.

Robinson, P.P. (1981). Reinnervation of teeth, mucous membranes and skin following section of the inferior alveolar nerve in the cat. *Brain Research.*, **220**, 241.

Rowe, N.L. (1960). The aetiology, clinical features, and treatment of mandibular deformities. *Brit. Dent. J.*, **108**, 45.

Sailer, H.F. (1976). Experiences with the use of lyophilized bank cartilage for facial contour correction. *J. Max-fac. Surg.*, **4**, 149.

Sailer, H.F. (1980). Reconstruction of the mandible by means of a similar allogenic lyophilized mandibular segment. *J. Max-fac. Surg.*, **8**, 303.

Schuchardt, K. (1959). Experiences with the surgical treatment of deformities of the jaws; prognathia, micrognathia, and openbite. In Wallace, A.B. (Ed.). *International Society of Plastic Surgeons, 2nd Congress*. London, E & S Livingstone.

Skaloud, F. (1951). New surgical method for correction of prognathism of the mandible. *Oral Surg.*, **4**, 689.

Sowray, J.H. and Haskell, R. (1968). Ostectomy at the mandibular symphysis. *Brit. J. Oral Surg.*, **6**, 97.

Steinhauser, E.W. (1972). Midline splitting of the maxilla for correction of malocclusion. *J. Oral Surg.*, **30**, 413.

Steinhauser, E.W. (1980). Variations of the Le Fort 2 osteotomies for the correction of mid-facial deformities. *J. Max-fac. Surg.*, **8**, 257.

Tessier, P. (1971). The definitive plastic surgical treatment of the severe facial deformities of craniofacial dysostosis, Crouzon's and Apert's diseases. *Plast. Reconstr. Surg.*, **48**, 419.

Tessier, P. (1978). Recent improvements in treatment of facial and cranial deformities of Crouzon's disease and Apert's syndrome. Chapter in Tessier, P., Callahan, A., Mustarde, J.C. and Salyer, K.E. *Symposium of plastic surgery in the orbital region*. Mosby.

Trauner, R. and Obwegeser, H.L. (1957). Surgical correction of mandibular prognathism and retrogenia with consideration of genioplasty. *Oral Surg.*, **10**, 677.

West, R.A. and Epker, B.N. (1972). Posterior maxillary surgery: its place in the treatment of dentofacial deformities. *J. Oral Surg.*, **30**, 562.

Winstanley, R.P. (1968). Subcondylar osteotomy of the mandible and the intraoral approach. *Brit. J. Oral Surg.*, **6**, 134.

Section 5: The Management of Special Clinical Groups

Brami, S., Lamarche, J.P. and Souyris, F. (1974). Treatment of facial asymmetries by one-stage maxillary and mandibular bilateral osteotomies. *Intern. J. Oral Surg.*, **3**, 239.

Caldwell, J.B. and Gerhardt, R.C. (1974). In Kruger, E. (Ed.) Oral Surgery. St Louis, C.V. Mosby, Co.

Converse, J.M. and Shapiro, H.H. (1952). Treatment of developmental malformations of the jaws. *Plast. and Reconstr. Surg.*, **10**, 473.

Freihofer, H.P.M. Jr. (1976). The lip profile after correction of retromaxillism in cleft and non-cleft patients. *J. Max-fac. Surg.*, **4**, 136.

Freihofer, H.P.M. Jr. (1977). Changes in nasal profile after maxillary advancement in cleft and non-cleft patients. *J. Max-fac. Surg.*, **5**, 20.

Henderson, D. and Jackson, I.T. (1975). Combined cleft lip revision, anterior fistula closure, and maxillary osteotomy; a one-stage procedure. *Brit. J. Oral Surg.*, **13**, 33.

Henny, F.A. and Baldridge, O.L. (1957). Condylectomy for persistently painful temporomandibular joint. *J. Oral Surg.*, **15**, 24.

Hovell, J.H. (1960). The surgical treatment of some of the less common abnormalities of the facial skeleton. *Dent. Pract.*, **10**, 170.

Hovell, J.H. (1962). Bone grafting procedures in the mandible. *Oral Surg. Oral Med. Oral Path.*, **15**, 1281.

Hovell, J.H. (1963). Conylar hyperplasia. *Brit. J. Oral Surg.*, **1**, 105.

Lavergne, J. and Gasson, N. (1978). Influence of jaw rotation on the morphogenesis of malocclusion. *Americ. J. Orthod.*, **73**, 658.

Longacre, J.J., Destefano, G.A. and Holmstrand, K. (1961). The early versus the late reconstruction of congenital hypoplasia of the facial skeleton and skull. *Plast. Reconstr. Surg.*, **27**, 489.

Obwegeser, H.L. (1974). Correction of the skeletal anomalies of otomandibular dysostosis. *J. Max-fac. Surg.*, **2**, 273.

Obwegeser, H.L. (1971). Deformities of the jaws, in Mustarde, J.C. (Ed.). *Plastic surgery in infancy and childhood*. Edin. and London, E & S Livingstone.

Sethi, S.S., Gupta, J.L. and Shriuastava, J.L. ( ). Ankylosis of temporo-mandibular joints. *Indian J. Plast. Surg.*, , 41.

Stark, R.B. and Saunders, D.E. (1962). First branchial syndrome. *Plast. and Reconstr. Surg.*, **29**, 229.

Towers, J.F.T. (1976). The management of congenital and acquired deformity of the mandibular condyle in children. *Cartwright Prize essay, Royal Coll. Surg. England.*

Wake, M. (1976). Paper read to the British Association of Oral Surgeons, unpublished.

Index

Numbers in **bold** type refer to pages on which illustrations appear. *Passim* means here and there throughout.